GROUPWORK WITH REFUGEES AND SURVIVORS OF HUMAN RIGHTS ABUSES

Groupwork with Refugees and Survivors of Human Rights Abuses describes, explores and promotes the power of groupwork for refugees and survivors of human rights abuses in a range of contexts.

Drawing on multiple theoretical approaches, the book features chapters from practitioners running groups in different settings, such as torture rehabilitation services, refugee camps, and reception centres. The voices of participants demonstrate the variety, creativity and value of group and community approaches for recovery. The editors have gathered chapters into three sections covering: community-based approaches; groups that work through the medium of "body and soul"; and group approaches that focus on change through the spoken word.

The book will be relevant to those working in rehabilitation, community, mental health, and humanitarian fields and are interested in using groupwork as part of their services.

Jude Boyles is a psychological therapist who specialises in working with refugees and survivors of human rights abuses. Jude established and manages a therapy service for UN resettled refugees for the Refugee Council.

Robin Ewart-Biggs is a systemic family therapist who works with survivors of human rights abuses with a focus on groupwork. He runs a charity for young people with cancer.

Rebecca Horn is an independent psychosocial specialist and senior research fellow at the Institute for Global Health and Development, Queen Margaret University, Edinburgh.

Kirsten Lamb worked as a clinical psychologist in NHS mental health services from 1981 to 2018. Kirsten works with refugee charities on a freelance basis.

W0113492

This is an exceptional and authoritative book that appears at the appropriate time, to help all of us grasp the complexities of human suffering resulting from the adversities of various forms of involuntarily dislocation and human rights violations, from a wide variety of perspectives. Its almost encyclopedic scope provides a broad vision of effective interventions in many different contexts and settings, all over the world. Combining theory and practice, the book is written by committed practitioners, generously sharing their expertise and experiences, but also their sincere reflections about their work. The book will be a welcome resource for everyone working in these fields as well as for the informed readers who wish to obtain a thoughtful update on the current developments of these interventions.

Professor Renos K Papadopoulos, *PhD, University of Essex. Clinical Psychologist, Family Therapist and Jungian psychoanalyst; author of* Involuntary Dislocation. Home, Trauma, Resilience and Adversity-Activated Development

Framing the injustices against torture survivors, including asylum seekers, as moral transgressions requiring moral responses, this book brings together a collection of varied and powerful group practice examples of such responses. Togetherness, in group-based and community-based work with survivors, is exemplified as both a metaphor and as a means to foster solidarity against injustice, human connection, awareness raising and collective action, towards the restoration of the human dignity of survivors and towards justice. In an era of individualising, pathologising psychological therapies being heralded as solutions to all forms of trauma, this book reminds us of the immense creativity and power of groupwork in enabling change beyond the individual. It is a timely and an invaluable resource for all those working with refugees and survivors of human rights abuses.

Nimisha Patel, *Professor of Clinical Psychology, University of East London and Director of International Centre for Health and Human Rights, UK*

As a practitioner based in Sri Lanka, this collected volume was one I wanted to immediately share with my colleagues. Drawing from practice across diverse contexts – from Zimbabwe to Tunisia, from the UK to Uganda – the book brings together a truly global set of contributions that are accessible, descriptive and genuinely inspiring. The chapters give us an account of the underlying theories of change and values that guide these processes. Crucially, many also provide us with vital details about how these are responding to the wider events and socio-political processes that the participants of groupwork have to navigate in their daily lives – and underscore the importance of organic connections between approaches, context and the people involved in this work. The voices and views of the people whose experiences drive the groupwork are consistently and actively represented throughout, as are the different traditions and epistemologies that the approaches draw from. The contrasts between the diverse settings and approaches are largely implicit, but are very present and tangible to the reader, greatly enriching their experience. This collected volume is truly relevant to a global audience, offering meaningful insights into therapeutic groupwork approaches that have a lot to teach practitioners in any context.

Ananda Galappatti, *Director of Strategy, MHPSS.net*

What a book! So much material, so many examples of hope emerging out of coming to terms with painful tragedy. The Contributors to this title have brought to life the challenges, and the joys of helping people to find their inner resources to cope with perhaps the worst of human experience – violent inhumanity. This is achieved by offering the reader examples of what has made a personal difference from groupwork projects around the world. The power of the group experience is revealed in many ways as people spend time together, seeking a way forward and offering each other support and encouragement. There is something fundamentally enhancing to the person through positive and constructive group experience. This title is impressive and inspiring, offering examples of how the best of human experience can help people to find new lives after experiencing the worst of humanity. And on a lighter note: from reading this book I now understand the therapeutic power of sprouting broccoli. You will have to read it as well to discover this.

Richard Bryant-Jefferies, *author,* Counselling Victims of Warfare

The absolute joy in this book is its accessibility and practical application for humanitarian practitioners engaged in groupwork with refugees and survivors of human rights abuses. The sheer geographic breadth of examples from Peru, Uganda, Rwanda, Zimbabwe, Kosovo, and the UK amongst other contexts, demonstrates the electric and creative work happening at a local level in countries hosting refugees – whether they are persons recently displaced, in transit or navigating legal asylum application systems in host countries. The case studies illuminate effective, culturally relevant and alternative group (therapeutic) approaches that counter-balance, and challenge, the harmful dominance of the "Western and individualised" medical mental health model. This book is recommended reading for anyone, working within and outside of humanitarian contexts, who wishes to harness the positive aspects of group approaches to support refugees and survivors of human rights abuses.

Sarah Harrison, *Mental Health and Psychosocial Support Practitioner*

This text opens us up to the power of collectiveness and how practitioners have applied the group approach to support individuals and communities heal and overcome emotional difficulties, suffered as a result of rights violations and abuse. The book is a rich collection of exemplars, showcasing the work of community-based practitioners that have been carefully selected from a diverse range of countries. The context where interventions were implemented, range from conflict, displacement and torture, hence enabling the reader to relate groupwork approaches with the unique needs of these communities. Each book chapter presents a very unique country context which enables the reader to broaden their understanding of groupwork and how it can be applied in multiple contexts. From Zimbabwe to Peru, the authors share lived experiences of survivors and their sheer will to overcome adversity, rebuild their lives and support one another to regain their esteem, by working together in groups. For a researcher looking to learn more about the collective healing power of groupwork, to the practitioner eager to deliver low-cost community appropriate interventions, *The Power of Togetherness* is an invaluable resource.

Patrick Onyango Mangen, *Chief Executive Officer, REPSSI*

This book is a very welcome addition to the literature; it is innovative in that it brings together a wealth of information from a number of countries about group and community work in relation to human rights. It is written in an accessible style, is broad in its scope and provides a range of diverse illustrative examples. The reader will learn a lot about varied projects and the power of this work. The chapters are written by people bringing a range of skills and creative thinking and it may encourage others to take part in this important work. The richness of the content of this book will be very useful to anyone concerned about human rights.

Rachel Tribe, *Professor of Applied Psychology, University of East London, UK*

GROUPWORK WITH REFUGEES AND SURVIVORS OF HUMAN RIGHTS ABUSES

The Power of Togetherness

Edited by
**Jude Boyles, Robin Ewart-Biggs, Rebecca Horn
and Kirsten Lamb**

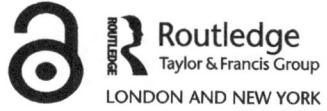

Routledge
Taylor & Francis Group

LONDON AND NEW YORK

Cover image: Story cloth made by Gloria Eugenia Santa, entitled: Arpillera Group. It was created in a Common Threads circle at La Federación de Mujeres de Sucumbíos in Ecuador.

First published 2023
by Routledge
4 Park Square, Milton Park, Abingdon, Oxon OX14 4RN

and by Routledge
605 Third Avenue, New York, NY 10158

Routledge is an imprint of the Taylor & Francis Group, an informa business

British Library Cataloguing-in-Publication Data
A catalogue record for this book is available from the British Library

Library of Congress Cataloging-in-Publication Data
Names: Boyles, Jude, editor.
Title: Groupwork with refugees and survivors of human rights abuses : the power of togetherness / edited by Jude Boyles, Robin Ewart-Biggs, Rebecca Horn, and Kirsten Lamb.
Description: Abingdon, Oxon ; New York, NY : Routledge, 2022. | Includes bibliographical references. | Identifiers: LCCN 2022022281 (print) | LCCN 2022022282 (ebook) | ISBN
9781032043883 (paperback) | ISBN 9781032043906 (hardback) | ISBN
9781003192978 (ebook)
Subjects: LCSH: Refugees--Mental health services. | Group psychotherapy.
Classification: LCC RC451.4.R43 G76 2022 (print) | LCC RC451.4.R43
(ebook) | DDC 616.89/14086914--dc23/eng/20220713
LC record available at https://lccn.loc.gov/2022022281
LC ebook record available at https://lccn.loc.gov/2022022282

ISBN: 973-1-032-04390-6 (hbk)
ISBN: 973-1-032-04388-3 (pbk)
ISBN: 973-1-003-19297-8 (ebk)

DOI: 10.4324/9781003192978

Typeset in Baskerville MT Std
by SPi Technologies India Pvt Ltd (Straive)

CONTENTS

WITNESSING RESILIENCE AND SUFFERING IN REFUGEES: A FOREWORD

As an old African proverb states:

> If you want to go fast, go alone.
> But if you want to go far, go together.

It was in January 1993 that I left war-torn Croatia for the Netherlands. I was a part of the team of Croatian therapists invited to participate in a Dutch project aiming to provide psychological help to concentration camp survivors from Bosnia-Herzegovina who arrived as refugees just a couple of months before. As a young psychiatrist/psychotherapist who spoke the language of the survivors, I had an idea about "how a war feels and sounds". My rudimentary knowledge of the impact of war and violence on the psychological wellbeing arose from my time in 1992 while assisting people displaced from the eastern part of Croatia who fled, upon the siege of the town of Vukovar, to the capital. Trying to make sense out of the engulfing chaotic war reality, I focused on the professional aspects of my training, reading scientific literature on psycho trauma and violence, finding many useful articles on Vietnam veterans in the US, and about Holocaust survivors. However, I could not avoid feeling somehow helpless since there was no literature on the war in ex-Yugoslavia, specific to that context, to those cultural characteristics of the people I would help, and to the particular influences of forced migration on survivors of war. What I could read in journals and books did not fully match with what I was experiencing and seeing at that time in my daily practice.

And yet, when I for the first time entered the refugees' reception centre in the Netherlands where a couple of hundred ex-concentration camp survivors resided with their families, just recently freed from "the hell", having been transferred to an unknown country with no clear idea about what their future will be, and with the war in their home country stubbornly continuing forcing these people to leave behind families and friends, my work had to be done. There were expectations, responsibilities, and a strong urge to help. This is when and where my quest started for an adequate culture- and context-sensitive approach to assist survivors of man-made trauma. This was the first time in my life to design and lead group treatment sessions.

Six months later, when my participation in the project ended, I looked back at the work done. The groups I led had been mainly supportive, and survivors had found it important to participate in the sessions and to share their memories and feelings to a certain extent. I had observed not only extensive suffering, but also tremendous resilience in survivors. Though most of them had spent similar time in the same camps being heavily tortured and mistreated, many came through these experiences without suffering from re-experiencing, nightmares and other complaints relating to post-traumatic stress disorder (PTSD). These people demonstrated that I must focus not only on psychological damage of survivors, but that I should also pay attention to different traits which made some of them less vulnerable, and which contributed to survival from atrocities in psychological ways.

A couple of years later, I was back in Eastern Croatia working in one village with the inhabitants who had suffered a lot during the war. In that community many men had been killed or captured by the enemy and had never returned home. They had "disappeared" with their families still waiting for them to return. Many females had been raped. My task was to engage with the male inhabitants and start group sessions, as they were in despair, abusing substances and abreacting aggressively in their families. However, these men were reluctant to engage with me, as they were suspicious about who I was; perhaps I was a spy working for the

International Tribunal for War Crimes in The Hague. They thought that I had come to investigate whether they had committed atrocities during the war. My efforts to convince them of my true identity and mission were unsuccessful. The power of a group manifested itself once again, but now in a negative and destructive sense led by fear. Clearly, the timing and the context of the intervention was wrong. It was the female inhabitants who stopped me from leaving the village with unfinished business. They expressed their wish to engage with group sessions. My colleague and I worked with them on and off in the subsequent two years. The women not only made use of a group setting to voice their feelings, fears, and doubts, but they also used it to organise themselves as a group and to start working on rebuilding the village through securing funding from different NGOs. I left that village with a renewed awareness of both a group's powerful destructive dynamics and its constructive capacities.

At the end of the 1990s, I set up a day treatment centre for people seeking asylum and refugees with psycho trauma in the Netherlands. Our clients came from different conflict zones in the world, most of them had been exposed to war and political violence, some of them were also torture survivors. All of them were dealing with the impacts of forced migration. Yet again, groups seemed to be a suitable treatment format. Through many years, together with my team I have developed different sorts of group treatments: groups with and without interpreters; male, female, and mixed groups; those combining group psychotherapy with experiential treatments (music therapy, art therapy, psychomotor therapy); groups with participants from the same country and those with participants with different cultures of origin. There were supportive groups, but also trauma focused group treatments. This was exciting work, which some considered pioneering. We conducted scientific studies to evaluate it and learn how and in which direction to proceed. During this time, I have learned about both the universal and the culture-specific aspects of psychological impacts of violence and also about the importance of traditional and cultural practices in healing and reconnecting with one's roots and positive pre-trauma experiences. I became aware of the power of combining "talking" with "experiencing by doing" in experiential treatments as the survivors cannot always find words to verbalise "the unexplainable" of the largely man-made human rights violations. I became more and more aware of the interplay of different contextual factors in my clients' daily lives with their psychological wellbeing. Although our main task was to help them to find peace with their painful past and to work through the traumatic events they had experienced, we realised ourselves that this works best by considering their current "real life" circumstances, their existential worries, uncertainties and doubts, and a lack of recognition for losses they have suffered. Advocacy became an integral part of our daily work. Boundaries of the therapist's professional role expanded, and we also became "human rights advocates" looking for partnership with the other professionals who could help our clients to deal with ongoing environmental stress and achieve recognition of their human and legal rights as refugees. Our framework for both understanding and healing of the impacts of violence has developed throughout the years into an integrative and a holistic one.

At the same time, the day treatment centre was a mental health facility in a highly developed first world country and we were expected to provide evidence-based PTSD treatment to our beneficiaries. Therefore, besides expanding our perspectives on the complexity of psychosocial impacts of man-made violence and forced migration, we continued developing trauma focused approaches in group treatment. Depending on resources available, both human and financial, we experimented throughout the years with imaginative exposure in a group format, and with a frequency of group sessions meeting one to three times weekly. We combined individual trauma focused treatments with those in a group and explored combinations of different forms of experiential treatments with group psychotherapy. Our research showed that the trauma focused group treatment with people seeking asylum and refugees in a host country can be efficient, despite ongoing existential uncertainties and an unstable daily life context of the participants. Moreover, we found out that adding experiential treatments enhances efficiency of group psychotherapy. However, evaluating this work from a historical distance I think that the most powerful therapeutic tool was the group format itself. It enabled survivors to re-attach emotionally with other humans in a safe space, to re-establish trust in others and a sense of belonging, to experience that the other is caring for them and that they still have a capacity to care for the other. The group enabled the participants to make the shift from being victim to becoming a survivor, and to re-invent playfulness, creativity, courage, and hope, which are so essential for future prospects.

In the past decades I have also had the opportunity to work together with colleagues in post-conflict zones in different parts of the world and to expand my knowledge and experience with groupwork in countries like Rwanda following the genocide, and Georgia shortly after the war in South Ossetia. I have learned from them about the significance of lay facilitators' work in a healing process and how important it is for survivors' wellbeing to take an active role in a community and rebuild "real life" opportunities outside of the "intimate bubble" of a treatment setting. Although I am primarily a clinician, I always remember the voices of survivors pointing out that upon mass human rights violations, like war, it is not mental health problems that are their top priority in life, but rather a collective acknowledgment of wrongdoings, the restitution of losses experienced, and experiencing existential safety. Unfortunately, in our world these top priorities of survivors are often unmet, and they are offered mental health treatments instead. However, group interventions, if designed and timed appropriately, can partly satisfy these survivors' needs and plant a seed of a full psychosocial recovery by enabling survivors to feel human and connected again and dare to start rebuilding their shattered lives.

To summarise, 30 years ago knowledge about group interventions with refugees was in its infancy. This long-awaited volume presents experience-motivated, well-considered and studied methods of providing group interventions to refugees in various settings. Its goal is to provide the professional community with a foundation for future development, and to enable continuation with the challenging endeavour of improving mental health and wellbeing of refugees worldwide.

Boris Drožđek, MD, PhD, psychiatrist/psychotherapist

De Hemisfeer

Den Bosch

The Netherlands

ACKNOWLEDGEMENTS

We would like to thank those who donated to our crowdfunding campaign and to those who contributed directly and anonymously to enable this book to be made freely available via Open Access.

The subtitle of the book, *The Power of Togetherness*, is taken from a stage in the Tree of Life Trust (Zimbabwe) community-based "trauma healing and empowerment workshop". This part of the group process focuses on the *power of togetherness*, showing participants how they are connected to each other and the world around them, even when they may feel isolated.

CONTRIBUTORS

Christine Adcock worked as a clinical psychologist in NHS learning disability services in the UK from 1981 to 1997. From 2004 to 2019, she volunteered for a torture rehabilitation charity, running a music group and offering individual therapy. Christine retired in 2020 and now offers supervision and mentoring in the UK and internationally.

Amanda Bingley, BSc (Hons) PhD, worked as a research fellow and then lecturer in health research at Lancaster University from 2001 until retiring in 2020. With a background in psychotherapy and cultural geography, she taught qualitative methods with a focus on narrative research and the use of creative arts. Her research explored therapeutic landscapes in relation to health and place in a wide range of contexts.

Leticia Biira Birungi is a clinical psychologist. She has worked in humanitarian settings since the beginning of 2019, offering community-based psychotherapy to both refugees and nationals in Uganda. She has worked for TPO Uganda since August 2020.

Jude Boyles is a psychological therapist and has specialised in working with refugees and survivors of human rights abuses since 1999. Jude manages a psychological therapy service for resettled refugees for the Refugee Council in Yorkshire, UK and is a clinical supervisor for practitioners working with refugees. She is the co-director of a small NGO, TortureID, that identifies and documents survivors of human rights abuses. Jude established Freedom from Torture North West in 2003 and managed the service for 14 years.

Ardiana Bytyçi is a clinical psychologist and has worked with people seeking asylum and refugees in Kosovo since 2012. She has dedicated her career to working with Kosova Rehabilitation Center for Torture Victims in mental health programmes for persons of concern to the UNHCR. She completed a Master's degree in Clinical Psychology and Health at University of Prishtina.

Victoria Cavero is a psychologist with a Master's degree in Global Mental Health (University of London). She is a researcher at Universidad Peruana Cayetano Heredia working on projects related to mental health and public policy. She is a member of the Research Group of Community Psychology at Pontificia Universidad Católica del Perú.

Dr. Bryan Cheng is the director of research of the GMH Lab at Teachers College, Columbia University, US. He provides oversight on various projects utilising interpersonal psychotherapy (IPT). He is also an IPT supervisor and trainer, and specialises in other forms of therapies, including CBT and DBT.

Rachel Cohen earned her Doctorate in Clinical Psychology in 1986. She is founder and director of Common Threads Project (CTP), an NGO collaborating with local organisations to promote trauma recovery for survivors of sexual violence, war, and displacement. CTP programmes exist in Ecuador, Nepal, Bosnia, the DRC and the US.

Jozef Corveleyn is an emeritus professor of clinical psychology and psychology of religion at the University of Leuven; Doctor Honoris Causa of Semmelweis University, Universidad Ricardo Palma and Universidad Femenina del Sagrado Corazon. Jozef is a professor honorario at the Universidad de Lima, Universidad Nacional Mayor de San Marcos and Pontificia Universidad Catolica del Peru.

Robin Ewart-Biggs is a systemic family therapist who has worked with survivors of human rights abuses since 2001 with a focus on groupwork. He is based in Cumbria in the UK, working with refugee organisations and running a charity supporting young people living with cancer.

Mark Fish has worked as a group therapist since 1992. In 2002, he worked in the conflict zone of Northern Uganda for two years. He worked at the Helen Bamber Foundation in the UK from 2006 until 2018, and at Room to Heal's therapeutic community, which he founded in 2007. In 2018, Mark set up Groupworks International to provide groupwork training to organisations in regions of greatest need.

Lucia De Haene is associate professor at University of Leuven, working on clinical and psychosocial migration research with refugees and immigrants. She leads the clinic transcultural trauma care for refugees at the Faculty Clinical Centre PraxisP, and co-leads the psychiatric day programme for refugee minors at the University Psychiatric Hospital.

Terry Hanley is a reader in counselling psychology at the University of Manchester in the UK. He is also an honorary psychological therapist at Freedom from Torture in Manchester. In this role he facilitates the football therapy group run in partnership with FC United of Manchester.

Aisling Hearns is a psychotherapist in Spirasi, a rehabilitation centre for survivors of torture in Ireland. She has several degrees in the area of mental health and is currently a psychology doctoral candidate in Trinity College, Dublin. Her role in Spirasi is to provide individual and group psychotherapy to survivors of torture.

Rebecca Horn is an independent psychosocial specialist. Her focus is primarily on community-based approaches to mental health and psychosocial wellbeing in humanitarian settings, particularly with populations affected by conflict and displacement. She is a senior research fellow with the Institute for Global Health and Development, Queen Margaret University, Edinburgh.

Ejona Miraka Icka is a clinical psychologist and social worker who joined KRCT in 2020. Ejona provides clinical treatment to people seeking asylum and refugees in Kosovo. She graduated in clinical psychology at "Albanian University" in Albania, as well as social work at "University Äleksandër Xhuvani" in Elbasan.

Rim Ben Ismail has worked as a project manager with the Reprieve "Life after Guantanamo" rehabilitation programme; as a therapist and consultant with torture survivors for the World Organisation Against Torture (OMCT); and as president founder of Psychologues du Monde Tunisie, developing projects for victims of institutional violence. Rim also provides organisational trainings with Groupworks International.

Kirsten Lamb worked as a clinical psychologist in NHS mental health services from 1981 to 2018 in the UK. From 2003 to 2021, Kirsten also worked in a torture rehabilitation charity as an individual/group therapist and medico-legal report writer. From 2021, she has been working with refugee charities on a freelance basis.

Elias Manirakiza is a regional coordinator with TPO Uganda in the south-western part of Uganda. He is a development worker with a degree in Development Studies and postgraduate diploma in Project Planning and Management. He has worked in the humanitarian field since 2012.

Laura Marchesini is a gender-based violence (GBV) in emergency specialist, collaborating with multiple NGOs and UN agencies since 2009, mainly serving as a cluster coordinator,

coordinator and advisor of GBV programming. She has two master's degrees, one in the management of non-profit organisations and a second master's degree in humanitarian emergencies.

Melanie Megevand has established and supported GBV programming in humanitarian emergencies worldwide since 2007. Her contributions include innovative programming to respond to and prevent violence against women and girls in urban displacement, co-authoring the WGSS toolkit and authoring EMPOWER: Preventing violence against women and girls in acute emergencies.

Enda Moclair brings extensive experience working with culturally sensitive mental health and psychosocial interventions in both emergency and developmental contexts. His background is in expressive arts therapy, clinical psychology, learning and capacities development, community and organisational development. He works for the World Food Program as a staff counsellor.

Eugenia Mpande is an experienced transcultural mental health and psychosocial (MHPSS) professional and counsellor. Since 2002, Eugenia has devoted much of her professional life to extensive work with individuals, families, community groups and members from civil society organisations who have lived both traumatic and traumagenic experiences.

Peggy Mulongo is a cross-cultural mental health practitioner, lecturer and researcher with a focus on women and young girls who experience mental distress related to male violence, specialising in work with women affected by female genital mutilation (FGM) and domestic servitude. She initiated several projects to promote health equality, including the Support our Sisters project at NESTAC in Greater Manchester, UK.

Lis Murphy is creative director and founder of Music Action International. She has pioneered the use of singing and song writing to support war and torture survivors to find peace through personal expression and collective experience. Lis is a professional performing musician with her bands, the glowe_ and Rubber Duck Orchestra.

Grace Obalim is a clinical psychologist with MSc. Clinical Psychology from the University of Nairobi and a Bachelor's Degree in Psychology, Guidance and Counseling from Nkumba University in Uganda. She has been the mental health and psychosocial support advisor for TPO Uganda since 2019.

Martha Orbach is an artist and community gardener, working with plants and communities since 2010. She has worked with Glasgow Botanic Gardens, UNESCO RILA, The Open Society Foundation, Maryhill Integration Network, Room to Heal, and Culpeper Community Garden, described by the UK's Royal Horticultural Society as "social and therapeutic horticulture at its best".

Mary Raphaely is a group analytic psychotherapist with extensive experience with victims of trafficking, torture and domestic violence. She is fluent in English and French and is drawn to issues facing our multicultural society in the UK, often using non-verbal methods. Mary has a special interest in vicarious traumatisation, working widely as an independent supervisor.

Annemiek Richters, MD, is an anthropologist and honorary professor in culture, health and illness at Leiden University Medical Center. Annemiek works at the Amsterdam Institute for Social Science Research, at the University of Amsterdam. From 2005, she has contributed to the development of community-based sociotherapy in Rwanda through capacity building and research.

Macarena Rioseco, PhD, is an associtae lecturer of Contemporary Arts at Universidad Metropolitana Ciencias de la Educación, Chile. Macarena is a scholar and art practitioner exploring the contribution of material creative practices for education and well-being. Her research is grounded on Deleuze and Guattari's work and the enactive approach to cognition.

Miryam Rivera-Holguín is a professor at Pontifical Catholic University of Peru since 2009. She is developing her PhD research at University of Leuven (Belgium). She has developed her practice in the fields of humanitarian emergencies, human rights and community mental health, focusing on public policies and vulnerable populations.

The **Room to Heal** chapter was truly a collaborative affair involving the Room to Heal team and community members. Jilna Shah led on the writing with significant contributions from members, Elli Free, director, and therapists Emily White, Bert-Jan Zuiderduin, Suzie Grayburn and Roro Ratih Ambarwati.

Emma Rose is professor of Contemporary Arts, at the Lancaster Institute of Contemporary Arts, Lancaster University, UK. Emma is a scholar-practitioner exploring the contribution of participatory arts for health and wellbeing, using qualitative and action research methods. She developed the theoretical lens of therapeutic landscapes in connection with art and wellbeing, self-identity and psychoanalytic theory.

Feride Rushiti is a human rights activist, founder and executive director of KRCT. She is mostly known for her work to secure legal recognition and institutional support for survivors of wartime sexual violence in Kosovo. Dr. Rushiti was honored with the US Secretary of State's International Women of Courage Award in 2018, in recognition of her work with survivors of torture and human rights advocacy.

Besnik Rustemi is a licensed social worker for social and family services with a Degree in Social Work at University of Prishtina, Kosovo. His career at KRCT started in 2019, and he provides group activities for young men in the Asylum Centres.

Emmanuel Sarabwe has an MA in Human Rights, Gender and Conflict and in Social Work and Social Administration. She is a staff member of subsequent community-based sociotherapy (CBS) programmes in Rwanda since 2005. From 2022, she has been head of programmes of CBS Rwanda. Her research interests include marital conflict, psychosocial support, forgiveness, and peacebuilding in post-genocide Rwanda.

Theophile Sewimfura is a healing, peacebuilding and reconciliation activist, and founder of Africa Restoring Bridges Initiative (ARBI). Since 2008, he has contributed to the development and adaptation of community-based sociotherapy in the Great Lakes of Africa, and is supporting the implementation of sociotherapy within displacement settings.

Caleb Tukahiirwa is a progressive student of psychology with an MSc. in Clinical Psychology from Makerere University in Uganda. He worked with TPO Uganda from 2019 until 2021 implementing MHPSS projects within refugee settlements. He is working towards contributing to the growth of MHPSS research, publications and building communities' capacity in MHPSS provision within Uganda.

Lynn Walker is the director of Tree of Life Trust Zimbabwe. She has a BEd. (hons) from Durham University and a MSc from University of Surrey in the UK. She taught in the UK for 13 years before moving to Zimbabwe in 1991. Lynn worked in Zimbabwean teacher education before joining the non-governmental sector in 1997, working for both local and international agencies.

Weihui Wang started her career in 2007, supporting survivors of torture and unaccompanied and separated minors. Weihui is a protection advocate with experience in child protection, GBV and MHPSS programming across the Middle East, West and Southeast Asia, and the Western Balkans. She holds graduate degrees in international human rights law and social work.

Micah Williams has served as International Medical Corps' senior GBV advisor and technical lead since 2010, supporting the design and delivery of GBV prevention and response programmes in humanitarian contexts across more than 25 countries. She has a Master's degree in International Relations, focused on gender and human rights.

Women Asylum Seekers Together (WAST) are a self-led women's group, all of whom are seeking asylum in the UK. The chapter is written collectively by WAST members.

Susan Wyatt graduated as an occupational therapist in 2009 in Australia, and is undertaking her Master's research in Zimbabwe in anthropology and development, specialising in conflict and development. She has expertise in transcultural mental health and trauma recovery. Susan is the founding director of Tana Consulting, and works part-time as the research and advocacy manager for Tree of Life, Zimbabwe.

Emmanuela Yogolelo is originally from eastern Democratic Republic of Congo and is a singer-songwriter, live performer, workshop facilitator, speaker, and cultural leader. In 2015, she co-founded the Manchester-based Amani Creatives, which promotes the arts and culture as a tool for community development, wellbeing and community cohesion. Emmanuela was a founding member of the Music Action International music facilitator team.

Malisa Zymberi is a psychologist with experience of working with refugees on the border with Syria-Turkey from 2015, providing psychosocial support for refugees through the Icelandic Red Cross. She joined KRCT in 2019 to provide group activities with people seeking asylum and refugees in Kosovo. Malisa graduated in psychology from University "Hasan Prishtina".

INTRODUCTION
The Editors

Human rights abuses are both deeply personal and broadly social. The impact is felt in the mind and body of the individual and yet the act of violation takes place within wider contexts, which include the families and communities that are also harmed. Similarly, recovery is a personal journey but the struggle may be part of wider community healing and is determined by social and political forces. The premise of this book is that group and community approaches are integral to those journeys and to those struggles.

The chapters that follow illustrate this commitment to the social context of recovery through 20 different accounts of human rights-based groupwork taking place across the world. The reader will see that local landscapes loom large in the descriptions of the approaches and provide relevant context for each piece of work. The focus is on adults and in some cases families but does not extend to groupwork with children and young people.

THE INTERNATIONAL REFUGEE CONTEXT

At the time of writing, in mid-2022, there are many reasons to be concerned at the global situation for those seeking safety and recovery. UNHCR reports 89.3 million forcibly displaced people at the end of 2021. This figure has more than doubled in a decade and rises dramatically to over 100 million in the May 2022 estimates, meaning "1 in every 78 people on earth has been forced to flee". The majority are internally displaced within the country where they are at risk; 72% of those outside their home borders are in a neighbouring country; and low-income countries are host to 83% of the world's refugees; women and girls make up around 50% of the refugee population, facing oppression and violence every day (UNHCR, 2022).

In the UK, where the editors of this book are based, the Nationality and Borders Bill has passed into law and has introduced increased levels of hardship, which appear to contravene the European Convention on Human Rights (ECHR). Beyond these shores, the physical manifestations of "fortress Europe" continue to grow along European Union borders long after the term was applied to immigration (Carr, 2012). This affects those recovering in the West but has a far wider impact, as the increasing politicisation of migration contributes to the lack of protection for growing numbers of migrants across the world. The Universal Declaration of Human Rights (UDHR, 1948) outlines the human rights that all people are entitled to, such as freedom from torture, freedom of expression, and the right to seek asylum. In reality, the universal right to "life, liberty and security of person" (UDHR, Article 3) is a privilege that only some benefit from.

BOOK VISION

Groupwork and community building are presented here as a response to the gravity of these circumstances. The work described in these chapters explores and promotes the ways in which groupwork can successfully engage and meet the broad needs of survivors wherever they are: in-country, where they have been persecuted; "on the move", when in flight or in transit; during temporary settlement, for example in refugee camps; and in places where survivors are seeking

DOI: 10.4324/9781003192978-1

asylum or settling as refugees. In any of these settings people may be going through different stages of survival, adjustment and settlement and facing complex circumstances relating to safety, destitution, rights, physical and psychological health, family separation and acute uncertainty about the future. All of these experiences are mediated through cultural and social values and the reader will see the ways in which groupwork provides rich opportunity for refugees and survivors to respond to the changed contexts that they face.

The book aims to provide a forum for survivors and practitioners working internationally to share their practice and learning. Some chapters present groupwork implemented in contexts where individual approaches predominate. Others highlight group approaches happening in places where groups are already the mainstream response. Both involve a move to collectivist values that are more common in countries where the majority of refugees and survivors both come from and are rebuilding their lives.

Groupwork places social reconnection at the heart of recovery, and opens the door to peer support and building community resources and resilience. These overcome the isolation and shame that human rights abuses intentionally cause and are also a more effective means of reaching and responding to the large numbers of survivors struggling across the world. Where persecution seeks to disempower, silence and isolate, group and community work bring together and connect survivor voices. This is more than a shift from individual work to helping individuals in a group context, and moves into supporting communities as a whole.

Considering its ambitious scope, this book will therefore draw on multiple theoretical approaches. It cannot cover the complete range of groupwork taking place internationally and is inevitably a partial representation. However, we have tried to bring together a collection of work showing some of the richness and diversity within therapeutic groupwork approaches in both humanitarian and rehabilitation settings.

THE PSYCHOSOCIAL CONTEXT

There are now many meta-studies and literature reviews focused on both the needs of survivors and the approaches used to support recovery, including efforts to evaluate the effectiveness of interventions. Despite the absence of agreed models, there are strong themes that recur. These make the case for acknowledging the multiple challenges facing survivors, the importance of considering the contexts within which these challenges are experienced, and focusing research on interventions and approaches that take place within these broader frameworks. Recommendations include: looking beyond post-traumatic stress disorder (PTSD) (Hamid et al., 2019); taking account of daily stressors experienced during recovery and the resulting need for an ecological perspective (Alfadhli et al., 2019; Miller and Rasmussen, 2016; Salo and Bray, 2016); the importance of socio-cultural knowledge (Hassan et al., 2016); and attention to issues of power and reliance on Eurocentric approaches (Patel, 2019a).

There is also a growing focus on social, group and community interventions and the importance of these for recovery. Bunn et al. (2016) literature review on group treatments for survivors of torture and severe violence, provides "a compelling conceptual rationale for using group treatment" (p. 45). Group approaches have long been part of rehabilitation services (Van der Kolk, 1993) and more recently these have been developed into formal group-based models, which are described in several chapters. Another, the Den Bosch model, has been written about by Boris Droždek (2010), who provides the Foreword to this book. Patel includes groupwork as part of a "whole systems recovery approach" (2019b, p. 20).

BOOK FRAMEWORK

The chapters that follow offer real-world interventions that have been delivered by practitioners running groups in different settings and respond to some of the challenges and recommendations referred to above. They describe a range of activities that practitioners and survivors have incorporated into groupwork in this field, including arts-based groups, culturally specific interventions and sports. They demonstrate the use of ecological perspectives, socio-cultural knowledge and attention to power dynamics. The voices of survivors are heard throughout, those who are active in peer groups or as therapy or activity group members.

The book is organised into three collections of chapters. The first section focuses on community-based and survivor-led approaches; Section 2 on groups that work through the medium of the "body and soul" (arts, sport, nature); and Section 3 explores groups that work primarily through the spoken word. Each section is followed by a narrative based on a discussion between authors from that section exploring groupwork themes and sharing the learning that arose through writing their chapters.

Women-only groups that are facilitated or self-led as a response to the impact of male violence are represented in all three sections. The power of mixed groups, and those for young male adolescents and men, are also explored. There are chapters that describe LGBTQ and faith-sensitive groupwork.

This book will therefore be relevant to those working in community, humanitarian, rehabilitation and social care fields internationally, who are interested in groupwork as part of their services.

EDITORIAL POSITIONS

We have emphasised the global, human rights-based values that shape the book and the ambition to emphasise survivor voices. However, this is not a neat fit with our position as four white, UK-based editors. There is clearly a tension here. A tension which potentially limits how widely these ambitions can be met.

This recognition has been a starting point, which we have used to guide our editorial decisions. It helped us to formulate our understanding of the centrality of power relations in work with survivors of human rights abuses and of group and community approaches as part of a response to these dynamics. It strengthened our determination to foreground learning from groupwork in low-income countries and international humanitarian settings.

Our guidance to prospective authors emphasised the human rights-based values and aims of the publication and the need to ensure that survivor's voices are present throughout. This framework positions rehabilitation as a process of empowerment in which survivors hold multiple roles, from service recipients and group participants through to service user involvement and survivor activism.

We have sought, in our editorial roles, not to get in the way of the individual voices of the authors and the approaches being described, and to support the unique qualities of those contributions; we have valued each chapter as a stand-alone piece of work. Many authors are not writing in their first language and different terminology is used to describe common processes such as seeking asylum/international protection. Where possible we have left authors to use the terms that reflect their values and context.

Equally, we have wanted to create a collective of authors to expand the knowledge and expertise so clearly articulated in the work that was submitted. This led to the three collaborative conversation pieces between the authors of chapters in each section.

We have ensured through generous contributions and funding that all chapters are freely available online as Open Access documents, so that colleagues and survivors can access them internationally.

We do not believe that any of this resolves the tension of our position. However, we present this work to you in good faith, hoping to create a community of interest in developing more co-produced groupwork with survivors.

REFERENCES

Alfadhli, K., Güler, M., Cakal, H. and Drury, J. (2019) 'The role of emergent shared identity in psychosocial support among refugees of conflict in developing countries'. *International Review of Social Psychology*, 32(1), p. 2. doi:10.5334/irsp.176.

Bunn, M., Goesel, C., Kinet, M. and Ray, F. (2016) 'Group treatment for survivors of torture and severe violence: A literature review'. *Torture Journal*, 26(1), p. 23. doi:10.7146/torture.v26i1.108062.

Carr, M. (2012) *Fortress Europe: Inside the War Against Immigration*. London: Hurst.

Drožđek, B. and Bolwerk, N. (2010) 'Evaluation of group therapy with traumatized asylum seekers and refugees—The Den Bosch Model'. *Traumatology*, 16(4), pp. 117–127. doi:10.1177/1534765610388298.

Hamid, A., Patel, N. and Williams, A. (2019) 'Psychological, social, and welfare interventions for torture survivors: A systematic review and meta-analysis of randomised controlled trials'. *PLoS Medicine*, 16(9), p. e1002919. doi:10.1371/journal.pmed.1002919.

Hassan, G., Ventevogel, P., Jefee-Bahloul, H., Barkil-Oteo, A. and Kirmayer, L. J. (2016) 'Mental health and psychosocial wellbeing of Syrians affected by armed conflict,' *Epidemiology and Psychiatric Sciences*, 25(2), pp. 129–141. doi:10.1017/S2045796016000044.

Miller, K. and Rasmussen, A. (2016) 'The mental health of civilians displaced by armed conflict: An ecological model of refugee distress'. *Epidemiology and Psychiatric Sciences*, 26(2), pp. 129–138. doi:10.1017/S2045796016000172.

Patel, N. (2019a) 'The mantra of 'Do No Harm' in international healthcare responses to refugee people', in Wenzel, T. and Drožđek, B. (eds.) *An Uncertain Safety. Integrative Healthcare for 21st Century Refugees*. Cham: Springer International, pp. 155–183.

Patel, N. (2019b) 'Conceptualising rehabilitation as reparation for torture survivors: A clinical perspective'. *The International Journal of Human Rights*, 23(9), pp. 1546–1568. doi:10.1080/13642987.2019.1612373.

Salo, C. and Bray, E. (2016) 'Empirically tested interventions for torture survivors: A systematic review through an ecological lens'. *Translational Issues in Psychological Science*, 2(4), pp. 449–463. doi:10.1037/tps0000097.

United Nations (1948) Universal Declaration of Human Rights. Available at: https://www.un.org/en/about-us/universal-declaration-of-human-rights (Accessed 7 June 2022).

UNHCR (2022) Global Trends. Available at: https://www.unhcr.org/62a9d1494/global-trends-report-2021 (Accessed: 17 June 2022).

Van der Kolk, B. (1993) 'Groups for patients with histories of catastrophic trauma', in Alonso, A. and Swiller, H. (eds) *Group Therapy in Clinical Practice*. Washington: American Psychiatric Press, pp. 289–305.

CHAPTER 1

GROUP AND COMMUNITY APPROACHES

A response to the barriers of institutional racism in the UK asylum system

Robin Ewart-Biggs

Those who seek support following human rights abuses face a range of physical, psychological, social, political and moral concerns. This chapter will look at the common features that survivors seeking asylum in the UK present with and the ongoing difficulties before them. In examining the day-to-day conditions in which they find themselves, it proposes that racism is the underlying condition responsible for the obstacles to rehabilitation, in the way that Andrews states it is for health inequalities, and that this creates a context in which the restoration of dignity is fundamentally compromised: "Once we connect the dots between health inequalities and wider racial oppression, then we understand that racism is the underlying condition" (Andrews, 2021b, p. 1343). Finally, it argues that group and community approaches based on liberation psychology offer a foundation for overcoming these obstacles.

I often think about a scene from a group that I co-facilitated at a UK rehabilitation centre, where I worked as a group and family therapist for 17 years. There were between 12 and 24 members; group analysts call this a 'median group', where social rather than personal issues are likely to be raised. It was a mixed-gender, multi-national group for asylum-seeking survivors of torture that combined orientation, general support and community therapy ideas, and aimed to address all the strands of a phased approach. One week, a colleague visited the group to discuss a country report that was being written about the Democratic Republic of Congo (DRC), and to gain lived-experience input from survivors. There was an animated discussion as was always the case when politics was the subject. This moved from curiosity to frustration, with several amongst the group becoming angry that the intended report was not encompassing the political realities that they experienced. They explained that a report highlighting the human rights abuses that were taking place in their country without examining the political and economic role of the West in the conflict was of no value. We will return to this as an example of the way in which services can unintentionally harbour Western colonial values.

Another memory is about one of the first survivors I interviewed. At the end of the assessment meeting, Claude[1] said that he wanted help to set up a radio station. Unfortunately, there was no scope for supporting this and he joined a group that I was running instead. Over the years the idea of the radio station never left me. I had presumed that he was wanting to resume his profession and regain the dignity that his torturers had tried to take from him. Listening to him in the group, the depth of his anger and the strength of his views, I realised that it was more than this; he wanted to create a platform to join with others and speak out against injustice. The group was a small starting point but hardly met the scale of his vision. Again, this is an example that will recur in the chapter as a reminder of the breadth of responses required for meaningful rehabilitation.

Finally, to set the scene, I share an extract from research (unpublished) into the experience of family therapy for asylum-seeking families in the UK, and one family member's words (using narrative analysis methodology) about the processes and hardships of rebuilding their lives:

> You see that hurts a bit, for people that you are embracing – you say to yourself, look this is me, this is me, this is my family, I'm building another world here, here I am, I am just with my children, I have no husband here, now I no longer have my mother, I no longer have my mother-in-law, I've got nothing left, nothing left, here's my family and now I'm making a family in

DOI: 10.4324/9781003192978-2

England, so I think here, okay, here's a friend, here's a friend here, so look here's a […], here's a […], so it's like that that you build another life – and then if you want to embrace this […] that is rejecting you, it's pretty disappointing, it's pretty disappointing, you turn back in on yourself and all the work you did before I don't know if it stays or else if it goes, and it's a shame, it's a shame, but that's how it is.

These words evoke a sense of the 'unlistened-to story' that Primo Levi writes about as the enduring burden of the survivor: "Why is the pain of every day translated so constantly into our dreams, in the ever-repeated scene of the unlistened-to story?" (Levi, 1958, p. 66). This experience of being shunned at moments of great need is one that we will consider both as an institutionalised process and for its relevance to group and community approaches.

The three case examples (the group engaged with the DRC country report, Claude and his 'radio-station' vision and the family's experience of the 'unlistened-to story') will help to illustrate how services can take account of the realities of survivors' experiences, understand the contexts within which they seek to rebuild their lives, and bring a 'radio station' breadth of vision that goes beyond therapy and creates a platform for solidarity and activism. They all relate in different ways to the silencing, and thus denigration, of survivor experience, and will demonstrate how group and community approaches promote the restoration of dignity as a guiding principle.

The Introduction to this book presented literature relating to survivor rehabilitation. It pointed to the variety and complexity of both the needs of survivors and of the work being carried out in different contexts. This complexity not only leads to a lack of clarity about what approaches are most helpful but also involves the issues of silencing raised by the three case examples. Lønning et al. state that "rehabilitation services for torture victims in Norway are fragmented, and the resulting practice is highly person dependent" (2021, p. 84). They go on to describe practitioners feeling "powerlessness when faced with a system that does not facilitate satisfactory rehabilitation". This introduces the notion that states do not just fail to adhere to the requirement to provide "as full rehabilitation as possible" (Convention against Torture (UNCAT), 1984, Article 14), but that they constitute an actual barrier to this realisation. The next section begins with reflections on the fragmentation of services before turning to the matter of obstruction.

FRAGMENTATION, DENIAL AND SILENCING

One explanation for this fragmentation is the nature of the challenges faced by survivors. High rates of post-traumatic stress disorder (PTSD), depression and anxiety are not the only problems. Papadopoulos has emphasised loss of home, rather than trauma, as the defining experience shared by all refugees (2002). Other losses, often involving violence, death or uncertainty about the whereabouts of loved ones, can lead to complicated grief or ambivalent loss. Human rights abuses frequently result in physical injury and impairment that cause chronic pain, which overlaps and becomes self-reinforcing with psychological pain. 'Enduring personality change after catastrophic events', now reframed in ICD-11 as 'Complex PTSD', reminds us of the severity and long-term nature of the harm that can be caused. Then there are the issues referred to as secondary or resettlement stressors: the significant hardships that survivors face in the aftermath of human rights abuses, whether as displaced people, in refugee camps, on the move or as people seeking asylum.

Forgetting

If the issues facing survivors are complicated, then so are the processes for providing support. This includes the idea that services take on features of the issues faced by the people they are working with (Cardona, 2020). Following this argument, the social and psychological fragmentation that are caused by human rights abuses can find their way into the fabric of organisations. Shephard (2002) and Herman (1992) write about the cycles of remembering and forgetting that psychological services in trauma fields go through, such that lessons learned are not integrated, are forgotten and have to be learned again, which Herman calls "a curious history … of episodic amnesia" (p. 7). Both fragmentation and amnesia relate to the vicarious impacts of trauma and the prevalence of denial as a response to atrocity.

Silencing

Denial as a way of avoiding distress is a common response and can be an instinctive part of trying to cope with overwhelming experiences and feelings. However, denial can also be an active process that is aimed at survivors in subtle or more direct ways. This may be the person who changes the subject when someone begins to talk about something traumatic or it could be the state response to an asylum application telling someone that they have fabricated their story. Both are acts of silencing. Again, it is Herman who writes about the need to "constantly contend with this tendency to discredit the victim or to render her invisible" (1992, p. 8). This is reminiscent of Levi's words about human rights abuses as 'unlistened-to stories'. Herman suggests that this challenge can only be met collectively: "In the absence of strong political movements for human rights, the active process of bearing witness inevitably gives way to the active process of forgetting" (p. 9). Group and community work can certainly provide witnessing, dignity and empowerment to its members, but a "strong political movement for human rights" sounds like the 'radio station' level of ambition that we heard from Claude at the outset.

The earlier group example describing the DRC country report is also relevant here, in showing the small acts of silencing that can take place in a rehabilitation context. The exchange in the group was multi-layered. Most immediately there was the meeting between Western advocates and the asylum-seeking people they were advocating for, and the moment when the former realised that their framework was not broad enough for the voices they sought to represent. In my experience, this is not an uncommon moment in this work. For the Congolese group members, it was another experience, even in the context of being offered support, where their reality was made invisible.

A MORAL TRANSGRESSION

Because human rights abuses are abuses of power, those working with survivors have a particular duty regarding further abuses of power, both in how power is enacted in their relationships with survivors, and how they respond to abuses of power that they witness in wider society.

Human rights abuses are often described as moral transgressions or injuries. This is easy to understand: the power of the state against the individual, the misuse of power, the inability of the victim to defend themselves, the supposed source of protection and redress being the persecutor, and the levels of cruelty from one human to another.

A moral transgression requires a moral response. Before describing what constitutes such a response, it is important to think about the secondary or resettlement stressors that asylum-seeking people encounter in the aftermath of these moral transgressions.

The establishment of safety for survivors is a cornerstone of trauma approaches. The ways in which the threat of forced return to the place of trauma obstructs recovery is well understood. As well as this, it is recognised that the burdens of seeking asylum, these secondary stressors, which include detention, no rights to work, enforced poverty, limited options for family reunion and an adversarial and bureaucratically broken asylum system, are barriers to feeling safe and therefore to recovery. Framing these as 'secondary or resettlement stressors' seems misleading and risks placing them in a mental health and wellbeing framework rather than in a moral dimension.

Survivors often use different language about this. They do not usually talk about secondary stressors; they commonly say that their experience of seeking asylum is one of *psychological torture*. Members of French-speaking groups I worked with described this as *torture morale* and, with a growing understanding of the culture they had arrived in, spoke of *polite torture*. This was at a time when politicians, the military and even some psychologists were talking about *torture lite* in relation to the 'war on terror' and the abuses taking place in such legal wastelands as Guantanamo Bay. These are not throwaway comments or exaggerations, but the descriptions chosen by people who know the reality of torture from lived experience. Stone Flowers (see Chapter 15) express this in their song, 'Double Torture':

People back home
Fathers and mothers
Listen, listen

At home there are tortures
Away there are tortures
Listen, listen

A Western psychotherapeutic response to such statements, which has been suggested to me in supervision, is that survivors are re-experiencing their primary trauma (the torture in their home country) through their current struggles in the UK. This interpretation becomes another instance of the 'unlistened-to story'. The silencing impact of this takes place within a racialised framework, whereby the White[2] therapist is ready to hear about the atrocities committed in 'foreign' countries but less ready to countenance atrocities closer to home.

Most stressors that researchers identify are a result of the systems that are deliberately put in place as part of immigration controls. The entire edifice of the 'hostile environment' in the UK, that was so clearly exposed in relation to the 'Windrush' generation (Institute of Race Relations, 2018), also targets survivors of human rights abuses. It is a system that: denies the traumatic experiences that people have survived and the rights to which they are entitled; imposes the indignities of detention; forces people into poverty; and encourages media and public views of asylum-seeking people as illegal. The negative impact of these measures on survivors is well documented (see Boyles et al., 2022).

This environment appears to be intensifying. In 2021, the UK Home Office began housing asylum applicants in former military barracks, which the Independent Chief Inspector of Borders and Immigration reported as "impoverished, run-down and unsuitable for long-term accommodation" (APPG, 2021, p. 16). Despite prior warnings from Public Health England, over 50% of residents contracted COVID-19. When challenged, the Home Office blamed residents for not socially distancing (an impossibility in the crowded shared sleeping and sanitation facilities) and issued its worn-out mantra that the UK has "a proud history of welcoming and supporting those in need of our protection" (Home Office, 2018). The more convincing description came from one of the residents, Kenan, speaking at the All-Party Parliamentary Group on Immigration Detention: "It would be difficult to design a system that more perfectly delivers despair and deteriorating human health and mental capacity than these asylum camps" (APPG, 2021, p. 10).

Those at the receiving end of this hostile treatment from the state, whether the 'Windrush' generation or those seeking asylum, are overwhelmingly Black and Brown people. Goodfellow concludes that "at its core, the nation's history on immigration legislation is a history of racism" (2019, p. 91).

From this perspective, the asylum system, the hostile environment and the context of institutional racism are ongoing moral transgressions. Survivors have experienced extremes of cruelty in which their dignity has been attacked. This is followed by further degrading treatment when exercising their right to seek sanctuary. UNCAT requires "that the restoration of the dignity of the victim is the ultimate objective in the provision of redress" (General Comment No. 3, 2012, p. 1, para. 4). Creating an environment and systems that survivors and multiple organisations, including the government's own investigators, have consistently over a period of decades reported as removing the dignity of survivors is clearly a failure to meet this requirement.

Part of the harshness of these measures is the level of denial about their existence. Not only are there parallels between the inhumane abuses that people suffer that lead them to seek asylum and the inhumanity of the systems that they encounter when seeking asylum, but there is also denial in both situations that the inhumanity has taken place. This is the kind of double-bind that, since the 1938 play *Gaslight*, is referred to as 'gaslighting'. More recently, Andrews has described this as the 'psychosis of Whiteness' (Andrews, 2018), whereby racial discrimination remains hidden and rational discussion about it is made impossible. In the example of the army barracks, with its COVID-19 risks and unfitness as accommodation, the fact that these transgressions were carried out by a private company contracted by the Home Office certainly fits with the view that the drivers of racism have moved from colonial to postcolonial to globalised mechanisms (Andrews, 2021a, p. 204). In this context, Claude's appeal for a radio station rather than therapy as a means of combatting these 'secondary stressors' makes complete sense.

The works of generations of writers on colonialism, racism and immigration (in this chapter, see: Dubois, Fanon, Andrews, Goodfellow, Mayblin and Patel) help to see the UK asylum system as institutionally racist. It is a system that has implemented and overseen an accumulation of acts that appear, as frequently expressed by survivors, to meet the UNCAT definition of torture [my italics]:

> *severe pain or suffering*, whether physical or *mental*, is *intentionally inflicted* on a person for such purposes as … or for any reason based on discrimination of any kind, when such pain or suffering is inflicted *by or at the instigation of or with the consent or acquiescence of a public official or other person acting in an official capacity.*
>
> (para. 4)

On both sides of the Atlantic, the treatment of child refugees bears out this analysis in particularly shocking ways: in the USA in 2018, children from migrant families were forcibly removed from their parents and, in many cases, without the means of being reunited; and in the UK in 2020, the government repeatedly rejected the Dubs amendments aimed at facilitating refugee children's reunion with their families. Mayblin, who has studied asylum and immigration in the context of colonialism, writes about this as "differential humanity" (2017, p. 5), whereby "some human bodies are simply more easily and acceptably degraded than others" (p. 3).

GROUPWORK AS PART OF A MORAL RESPONSE

People's lives are therefore at stake in this legal and bureaucratic territory within which human rights conventions are contested. Our interest here is in how the mechanisms of trauma and power, and the inhumanity and degradation inherent in the asylum system, influence recovery; and how services should be organised to mitigate and overcome these influences.

Writing during colonial rule, Fanon described its subjects as being left with "no choice save between inferiority and dependence" (1952, p. 69). Whilst discrimination is an imposition of inferiority, there are also many ways in which survivors are positioned into dependency. Some of these arise within the services set up to support them, which are after all members of the host society and, as such, in positions of power and prone to institutional racism. Fanon goes on to talk about individualism as an obstacle to the process of liberation. The rest of this chapter will look at steps that move away from individualising processes and towards processes of liberation.

There is often an assumption amongst Western practitioners that survivors need individual support to regain a sense of safety. Indeed, a survivor may often choose individual support if offered the choice. This is unsurprising, given their multiple needs, the sense of exposure in a new environment, the humiliation that is such a central part of abuse and the wish to avoid exposure to further feelings of vulnerability. The offer of a group can be daunting. But equally, in my experience, most survivors who are encouraged to join a group or community, and who experience the benefits of a carefully organised social intervention, choose to continue with this.

As highlighted in this book's Introduction, attending to the social part of a bio-psycho-so-cial model is increasingly recommended. At its most basic level this is a response to the iso-lation that is a consequence of abuse, whereby people retreat through shock, altered mood, shame and other psychological impacts, and due to the disruption to the main strands of their lives, such as family, home, work and community. The approach proposed here emphasises the importance of social approaches from the outset, as a way of ensuring that 'the restoration of the dignity of the victim' is paramount, and that the relationships offered are ones that will not fall into the false dichotomy of 'inferiority and dependence'.

The advantages of groupwork identified throughout this book offer clear steps away from the risks associated with individualising processes. They begin as a response to the human urge to come together in adversity and build resilience.

I remember seeing this most vividly in psychoeducation groups for recently arrived asy-lum-seeking people. The aim was to share information that would assist group members to orient themselves and navigate the new society they were encountering. The evaluation of these groups concluded that social connection was as valuable as the psychoeducation. A turn-ing point was often the week when a former service-user was invited to speak with the group. One such visitor would always start by talking about the terrible British weather. He was partly breaking the ice but at the same time he was being serious; those first cold winters were often a shock for which people were unprepared. And at a further level, he was opening a metaphorical discussion about the terrible welcome in the new country, which group members responded to with stories of the high hopes and expectations that they had arrived with, and how these had disappeared in the rain and on the cold shoulders they encountered.

The most striking aspect of these groups was the different kinds of story that emerged. In the early weeks, members would share tales of adversity and speak about their current pressing needs. These showed the value of general group concepts such as universality, sharing infor-mation, rebuilding social skills and interpersonal learning. These were important and remained a central focus for the duration of the groups. However, during the sessions with the former service-user, different stories were told. These were about survival in the face of hardship, over-coming the odds, and hope over despair. Members would speak about standing up in asylum hearings and successfully representing themselves; about support they had given to others in the community; or of the value of the family and professional roles they previously held. Again, these related to general group concepts, such as re-finding hope and building collective resil-ience. However, they also related to the experiences of powerlessness and dehumanisation that are imposed by both perpetrators and then within the context in which survivors attempt to recover, and demonstrated the group's efforts to resist such impositions through creating trust, connection and belonging.

This relates to the idea of building social identity, whereby social interventions can create a 'trauma membrane' that helps survivors to cope with the impacts of past experiences and that acts as a buffer to the secondary stressors of refugee life. Alfadhli et al. (2019) present these ideas as important parts of effective interventions to boost collective resilience. Others have written about developing whole integrated models around group and community approaches (see Introduction).

COMMUNITY, LIBERATION AND SOCIAL ACTION

The earlier example, in which group members contributed to the DRC country report, showed an integrated groupwork approach. There was an effort to address the specific needs of survivors, taking a human rights approach, with awareness of the adverse contexts within which rehabilitation was taking place. However, this went beyond these group, community-building and social identity ideas to ones of advocacy and social action. There was an effort to join with survivors in taking action (writing a country report) concerning the adverse conditions they were experiencing (poor immigration decision-making).

This draws from the traditions of liberation social psychology, which were developed in the politically repressive environments of Central and South America from the 1970s through the work of Martín-Baró and then Paulo Frere, and which have since been extensively written about in the UK context (Burton and Kagan, 2005). These combine group and community-based models with liberation practices and social action components that move out of the 'inferiority or dependence' positions and into dignity positions through an emphasis on empowerment and consciousness-raising. They propose a form of collectivism that is transformative rather than simply ameliorative. They move from thinking about community as the context in which individuals recover from adversity to considering the health and power of community as a whole.

Conscientização

Looking at the works of liberation theory and other writers already referred to, it is noticeable how much they highlight consciousness-raising. Du Bois refers to emancipation through understanding the ways of oppression (1903); Fanon writes about helping patients to become conscious of the unconscious wish to "turn white or disappear" (1952, p. 75); Freire frames his ideas around the word conscientização (1970); whilst Martín-Baró makes the links between personal distress and social oppression (1996). Consciousness-raising is also at the heart of the women's liberation movement.

As Afuape and Hughes (2015) remind us, this does not lead to a clear model for working with survivors, as this would fall into the same orthodoxies that were being challenged, but instead holds up a frame with which to challenge ourselves about the positions we take in relation to marginalisation and oppression within society and how we position our work through our values and practices.

Returning again to the DRC country report group example, we can see deeper layers of power and racialisation that involve these positionings. The report was positively intentioned. The (White) report writers planned to provide information to (White) decision-makers, about (Black) human rights abusers, so that their (Black) victims stood a better chance of gaining the right to asylum. Claiming asylum is a dependent position and one where institutionalised racism can confer inferiority to deny the right being supposedly upheld. The report writers were asking survivors to narrate the persecution inflicted on them, whilst denial was maintained about the ongoing Western economic and political interference that played a role in the country context. There was also silence about the legacies in modern society of the atrocities that were committed by the White protagonists' ancestors towards the Black protagonists' ancestors in the form of colonialism. And so, a situation in which report writers sought to ally with victims, to resist unfair asylum decision-making, contained more hidden relationships.

The advocates (and the groupworkers) saw that their intention to use the power of their voice to positively influence the asylum system was not well-received. This was followed by a second realisation about the globalised context of the conflict taking place in the DRC that involved the precious metals so important to the mobile phones sitting in their and everyone else's pockets. In this way, a piece of advocacy work became fraught with the postcolonial and therefore racialised context for asylum-seeking and risked perpetuating further silencing, and invoking another moment of choosing between inferiority or dependence.

The opportunity that the group gave was for this set of circumstances to be brought to light, for the challenge to be made and the silence broken. This could not have happened in the same way in a series of individual meetings to take people's testimonies and relied on a group committed to making space for such conscientização.

Social action

This consciousness-raising has a natural link with social action. The power of social action as a part of recovery is demonstrated by groups such as Women Asylum Seekers Together (see Chapter 3), community support in Peru (see Chapter 4), Voices Network (British Red Cross) and Survivors Speak Out (Freedom from Torture). In their interventions and actions, they show the value of campaigning and advocating on the issues facing them, including through demands for changes to oppressive asylum systems and calls for placing dignity at the heart of the state's response to immigration and asylum. These are embodiments of the principles of conscientização.

However, such direct action is not the only kind of social action that can be part of reha-bilitation approaches. It is possible to create environments within rehabilitation, psychosocial and other support activities that survivors can engage with and co-create.

Groups that offer participants a meaningful role in the ways in which they operate and over the conversations that can be had promote conscientização and lead to such forms of social action. I saw this clearly from a time-limited group I was working with, who, at the end of the six-month intervention, arrived together at the director of the organisation's door and demanded that the group continue. At the close of a different 18-month group, its members made a proposal for a survivor-led peer-support project. They were far ahead of the organisa-tion in their vision and their proposal was not taken up, but they had set down a challenge that eventually led to senior survivor representation in the organisation – Claude's 'radio-station' vision in action.

This moves us the whole way from individualising processes (that impede the processes of liberation) via groupwork, peer support, community-building, social identity, and social action through to liberation practices.

Why is this full cycle so important? We understand the loss of dignity that is an inherent part of abuse and, in the case of human rights abuses, is a deliberate aim of the perpetrator. We recognise the importance of the restoration of dignity as part of recovery and the extent of the challenges involved in recovery. The debilitation and stigma of mental health problems associated with trauma involve their own indignities. The compounding features of chronic pain present major obstacles to carrying out the tasks of confronting the past and reconnecting with a meaningful future. Avoidance predominates as both a feature and a consequence of these challenges. Together, these cumulatively hinder access to support and community.

Avoidance is usually framed as an individual process that occurs as a consequence of trauma; it is one of the core features of PTSD. Avoidance by survivors is understandable due to lack of trust, through anxiety and shame, and through repeated experiences of rejection and denial of opportunity. However, avoidance is not just the preserve of the trauma victim. Witnesses, helpers, communities, organisations and societies can also enter into the dynamics of avoidance. And at organisational, social and political levels this can move into processes that, both unwittingly and deliberately, involve the silencing and further oppression of survivors. This is institutional avoidance, which takes place and is driven within the context of racial discrimination. These are not conditions that are conducive to the restoration of dignity and are barriers to rehabilitation that services have a responsibility to address (Patel, 2021).

Groupwork can bring people together, help build feelings of belonging and resilience, and can support people to deal with the traumas of the past. It can be ameliorative and buffer some of the stressors that survivors contend with. However, group approaches can only become transformative when they move through the full cycle referred to above. This is how they can challenge the framework of oppression, including institutional racism, that survivors continue to endure in host contexts, when they address institutional avoidance and when they incorporate the consciousness-raising practices of liberation approaches. This is a 'radio station' level of ambition.

SUMMARY

The human rights abuses that lead people to leave their homes behind and seek safety as refugees are both extreme and commonplace, often hidden but widespread, private to the lives of those affected but impacting the communities where they occur, local and yet framed within the global political contexts that drive them. Many victims do not survive. At the heart of human rights work is the necessity to bear witness, to not turn away from the 'ever repeated scene of the un-listened to story'. One of the un-listened to stories that won't go away is the racism that is embedded in colonial history, compounding the injuries of prior persecution and abuse, and blocking people from the recovery that is their right.

Human rights-based approaches (Boyles, 2017; Patel, 2019) challenge us to make every aspect of our practice work towards the restoration of dignity. Liberation social psychology helps to make the link between human rights and social approaches. And critical race theory allows us to see the racialised contexts within which survivors seek to regain dignity and within which services seek to engage in meaningful and effective support. The combination of these powerful intellectual positions makes a convincing argument for group and community approaches as the main framework for models based on the restoration of dignity.

NOTES

1 Anonymised name.
2 The term White is used to refer to a system – an "enduring system of invisible, racialised advantage (where darker, 'not White', skin colour is constructed as a marker of inferiority)" (Patel, 2021, p. 4).

REFERENCES

Afuape, T. and Hughes, G. (eds.) (2015) *Liberation Practices: Towards Emotional Wellbeing Through Dialogue*. London: Routledge. doi:10.4324/9781315758244.

Alfadhli, K., Güler, M., Cakal, H. and Drury, J. (2019) 'The role of emergent shared identity in psychosocial support among refugees of conflict in developing countries', *International Review of Social Psychology*, 32(1), p. 2. doi:10.5334/irsp.176.

All-Party Parliamentary Group (APPG) on Immigration Detention (2021) *Report of the Inquiry into Quasi-Detention*. Available at: https://appgdetention.org.uk/wp-content/uploads/2021/12/211209-APPG-on-Immigration-Detention-Report-of-Inquiry-into-Quasi-Detention.pdf?x72338 (Accessed: 13 January 2022).

Andrews, K. (2018) *Back to Black: Retelling Black Radicalism for the 21st Century*. London: Zed Books.

Andrews, K. (2021a) *The New Age of Empire: How Racism and Colonialism Still Rule the World*. London: Penguin.

Andrews, K. (2021b) 'Racism is the public health crisis', *The Lancet*, 397(10282), pp. 1342–1343. doi:10.1016/S0140-6736(21)00775-3.

Boyles, J. (ed.) (2017) *Psychological Therapies for Survivors of Torture: A Human-Rights Approach with People Seeking Asylum*. Monmouth: PCCS Books.

Boyles, J., Ewart-Biggs, R., Kazembe, J., Miller, J. and Oliver, K. (2022) 'Seeking Asylum in the UK', in: Maloney, C., Nelki, J. and Summers, A. (eds.) *Asylum Seeking and Mental Health Services*. Cambridge: Cambridge University Press, pp. 29–49.

Burton, M. and Kagan, C. (2005). 'Liberation social psychology: Learning from Latin America', *Journal of Community and Applied Social Psychology*, 15(1), pp. 63–78. doi:10.1002/casp.786.

Cardona, F. (2020) 'The Team as a Sponge*: How the nature of the task affects the behaviour and mental life of a team', in *Work Matters*. London: Routledge, pp. 27–38. doi:10.4324/9780429317439.

Du Bois, W.E.B. (1903) *The Souls of Black Folk*. Reprint, New York: Dover Publications, 1994.

Fanon, F. (1952) *Black Skin, White Masks*. Reprint, London: Pluto Press, 1986.

Freire, P. (1970) *Pedagogy of the Oppressed*. New York: Seabury Press.

Goodfellow, M. (2019) *Hostile Environment: How Immigrants Became Scapegoats*. London: Verso.

Herman, J. (1992) *Trauma and Recovery: From Domestic Abuse to Political Terror*. New York: Basic Books.

Home Office (2018) *Factsheet: Asylum and resettlement*. Available at: https://homeofficemedia.blog.gov.uk/2018/01/19/fact-sheet-on-the-uks-support-for-asylum-seeking-and-refugee-children-in-europe/ (Accessed: 13 January 2022).

Institute of Race Relations (2018) *The Embedding of State Hostility: A background paper on the Windrush Scandal*. Available at: https://irr.org.uk/app/uploads/2018/11/Embedding-State-hostility-v4.pdf (Accessed: 19 January 2022).

Levi, P. (1958) *If this is a Man*. Reprint, London: Abacus, 1987.

Lønning, M. N., Bringedal Houge, A., Laupstad, I. and Aasnes, A. E. (2021) '"A random system" The organisation and practice of torture rehabilitation services in Norway', *Torture Journal*, 30(3), pp. 84–100. doi:10.7146/torture.v30i3.119875.

Martín-Baró, I. (1996) 'Toward a liberation psychology', in: Aron A. & Corne S. (Eds.), *Writings for a Liberation Psychology*. New York: Harvard University Press.

Mayblin, L. (2017) *Asylum After Empire: Colonial Legacies in the Politics of Seeking Asylum*. London: Rowman & Littlefield International.

Papadopoulos, R. (2002) 'Refugees, home and trauma', in: Papadopoulos, R. (ed.) *Therapeutic Care for Refugees*. London: Karnac, pp. 9–39.

Patel, N. (2019) 'Conceptualising rehabilitation as reparation for torture survivors: A clinical perspective', *The International Journal of Human Rights*, 23:9, pp. 1546–1568. doi:10.1080/13642987.2019.1612373.

Patel, N. (2021) 'Dismantling the scaffolding of institutional racism and institutionalising anti-racism', *Journal of Family Therapy*, 2021(00), pp. 1–18. doi:10.1111/1467-6427.12367.

Shephard, B. (2002) *A War of Nerves*. London: Pimlico.

United Nations Committee Against Torture (2012). General comment No. 3: Convention against Torture and Other Cruel, Inhuman or Degrading Treatment or Punishment: implementation of Article 14 by States parties, 19 November 2012, CAT/C/GC/3.

United Nations Convention against Torture and Other Cruel, Inhuman or Degrading Treatment or Punishment (1984) Available at: https://treaties.un.org/doc/Treaties/1987/06/19870626%20 02-38%20AM/Ch_IV_9p.pdf (Accessed 24 January 2022).

SECTION 1

BUILDING COMMUNITIES

CHAPTER 2

TREE OF LIFE ZIMBABWE

Community-based trauma healing

Lynn Walker, Eugenia Mpande and Susan Wyatt

> Who thought of the tree analogy? It is so brilliant. That was the tipping point for me. When I did the tree meditation, I began to find myself for the first time for a long time.
>
> (Workshop participant, 2016)

A former freedom fighter in the Zimbabwean Liberation struggle in the late 1970s, and then a victim of torture and abduction, Collin struggled with the impact of the multiple distressing events he had experienced and witnessed. This deep and continuous trauma was affecting every aspect of his life, and he was grappling with his mental health. Collin was invited to take part in a Tree of Life trauma healing and empowerment (THE) workshop in 2014, and later told us that this was the start of his long journey to restoration and recovery.

Tree of Life Trust is a Zimbabwean non-governmental organization (NGO) which provides community-based mental health and psychosocial support for survivors of torture and collective violence. In this chapter the authors, who are all staff at the Tree of Life Trust, will show how the use of groupwork is key to the restorative process in our context, and how we are using the tree as an analogy for healing and as a tool which enables survivors to reconnect with themselves, their families, and communities.

HISTORY AND CONTEXT: UNDERSTANDING THE CYCLES OF VIOLENCE

Zimbabwe has faced decades of systematic political and structural violence, including colonisation and a civil war leading up to the country gaining its independence in 1980. These cycles of violence have continued and span across different generations, tribes, ethnicities and political factions. The regular and methodical use of organised violence and torture by authorities over the years, on activists and civilians alike, has instilled deep-seated fear across all levels of society. This has resulted in fragmented social support structures and disempowered communities.

At the time of writing in 2021, Zimbabwe continues to be in a protracted state of political and economic instability with few accountability or justice measures to combat human rights abuses. Tree of Life Trust was founded when ongoing violations were happening, and we continue to operate under some of the conditions described above. The Trust remains politically neutral, providing trauma healing measures to both individuals and communities, regardless of their background.

Collective healing

Collective trauma refers to "collectively experienced extreme situations [that] have unique social and psychological trajectories … impacting on the social dynamics, processes, structures and functioning of a collective" (Reimann and König, 2017, p. 5). In order to combat the effects of collective trauma, a critical focus must include restoration of social support systems and assisting people to feel connected to each other (Bubenzer and Tankink, 2017).

DOI: 10.4324/9781003192978-4

> Trauma does not occur in a vacuum. Individual trauma occurs in a context of community.
> … How a community responds to individual trauma sets the foundation for the impact of the
> traumatic event, experience, and effect. Communities that provide a context of understand-
> ing and self-determination may facilitate the healing and recovery process for the individual.
> Alternatively, communities that avoid, overlook, or misunderstand the impact of trauma may
> often be re-traumatising and interfere with the healing process.
>
> (SAMHSA, 2014, p. 17)

Research done in 2009, across 40 countries, examining the types and severity of mental illnesses experienced due to national-level conflicts revealed that the only difference between those directly tortured and those living in constant fear (indirect victims) were the types of psycho-logical disorders experienced. Survivors of direct violations and/or torture experience higher levels of post-traumatic stress disorder (PTSD) and anxiety, while those indirectly affected due to social proximity or vicarious trauma and/or exposure to the events experience higher levels of depression (Steel et al., 2009).

Local research in Zimbabwe (Parsons et al., 2011) demonstrated similar trends and high-lighted the need to address collective trauma experiences in the country, in addition to pro-viding individual psychological rehabilitation processes for direct survivors. With this working knowledge of Zimbabwe and its specific healing needs, Tree of Life was formed, targeting both individual and collective trauma and its impacts.

THE HISTORY OF THE TREE OF LIFE TRUST

During a period of election-related violence and abuses in Zimbabwe in 2003, Bev Reeler, the founder of the Tree of Life Trust process, relocated temporarily to South Africa. There she met up with exiled Zimbabwean activists, most of whom were survivors of torture and politically moti-vated violence. She was moved to support them in overcoming their trauma and, after a number of conversations with exiled survivors, adapted the Tree of Life workshop, which was originally being used with young people in environmental education activities, as a healing and empowerment tool.

The very first trauma healing and empowerment workshops were held in South Africa soon after, with a small number of Zimbabwean survivors being trained as facilitators. In 2004 the process was brought back to Zimbabwe.

With a surge of violence during the 2008 presidential election re-run, the Tree of Life project was asked to roll out healing workshops for torture survivors. Later the approach was extended to help survivors of collective violence and those who live in fear of human rights abuses. The project grew very rapidly and in 2010 the trust was formerly registered. In 2021, Tree of Life Trust operates in over 20 Zimbabwean communities and has reached over 15,000 survivors of collective violence and torture.

THE PRESENT DAY STRUCTURE OF TREE OF LIFE: BIG TREE AND SMALL TREE

Tree of Life Trust consists of two main therapeutic teams known as the 'Big Tree' and the 'Small Tree'. The Small Tree comprises the core team of 15 field officers, who are mostly sur-vivors of organised violence and torture, complemented by a network of over 150 community facilitators who make up the Big Tree. These community facilitators are either direct or indirect survivors of torture and organised violence who have all gone through the trauma healing and empowerment workshops prior to becoming community facilitators and have varying levels of technical skills in psychosocial support work.

Both teams receive ongoing training, skills development and capacity-building activities guided by identified needs. This process includes, as a matter of routine, restorative debriefing, supervision sessions and case conferences.

The identification of survivors in the community who have the qualities and the mental resilience to become community facilitators is undertaken through a rigorous assessment and selection process. Those who do not have these qualities are trained to take on other complementary roles, as workshop organisers or negotiators with the authorities. The Big Tree members undergo an ongoing training process, where they continue to explore their own healing and reflect on how to embody our key principles of honesty, integrity, trust and respect.

Trauma healing and empowerment workshop facilitators undergo a two-year phased training, coaching and mentoring process. This training places as much importance on the cohesion of the whole facilitation group, and on self-care and wellbeing, as we do on specific technical skills. The community facilitators are encouraged to form their own groups in their geographical location to further integrate peer support and create a safe space to share experiences. Several of these community groups have later registered as community-based organisations and have extended their networking activities with other NGO's to provide complementary services and support for the community.

Our experience and commitment to building a network of local facilitators at community level helps to build ownership and ensures continuity of care and support. The community facilitators are able to identify individuals for referral to the trauma healing and empowerment workshop and provide a gentler and more acceptable initial pathway into the formal health system. They also support the Tree of Life team to offer longer-term support, and systematically provide follow-up sessions with individuals or communities after conducting any type of workshop.

TREE OF LIFE INTERVENTIONS

In Zimbabwe, like most of Africa, the collective nature of the culture and the importance of relationships is key to effective healing interventions. Building on the understanding that in Zimbabwe wellbeing is a collective state of healthy connections, an individual does not exist in isolation from a community, everyone is interconnected with each other (*ubuntu*). The greeting, *"I am well, if you are well"* is used across the region, Zimbabwe included, and the concept of ubuntu resonates in many African communities. The group is, therefore, a vehicle for reconnecting.

Tree of Life's work aims to tap into existing community resources and strengths and to draw on local knowledge and capacities. We have a range of activities to facilitate trauma healing at the individual and collective level, which are community-rooted and community-driven, and aimed at restorative justice. These interventions promote personal agency and unlock the innovation and creativity which is needed to address the challenges of one's life and those of one's community (Colletta and Cullen, 2000; Curling, 2005; Higson-Smith, 2002). Tree of Life works in a careful, gradual and protracted process of engagement, aiming to create sufficient safety, and to promote ownership of the outcomes. *"Tree of Life uses a gentle and humble approach. You do not hit direct. You give us time and space to share and to gradually enter the process"* (Community Leader, Nkayi district).

Tree of Life signature group activities include the trauma healing and empowerment workshops, which address individual trauma, and the psychosocial awareness and coping skills workshops, which work at the community and collective level. We also facilitate a trauma informed art therapy programme and psychological first aid activities. Additionally, we support and train other civil society organisations in trauma awareness and trauma-informed practice and self-care, also employing groupwork as the main delivery model.

TRAUMA HEALING AND EMPOWERMENT WORKSHOPS

Trauma healing and empowerment processes are based on the rationale that if survivors are able to narrate their experience to a group of respectful and understanding witnesses, they will find relief from the emotional burden of their distressing experiences. This witnessing also affirms dignity and respect, builds lasting support between people, and helps to lay the foundations for reconciliation and a healthier community in the future. The workshops help survivors to recover their power through connectedness, by working together to reclaim a sense of community (Reeler et al., 2009).

The workshops provide personal healing for survivors of torture and organised violence measured in terms of a reduction in symptoms. At the interpersonal level, this is measured by an increase in reported engagement with other members of the community, active concern for the wellbeing of others, and more positive attitudes toward community healing. The process is based on a group narrative approach using the tree as an analogy for resilience, healing and restoration.

Tree of Life trauma healing and empowerment workshop structure

In this three-day residential workshop, the tree is used as a metaphor to represent the different aspects of a person's life, and as a tool to structure storytelling and bonding within the group. The workshop is carefully planned to support participants to slowly and gradually build their story.

The participants are put into small groups (circles) of no more than ten people and the circles are guided and supported by a minimum of two experienced facilitators. The circle ensures that everyone can see each other and that everybody has equal status. A talking piece is used, usually a culturally appropriate, meaningful or significant object. Holding the talking piece empowers the person to talk and encourages the others to listen without interrupting. At the centre of the circle the group construct a mandala, a circle of plant material (flowers, leaves, etc.) which strengthens connection with nature and serves as a witness to the stories.

The workshop is structured into eight circles. The first welcoming circle aims to familiarise the group with how the circle process works. The group then forms its own set of agreements about how they would like to live and work together over the period of the workshop (such as respect, confidentiality, non-judgement). This process helps to make the participants feel welcome and safe and builds their readiness to witness other people's stories.

Firstly, the *roots* are used to enable participants to honour their origins and connect with and acknowledge their own history, to understand that their stories began a long time ago and will continue long after their lives have passed on. It shows them how their history, for which they were not responsible, has shaped who and where they are at this moment in time.

The second circle, *the tree meditation*, extends the participants' view of themselves by connecting with the world of nature around. Here the participants identify a tree which they feel a connection with and they sit alone, observing this tree in great detail. The tree meditation is done in two parts. In the first part, the participants consider what impact being silent in nature and paying attention to what they observe has on them. The participants then undertake *the tree inquiry* (the third circle) where they are invited to observe how the tree resonates with their own life story and what they observe about the cyclical and interdependent nature of life. This shifts their attention from the chatter in their minds to the peaceful sounds of nature and they begin to recognise how they are a part of a larger natural system, and that nature has cycles of growth and periods of trauma that shape it. This process establishes the connection with the natural environment that is deeply embedded in Zimbabwean culture and spirituality and provides a tool that participants can take away after the workshop. *"When I struggle, I go to my tree and it helps me to be calm. I remember that I am like the tree, I can grow even with wounds"* (Workshop participant at closing ceremony).

Having noted how the tree shows the scars of past traumas, but continues to grow, thrive and blossom, the following group circles will then focus in on the parts of the tree. Each participant is given a large piece of paper, and over the course of the subsequent circles will build up a drawing of the tree that symbolises the story of their life.

The fourth circle, the *trunk*, focuses on the important stories of their upbringing and childhood. The approach brings the value of listening, and being listened to, as well as guiding the participants to remember important stories from their childhood and upbringing.

These four stages in the process are a graduated lead-up to the moment when participants tell their trauma stories, and also witness the stories from other members of the circle. Prior to this fifth circle, the participants are first taken through a series of relaxation exercises. The aim of this is to create a trusting and secure environment in which participants feel able to tell the stories of the difficult parts of their lives. As well as the group approach in the workshops, we also provide a facility, called the *compassion corner*, where participants can talk to a trained counsellor from the team on an individual level.

Circle six, focusing on the *power of togetherness*, shows participants how they are connected to each other and the world around them, even when they may feel isolated. This session explores how hard it is to achieve things without support and participants are encouraged to think about ways to be more powerful as individuals as well as a group, family or community.

At this point, the participants look back and think about what they have learned and gained through the difficulties they have faced, and they are invited to recognise and acknowledge where they have received support and recognise what gifts (*leaves* and *fruits*) they have to contribute to the *forest*.

These circles are interspersed with body work; a mixture of exercises, yoga moves, games, dancing and breathing exercises that help the participants regain connection with their bodies and feel the joy of movement and learn ways to regulate the physical reactions they have due to the impact of trauma.

At the *closing circle* ceremony, the journey people have travelled is validated and what they would like to celebrate is made the central emphasis. Participants identify what they would like to leave behind, and what they would like to take forward in themselves. This part of the workshop aims to address the powerlessness that many victims of torture and organised violence experience. The different forms of power are explored, and participants are supported to find their own power and the power that comes from togetherness.

Hence, each element of the tree represents part of the story; the roots symbolise the connection with our histories; the trunk our childhood and adolescence, which shapes our resilience and capacity to cope with potentially traumatic situations; the branches, which represent the system and networks of the community we live within, and the leaves and fruits, which represent our strengths and the gifts we possess, and how we can begin to build on these in our families and communities. The scars and broken limbs are symbols that it is possible to thrive and blossom whilst still wounded and scarred. This analogy has real resonance in the Zimbabwean context and has been repeatedly mentioned in feedback from participants as being a key part to the start of the journey of healing.

> Whenever I feel that I am not coping, or I start to lose my strength I go and sit with my tree. It reminds me that even when I get difficulties, I can heal just like the tree does when cut.
>
> (Participant at follow-up)

After the three-day workshop, the facilitators provide ongoing follow-ups, and may make referrals for specialist counselling when needed. We also work closely with various other organisations who provide legal services, medical treatment and support to survivors of organised violence and torture.

The feedback from participants, our internal monitoring data and an external evaluation (Mpande et al., 2013) has shown that the process has a clear impact on mental wellbeing with significantly reduced trauma symptoms.

> … after sharing my story and witnessing other participants' stories, I felt I had off-loaded. … I felt relieved emotionally and relaxed physically and the understanding that I was not the only one who has survived torture empowered me internally.
>
> (workshop participant)

Workshop facilitators are often members of that community, as research recognises that victims and witnesses are more likely to work through their grief in a community that is familiar to them, one that recognises and identifies with the nature of their pain (Hutchison and Bleiker, 2008). It also encourages access to local mental health and psychosocial support, reducing the stigma and discrimination often associated with mental illness, providing a more acceptable initial pathway into the health system.

Where appropriate we hold the workshops in the community, in a safe and natural place, and involve members of the same community. But, where it is not safe, feasible or relevant the workshops take place in an alternative location. This is often the case when we work with special focus groups, bringing together participants with similar experiences, such as sexual assault survivors, war veterans or victims of abduction or trafficking.

Psychosocial awareness and coping skills workshops

The psychosocial awareness and coping skills (PACS) workshops are a complementary intervention and strengthen resilience and mental wellbeing for community members. These workshops can be used as an entry point when working with new communities, or prior to the trauma healing and empowerment workshops.

The PACS workshop explores the nature of trauma in the community and educates community members to recognise the signs of individual and collective trauma, to identify the nature and causes of trauma in their community, and then plan collective action to address both the symptoms and, over time, the causes. The meeting also generates awareness of the importance of supporting others to build resilience at community level.

PACS workshops bring together between 40 and 200 community members at one time. The participants are from all walks of life and involve the leaders and those who are powerful in the community, as well as the most vulnerable, including survivors of human rights abuses. Some of the participants have recognised positions of authority or professional roles in the community. These positions or roles bring with them a level of power or influence which potentially could inhibit inclusive, equitable participation by the whole group. Hence, we encourage all participants to de-role during the workshop. Each person writes their title on a piece of paper and puts the paper in a box at the start of each day. By doing this they also place the perceived authority their role encompasses and the expectations and assumptions that come with their role into the box. They are then able to step out of the role and participate in the workshops as themselves, contributing in an authentic way and enabling other participants to also speak more freely. At the end of the day, each participant is able to revert to their role when they retrieve the paper from the box.

The guided conversation takes place over two days and utilises groupwork in a very similar way to the trauma healing and empowerment workshops. Agreements are made the circle and talking piece are used and report backs are made in a mutually respectful environment. Skilful facilitation and the use of facilitators from the community intensifies the impact

UNDERLYING PRINCIPLES OF THE TREE OF LIFE INTERVENTIONS

The foundation on which the success of Tree of Life's interventions has been built is the result of years of continuous relationship building that has been cautious, non-partisan, transparent, inclusive and persistent.

Community-led, community-owned and culturally appropriate

One of the key principles underlying Tree of Life's healing approach is that the process has to be rooted in the community, tapping into existing community resources and strengths. The approach draws on local knowledge and social networks to promote ownership. This way of working offers us a powerful, culturally grounded understanding and invites community action which begins with conscientisation. The process entails an awareness of ourselves in a historic context, setting the stage for a healing trajectory (Summerfield, 2003; Templar, 2010).

In Zimbabwe, wellbeing is closely related to context: it is not necessarily the same across communities. Because people's ideas are shaped by their culture, religion and history, we make great efforts to understand and incorporate cultural understandings in our approach and rec-ognise that it is important not to gloss over the fact that some of the cultural/traditional ideas may be problematic. These may include values and beliefs held by community members for periods spanning generations that are harmful to a particular group. Examples are the stigma surrounding rape and sexual violence against women and girls, the use of violence by men in the home, early/child marriages of girls and the labelling of men and women with mental health problems as witches.

The PACS workshops support communities to look critically at the traditional rituals which may be in use, and encourages them to identify those which promote healing, whilst discour-aging those practices that are disempowering and which abuse or exploit others. The circle is used in many traditional cultures. For the Tree of Life workshop, it is used simply to ensure fairness and respect. Everyone can see each other, and nobody is more important than anyone else, they are all different and equal regardless of their background. "*With the Tree of Life, we are all the same. We are all participants. No one can tell who are the participants and who are the facilitators*" (Workshop participant).

This is made possible through a gradual and intentional process of engagement at a local level. Taking the time to engage with cultural and religious community leaders, and later with powerful people who are often seen as complicit in violence and abuse. Tree of Life are careful not to be seen as experts and each step is taken with careful consultation across the community. At times, communities need time to decide if they are ready to invite the programme in.

Once confidence has been established, we work with trusted community members who organise the workshops and identify individuals who they feel would benefit from them. All of these organisers have been through the process themselves which enables them to effectively and appropriately identify participants.

Social relationships

Tree of Life facilitators are trained, mentored and supported to remain cognisant of individual or collective identity factors, including their history, experiences of previous and current discrimination, access to power, and/or privilege dynamics (Ratts et al., 2016). This is critical for how the project builds rapport and maintains relationships with communities.

We orientate service delivery around the survivor and/or community, placing them at the centre of the healing process, ensuring they have a level of choice and control over the journey. This requires a genuine acknowledgement that healing processes are not the exclusive provenance of clinicians, psychologists and psychiatrists, but that cultural and collective processes in the community are a vital part of trauma healing. The family, neighbours, the traditional healer, church, school and the health centre all have their part to play.

SURVIVOR IMPLEMENTED

Zimbabwean survivors of torture, in particular, but often also survivors of other violations, frequently say that a conventional counselling approach is not only ineffective but often exacerbates their trauma.

> Before the workshop I was feeling very lonely, I had lot of anger, I wanted to revenge and I was scared at the same time. I did more than 10 sessions with my counsellor. … One-on-one counselling was ok, but I felt like I was treated like someone who was losing her mind. I felt every time I visited my counsellor; I was repeating my story again and again. I felt uncomfortable when she was taking notes as I was talking.
>
> (Workshop participant who later became a Tree of Life member)

> The Tree of Life workshop was very different from the counselling I had received… the counselling reminded me of my interrogation. I was in a room similar to the interrogation room, in a building very like the one I was interrogated in. The counsellor was professional and caring but being alone, in a closed room, being asked questions gave me flashbacks to my interrogation … it brought back the fear I had felt. … This counselling focused on my memory of my interrogation and I was not connected emotionally, it did not touch my soul.
>
> (Participant in the first healing workshop)

These survivors and many others reported that being in a group with other people who had been through similar experiences was instrumental to the healing impact of the approach. The group members themselves knew what it felt like to be in the darkest of places, to be humiliated and demeaned, harmed and to lose all hope.

> At the workshop there were other people who were coming from different places in Zimbabwe. I was very comfortable to be with other victims of torture. I felt like we had gone through the same ordeal and it made me open up and share my experience. As the workshop proceeded, I felt connected.
>
> (Participant of an early workshop in South Africa)

Crucial to the process is that most of the facilitators of the process are survivors of torture and organised violence. We ensure that we have a gender balance in the facilitation teams and that they all have been through the process themselves. These women and men genuinely know what it feels like, and they understand the importance of peer support and mutual self-help, which are key vehicles for establishing safety, hope and in building trust. They are highly skilled in supporting shared decision-making that promotes recovery in a non-controlling way. They are also the living embodiment that it is possible to restore and move on in life with hope.

Tree of Life has also noted how helping others heal and restore is an integral part of the healing process for the individual. Consequently, workshop participants are encouraged to undergo training with Tree of Life to become community facilitators.

Working with survivors of torture has helped me to heal from my trauma, and the process has helped me to under-stand that the journey of healing is not a one-day thing but it is a process.

(Tree of Life field officer)

Group-based

Working in groups in all of our interventions is an intentional way to build on *ubuntu*; to build connections. We recognise that each community is different, so although the structure of the workshops and activities remains the same, the way workshops are delivered, the tools, anal-ogies and language used are carefully chosen to be appropriate to the specific culture of the community in which we are working. The way we greet, how the body work is structured, and the celebrations and honouring ceremonies are all selected to reflect the local culture.

The members of the group, who frequently come from the same community, are helped to build an understanding of their connection, which is both historical and current. The telling and witnessing of stories helps participants understand that they are not the only ones who went through distressing experiences. They learn that their neighbours also had similar, often worse, experiences. This breaks down the sense of isolation, and also the shame and stigma invariably felt by victims of violence and torture; it helps participants to normalise their experiences.

This has been particularly powerful when working with groups of women who were sub-jected to sexual violence as part of their torture. It is significant how often women who are neighbours, who go to the same church and meet daily, learn for the first time that they have had the same distressing experience. This revelation can often be life changing and lead to sexual violence survivors forming their own support groups and sometimes collaborating in livelihood projects supporting other women survivors of sexual and domestic violence.

This use of groups in the workshop setting facilitates the natural formation of peer-support groups after the workshop. The community facilitators remain in the community and under-take follow-up and ongoing support for the participants. But the group members themselves often continue to support each other and, in many cases, continue to meet independently.

MONITORING AND EVALUATION

Tree of Life monitors the impact of our interventions through the use of two tools, a World Health Organisation developed Self-Reporting Questionnaire 20 (Beusenberg and Orley, 1994) which assesses trauma symptoms, and a locally developed Zimbabwe Community Life Ques-tionnaire 20 (Mpande et al., 2013) which measures social engagement. These tools are admin-istered prior to the workshop, and then at follow-up, three months later.

The PACS workshops use pre- and post-workshop evaluations and follow-up visits, to mon-itor the community action plans developed and to measure impact. Monitoring data from these workshops, anecdotal evidence from facilitators by way of observation and feedback, and com-munity development initiatives also indicate more cooperative relationships, with well-function-ing community networks and reinstated social support mechanisms.

The feedback has also noted that the process contributes to reconciliation at community level and builds motivation to engage in development activities. *"People in this community used to fight a lot. We now sit down and talk and stay together in peace. We have come together and we are now a 'society'"* (Community leader, Nkayi).

ADAPTABILITY DURING THE COVID-19 PANDEMIC

The COVID-19 pandemic meant that for a prolonged period, face-to-face activities were not possible. As Zimbabwe, along with much of the world, entered a series of lockdowns which prohibited social interaction, we were challenged on how to continue to support our beneficiaries and care for our staff and community facilitators.

Although it was possible to provide individual follow-up and support to beneficiaries on the phone, there was a risk that the healing power of collective engagement would be lost. Consequently, we were forced to depart from our simple, low-cost and personal model of working and embrace technology. Initially, WhatsApp groups of community facilitators were formed to foster communication pathways across the entire Tree of Life network. These groups were provided with initial learning resources and restorative debriefing mechanisms to provide support and care. After initial feedback from the groups on what they were witnessing, and after gaining their feedback on the learning materials, we developed a range of virtual training materials. We employed action learning cycles (action, reflection, learning and planning) (The Barefoot Guide Connection, 2012) to adapt and revise the materials to fit the context and to respond to the changing environment. Virtual supervision and support sessions incorporated self-care and coping strategies, and later included psychological first aid tools (WHO, War Trauma Foundation and World Vision International, 2011).

This approach has helped to retain some level of engagement and connection during the pandemic, as well as to increase knowledge, and to strengthen coping capacities in communities. The success of this was due in large part to the sound foundation of skills and connection that had been established prior to the crisis. The strength and skills of the Big Tree groups, built on relationships of trust and attitudes of listening, respect and empathy, provided the springboard to continue to reach out and connect with the communities at a time when other social networks were fragmenting.

CONCLUSION

The Tree of Life's model of trauma healing and empowerment, which is primarily a group-work approach, provides both an individual and collective trauma healing mechanism. As practitioners in this process, with both clinical and community development experience, we have learnt that the healing process is dependent not only on what you do, but how it is done. It is not just the process or structure that facilitates healing, but the way in which the facilitators work, and the connection back to self and with others that is transforming.

As a practitioner or facilitator in trauma work, one needs to be anchored and self-aware in order to hold the space for others as they progress through their healing journey. Our experience of working in and with communities which have experienced deep and sustained trauma has taught us that leading by example, that living and embodying healing and growth after trauma is the starting point for this kind of work. But we have also learnt that everyone can play a role in collective healing, that we are social creatures and relationships are critical for our wellbeing. Through *ubuntu*, we together contribute to each other's restoration.

May we grow back, not to what was, but instead toward what we can become.
Jen Bloomer, Radici Studios

REFERENCES

Beusenberg, M. and Orley, J. (1994) *A User's Guide to the Self-Reporting Questionnaire (SRQ)*. Geneva, Switzerland: World Health Organization. Available at: https://apps.who.int/iris/handle/10665/61113 (Accessed: 11 May 2020).

Bubenzer, F. and Tankink, M. (2017) 'Introduction to special issue: Linking mental health and psychosocial support to peacebuilding in an integrated way', *Intervention*, 15(3), pp. 192–198

Colletta, N. J. and Cullen, M.I. (2000) *Violent Conflict and the Transformation of Social Capital: Lessons from Cambodia, Rwanda, Guatemala and Somalia*. Washington DC: The World Bank. Available at: http://documents.worldbank.org/curated/en/799651468760532921/Violent-conflict-and-the-transformation-of-social-capital-lessons-from-Cambodia-Rwanda-Guatemala-and-Somalia (Accessed: 11 May 2020).

Curling, P. (2005) 'The effectiveness of empowerment workshops with torture survivors', *Torture*, 15, pp. 9–15.

Higson-Smith, C. (2002) *Supporting Communities Affected by Violence: A Casebook from South Africa*. Oxford, UK: Oxfam

Hutchison, E. and Bleiker, R. (2008) 'Emotional reconciliation: Reconstituting identity and community after Trauma', *European Journal of Social Theory*, 11(3), pp. 385–403. doi: 10.1177/1368431008092569.

Mpande, E., Higson-Smith, C. and Vinson G. (2013) 'Community intervention during ongoing political violence: What is possible? What works?', *Peace and Conflict: Journal of Peace Psychology*, 19(2), pp. 196–208. doi: 10.1037/a0032529.

Parsons, R., Reeler, T., Fisher, J, and Mpande, E. (2011) Trauma and mental health in Zimbabwe, Research and Advocacy Unit, Harare. *Zimbabwe*. Available at: https://www.academia.edu/976195/Trauma_and_mental_health_in_Zimbabwe (Accessed: 5 May 2020).

Ratts, M., Singh, A., Nassar-McMillan, S., Butler, S, and McCullough, J. (2016) *Multicultural and Social Justice Counseling Competencies: A Leadership Framework for Professional School Counselors*. Alexandria, VA: Association for Multicultural Counseling and Development.doi: 10.1177/2156759X18773582.

Reeler, T., Chitsike, K., Maizva, F., and Reeler, B. (2009) 'The tree of life: A community approach to empowering and healing survivors of torture in Zimbabwe', *Torture*, 19(3), pp. 180–193.

Reimann, C. and König, U. (2017) 'Collective Trauma and Resilience. Key Concepts in Transforming War-related Identities' in Austin, B. and Fischer, M. (eds.) *Berghof Handbook Dialogue Series No. 11*. Berlin: Berghof Foundation.

SAMHSA. (2014). Substance Abuse and Mental Health Services Administration. SAMHSA's Concept of Trauma and Guidance for a Trauma-Informed Approach. *HHS Publication No. (SMA) 14-4884*. Rockville, MD: Substance Abuse and Mental Health Services Administration. Available at: https://ncsacw.acf.hhs.gov/userfiles/files/SAMHSA_Trauma.pdf (Accessed: 11 May 2020).

Steel, Z., Chey, T., Silove, D., Marnane, C., Bryant, R.A., and van Ommeren, M. (2009) 'Association of torture and other potentially traumatic events with mental health outcomes among populations exposed to mass conflict and displacement', *A Systematic Review and Meta-analysis, JAMA*, 302, pp. 537–549. doi: 10.1001/jama.2009.1132.

Summerfield, D. (2003) 'Fighting "terrorism" with torture', *British Medical Journal*, 326, pp. 773–774. doi: 10.1136/bmj.326.7393.773.

Templar, S. (2010) 'Integrity of process: How tree of life is taking root in Zimbabwe', *Africa Peace and Conflict Journal*, 13(2), pp. 106–112.

The Barefoot Guide Connection. (2012) The Barefoot Guide 1 Working with Organisations and Social Change. Available at: https://www.barefootguide.org/ (Accessed: 6 May 2020).

World Health Organization, War Trauma Foundation and World Vision International. (2011) *Psychological First Aid: Guide for Field Workers*. Geneva: WHO. Available at: https://www.who.int/publications/i/item/9789241548205 (Accessed: 11 May 2020).

CHAPTER 3

LISTEN TO OUR VOICES

Women Asylum Seekers Together (WAST)

Together with love we are like a family
Together with humility respect plays a big role between us
Together with compassion we support each other
Together in unity we can build a better future
Together with honesty we can share our problems
Together without shame
It is together that we say unity is strength

Women Asylum seekers Together (WAST) was founded in 2005 in Greater Manchester by and for women seeking protection in the United Kingdom. WAST is made up of women who have had difficult lives in the countries we have come from. We are women of all ages, nationalities, ethnicities, sexual orientations and disabilities. We speak many languages, practice many religions and accommodate all women. Some of us have children and spouses or partners with us, others have been separated from our families by deportation. Many of us are alone.

The aim of WAST is to support each other to rebuild our lives, and to help us manage the difficulties we face as women in the asylum process. We are a self-organised group and campaign for the rights of women seeking asylum, seeking to make changes in the policies that affect us. We do this through lobbying MPs, taking direct action, building coalitions, taking part in research, speaking out and supporting one another.

People talk about the asylum process in general, but not the hidden struggles we face as women when we seek asylum. Seeking asylum is not just one process but a collection of challenges that we have to go through and overcome. There is the worry we go through about our asylum claims and the problems with housing and finance. Those difficulties are the most visible. What we don't talk about in the UK is the mental struggle we go through as part of the asylum process. More than anything, the hardest part, for most of us, is keeping our mental health stable.

When I came to this country in Nov 2019, I thought I was ready for the asylum-seeking process. The people I met before, during and after the process had told me that it is hard. But what does it mean when someone says it is hard? Does it differ from person to person? Does it differ from case to case? For me personally, I thought I was ready and felt strong enough to do it alone. But in reality, I needed people to support me, guide me and be there when the going got tough. The process gets extremely lonely. And if you are not careful you get depressed. It doesn't matter how educated you are or how strong you think you are.

I started this journey on my own. I was heavily pregnant with two young children. The process was so frustrating, I got so confused that I needed to have a family who I could talk to. And then I found this wonderful family called WAST. The women have been so supportive; the smile has been restored back to my face.

The quotes above and within the chapter are all from WAST women. We have chosen not to identify the author of each quote to retain our anonymity, as many of us are still in the asylum process.

DOI: 10.4324/9781003192978-5

HOW WAST STARTED AND OUR STRUCTURE

In 2005, our WAST founder was a woman seeking asylum from Pakistan who was facing deportation. She had fled her country because of domestic violence. She started a campaign to stop her removal and during that process, she met lots of other women who were in the same situation. This group of women organised a big meeting and many women came. They began to meet together to support each other.

The group was very informal at the beginning, but gradually became more structured, setting up a weekly group meeting in Manchester city centre. After 10 years, the group recruited a volunteer to help us develop an organisational structure and support us to apply to become a charity. We applied for funds to cover women's bus fares and venue hire, as well as food and childcare for the group.

We decided to set up a management group so that this team of women could oversee the running of the group and do all the associated tasks. The WAST women members elect this group and there is an election every two years so that all WAST women are given the opportunity to take more responsibility and learn new skills. Each management group member agrees to take on different tasks to ensure WAST runs smoothly.

There is a creche every week that is staffed by childcare workers. We do not use interpreters but interpret for each other. We have a confidentiality policy and so we all feel secure when we translate private information.

In 2018, we employed a grassroots coordinator, and in 2021 a development worker. Both roles help WAST sustain our organisational structure and ensure that we continue to develop in the long term. Both women are WAST women and work alongside the management group to do all the administration and organisational work that keeps WAST running.

> I was an asylum seeker with two children. I started as a member of WAST and then I joined the Board and was a management member. I learnt how to run the organisation, sorting out bus fares for women, arranging the food and activities. Then I got my leave to remain and I had the opportunity to apply for this new role of grassroots co-ordinator. We are in a good position now to develop WAST.
>
> (Eunice Manu, 2021)

HOW WAST WOMEN SUPPORT EACH OTHER

We share our experiences, empower and support one another whilst fighting for our rights. We all have different skills and knowledge, and we share these with each other too. We help each other take forward our asylum applications and run anti-deportation campaigns when one of us is in that desperate situation.

As women seeking asylum, we can often feel vulnerable due to isolation, trauma, ill health, destitution and the fear of deportation. At WAST we have a safe space where we can be ourselves.

WAST members come together weekly for a safe social place that is women only. We share our joys and sadness as a group and this brings us closer, knowing that we are each sister's keeper.

Each week we find out about other activities happening in the region that we can get involved in and every month women can receive legal advice from an asylum and immigration solicitor regarding their asylum cases. There is one to one support for women who have experienced FGM through Support Our Sisters (see Chapter 22) as well as a food bank, a domestic abuse self-help group and a basic English language class. At every drop-in, we share a hot meal together prepared by one of our women.

We have our own choir and a sewing class fortnightly. In the choir, women compose their own songs that have messages about what is happening to us, so we raise awareness of the challenges we face day to day.

> To be heard in that way when we are performing, well it is phenomenal. The songs we sing are so peaceful and we sing out strong with all our emotions. It's a healing process, it's pain relief and we are being listened to, we are raising awareness.

The sewing class involves women who were seamstresses back in their native countries teaching women who are interested in sewing. We sell the pieces we create to our supporters and raise a little money for the organisation.

WAST consists of a diverse community of women from different backgrounds. Our ethos is that we respect all women and accept each other's values and differences. Our ground rule is that we create a safe space for each other and are a welcoming and warm organisation. We have a shared experience that has brought us together, that we are all women seeking safety.

> I am so grateful to have known so many wonderful women during the asylum process. They made the waiting period so much easier. But more than that, they made an impact on my life. They have given me strength, courage and made me determined not to be silent and to share my story with others so I can also help.

> WAST is the true meaning of a support group that meets our needs. I have struggled with pain and depression for as long as I can remember. I have cycled through many ups and downs. Depression was a constant struggle until I was introduced to the WAST Group. It's a life-changer, it's been so healing, soothing, and reviving. I feel happy with WAST, when I see the people from different countries, you can talk with each other, you can find some friendship and get more experience.

WHY WAST MAKES SUCH A DIFFERENCE TO OUR LIVES

WAST is women only and is run by us. We empower each other, support each other and show empathy to one another.

Practically, women get advice and are signposted to other organisations that can support them further. We have women in the group who are skilled, and they share their knowledge and skills with the other women. WAST helps us because it has created a safe space where women who are vulnerable can come and feel comfortable and relaxed when they have been failed by the system. We can feel part of society. In WAST, women restore their confidence and gain trust in others again.

> Being introduced to WAST by a good friend of mine, was a God-given gift. WAST was founded by strong and inspiring women from diverse backgrounds. They are ready to help and support you when you need it. Because all the women are still in the process or had gone through the process in the past, the support and advice you get is firsthand, which makes it so much more helpful. They tell you how to cope with waiting. They have the courage to share their story and their journey and be there in any way they can to help you.

> When things were difficult and really rough, WAST gave me refuge and strength. WAST gave me a listening ear, a gentle shoulder to lean on. Even now that I have my status, I will forever be grateful to WAST.

In addition to the drop-in support and our other activities, we support women who are having to report. In the UK, anyone who is waiting for a final decision on their application to live in the UK can be required to regularly travel to report at an immigration reporting centre (IRC). Every appointment carries the risk of being randomly taken to a detention centre. When our members go to report, we have a phone tree so that we can ring one another as we go in and out of the IRC to reduce the stress and to support any woman who is detained.

> I remembered the first time I came to WAST. I was stressed and worried, but after sharing my problems the love, advice and support I got was tremendous and I knew this is the place I should be. You've cared and supported us through these difficult and challenging times, and we are honoured and thankful to everyone for their support in diverse ways.

WAST CAMPAIGNS – LISTEN TO OUR VOICES

One of our main aims is to raise awareness about the issues that force women to seek international protection, such as gender-based violence and the impact on us of the injustices experienced through the UK asylum and immigration process. Outlined below are some examples of our campaigning and partnership work.

WAST aims to raise awareness about the enormity of the stress we go through in the asylum process, both mentally and physically when we have been or still are traumatised by past experiences. Despite this, we have not always been well treated by services when we ask for help. In April 2008 we produced a set of guidelines for services in our region: WAST Recommendations for Good Practice for Agencies Working with Women Asylum Seekers. In these guidelines we set out some core principles for how we should be treated, as well as giving us our rights and sharing our ideas about what would help us, for example specialist women solicitors.

WAST has been part of the nationwide campaign to shut down Yarl's Wood detention centre in the UK where the Home Office detains asylum-seeking women indefinitely. On the 21 February 2018, 120 women in this 'immigration prison' went on hunger strike to highlight the dehumanising conditions and to call for an end to detention. Many WAST women have experienced detention, and so as a symbol of our solidarity with the hunger strikers, WAST women wore purple armbands. The armbands helped raise awareness and support for our sisters on strike and were sold across Manchester and at The Safety4Sisters conference on Migrant Women's Rights in March 2018. (Safety4Sisters is a support group for women who have experienced domestic violence). The strike ended but our campaign goes on to end detention.

As well as our local work, we join together with other national campaigns in the UK that campaign against inhumane policies that affect women seeking safety in the UK, such as destitution and reporting to immigration reporting centres. We will also take up individual cases where one of us is at risk of being sent back to the country they fled from.

In 2021, a group of WAST members began working with Manchester University, learning research skills and taking part in research on how we survive and the reality of our lives in the asylum process. That same year we stood alongside 70 leaders working with refugee women to highlight how the UK Government's new piece of legislation, the Nationality and Borders Bill will harm women. Sadly this Act was passed in May 2022, but we will continue to raise awareness about its impact.

WAST has gained a national reputation for our work and NGOs and asylum and immigration solicitors recommend us to their women clients.

WHAT HAVE WE LEARNT DURING WAST?

If women are setting up a group, we would advise them to be inclusive and accepting of women with all their differences. It is important to set a ground rule that despite our differences, we need each other. Respect should be first on the agenda.

There can be challenges in the group because some women are more skilled or educated, while others have had less opportunities. So, there can sometimes be a division between the educated and less educated members. One common factor that really binds us together is our experience with the asylum and immigration process.

SUPPORTING EACH OTHER DURING A PANDEMIC

WAST continued to run during the COVID-19 pandemic. It was not possible to do all our usual activities, such as choir practice and sewing, but we still met weekly as a group. This was helpful as most women felt lonely and isolated, and continuing to meet online was good for our mental wellbeing. Women also received practical and legal advice through a caseworker who would get referrals from WAST's grassroot coordinator.

During the pandemic a WhatsApp group began, made up of 183 women. We used the group to chat, share our pictures of celebrating birthdays and new-born babies. We encouraged one another and during this time we have become even closer.

> In 2020, a few months after claiming asylum and moving to a new town, COVID 19 hit. It was a strange time, when the government declared the lockdown rule for the first time. I didn't know what to do with myself nor how to kill the time. I was at home with limited activities and nothing much to do. It was quite hard on top of my constant worry of what will happen to my claim. I felt like my mind was going to explode with worry. Am I going to get it [be granted asylum]? If not what is going to happen to me…. The worry was endless.

> I joined WAST during the pandemic. Sometimes I feel like lockdown was a blessing in disguise. It made us use Zoom and helped us create a network. It feels weird in some way to have a great connection with others while you only know them via the online platform. But saying that, in WAST this didn't make any difference at all. I feel like I know them personally though I haven't met them in person.

SUMMARY

WAST has given women a platform where we can speak out about the challenges we are facing as refugees in a foreign land. Some women have developed skills through WAST, as well as built their confidence and self-esteem. Women have found a safe space which they call home away from home. We have made friends. We are sisters.

> Truly I tell you, I am very happy to be in this WAST group, it has helped me a lot, I intend to stay in it always. I am very much counting on it for ever.

> WAST has helped women discover their talents. I for one discovered a talent of writing poems. I developed this by expressing my feelings on paper.

> I'm writing to share with you my profound gratitude for all the help WAST has given me during this trying process. I am ever grateful for all the support and kindness you have shown me, and for supporting me when things were very difficult and frustrating. You have proven to be a blessing in my life. I have been granted my refugees status!

Once I was lost
Not knowing where to go
Until I was directed to this place
Where I found sanctuary
Where I found laughter and support

During this difficult journey
To all the women who supported me
I say thank you

Without your help and support
This journey wouldn't have been easy
This journey would have been so lonely

I am thankful that I found WAST
Women who inspire and encourage me
Make me laugh though the journey is hard
Made me hopeful when the process is tough
Now the waiting is over

To contact WAST, go to our website: https://www.wastmanchester.com

REFERENCES

Women Asylum Seekers Together, 2008 WAST Recommendations for Good Practice for Agencies Working with Women Asylum Seekers. Unpublished paper. WAST. Manchester, UK.

CHAPTER 4

"WE ALL TOGETHER CARRY THE SUFFERING NOW"

Community supports after enforced disappearances in Peru

Miryam Rivera-Holguín, Victoria Cavero, Jozef Corveleyn and Lucia De Haene

During the internal armed conflict in Peru (1980–2000) approximately 70,000 lives were lost; more than 20,000 people were disappeared and about one million fled from rural areas to the cities. During 2001–2003, the Truth and Reconciliation Commission (TRC) provided victims with the opportunity to officially talk about what they went through. The largest number of fatal victims were Andean men, Quechua speakers whose main occupation was farming (TRC, 2003). In this conflict, people were victimised not only by the Shining Path (Revolutionary Communist Party) but also by Peruvian army forces. This led to thousands of people experiencing human rights violations, but only 42 files were able to convert into judicial cases (International Center for Transitional Justice, 2013). Most of the victims had little legal evidence to support their search for justice. Peru is a culturally and geographically diverse country, characterised by social fragmentation in which postcolonial legacies and current social inequities among Peruvians are evident. It is common for relationships to be mediated by filters of social class and race (Jenner, 2018), so that indigenous, rural populations are particularly likely to face challenges in accessing health, education and justice.

Forced disappearances in Peru were not isolated events but formed part of systematic human rights violations that sowed terror in thousands of families, leading them to flee from their communities to preserve their lives (TRC, 2003). Lima, the capital of the country, was among the cities that hosted the largest number of people fleeing from the rural areas. Those who fled to cities encountered significant challenges, in the absence of institutionalised support systems, the new arrivals collectively organised to share key information, housing facilities and, sometimes, to connect each other to short-term jobs.

In this chapter, we will focus on the experiences of women whose family members were forcibly disappeared by the State. Forced disappearance involves actions of kidnapping and disappearance carried out by governments which aim to eliminate the person, but also to conduct forced interrogations, torture practices, concealment of evidence, disappearance of human remains and hindering the complaint and access to justice (Grupo de Trabajo sobre las desapariciones forzadas o involuntarias, 2015). More than three decades after the events, these women and their families continue to collectively search for their relatives and to struggle within a judicial system that limits the rights of the Andean Quechua population (International Committee of the Red Cross, 2019).

We will explore the ways in which the informal, spontaneous groups formed by these women function and impact on their emotional, social, material, and cultural wellbeing. In this chapter, we find that the strength of these women's capacities relies on their cultural background, which leads them to act as a community. Their collective self allows them to transition from the experience of being individual victims into collectively accompanying each other to advocate for human rights and democracy. Here, we aim to explore one angle of their transition from "victims" to "human rights activists and peace builders". They share the claim for truth and justice while building a collective memory for society to prevent repetition.

We met these women in the frame of the first author's PhD research project on family dynamics and enforced disappearances during the armed conflict. During the fieldwork, the Directive Committee of this women-led organisation requested a series of training activities

DOI: 10.4324/9781003192978-6

to strengthen their organisation and we began a process of psychosocial accompaniment with them. We will draw on group discussions conducted during the months we accompanied these women in their group activities.

WOMEN-LED PEER SUPPORT NETWORKS IN THE AFTERMATH OF THE CONFLICT

During the 1980s and 1990s, family members of the enforced disappeared contacted church-based organisations or human rights institutions so they could access legal aid. Only a few of them were able to access judicial processes because the majority did not have sufficient evidence to file a case with the Peruvian judicial system. Nonetheless, those family members took the opportunity to build their own social platforms which allowed them to accompany each other in their struggle for truth and justice.

At that point in time, these networks also allowed for support in a context of social marginalisation: Andean families were not only challenged by the consequences of economic constraints after fleeing from their rural hometown, but also by the social stigmatisation in the city. Most people coming from rural areas were unfairly labelled as supporters of Shining Path and were subject to raids and harassment. Therefore, many people felt forced to change their address on their identity cards, refused to talk in Quechua (their mother tongue), were hesitant to gather together and tried to hide themselves in order to avoid being victims of unjust detentions, torture and prison (Rivera-Holguín et al., 2019).

These migrant women, while trying to maintain connections with their hometowns, organised mutual support platforms in the city to search for their disappeared family members, to support others in fleeing from violence, and to contact human rights organisations.

BERTHA: For all the paperwork, everything, we must collect money, go to the commissions in another city, all that. We don't have much support from other family members, so there isn't enough money, resources

GABRIELA: There is also no strength but when you are among several, one walk in a group

CARMEN: And it gives me strength. To know the truth and seek justice.

This mutual support allowed them to continue gathering together to search for their loved ones, but also to address the daily stressors they had to deal with in the aftermath of a family network destroyed by the conflict. Whilst they continued to care for their children and elderly relatives, the women took on traditionally male roles which involved new responsibilities in working for the survival of their families (suarez, 2015). This created changes in family dynamics, as women were more often absent from home, working in precarious conditions, involving older daughters in the care of their younger siblings, and often neglecting their own safety and health.

At the family level, relationships were fragmented by loss, chronic suffering, hopelessness, distrust, and frustration. On an emotional level, these disappearances left families in the situation of having to deal with an ambiguous loss (Boss, 2017), meaning that there is uncertainty about the fate of the loved one, there is no evidence of the person being either alive or dead. This uncertainty makes it very difficult to experience uncomplicated grief or to perform traditional burial rituals, as one woman explained:

JUANA: It has been thirty-two years, but (…) I can't! No, no, no, I can't stand it! I can't stand it! No (…). It's like it happened just yesterday, as if it had just happened (…). I can lose some other relatives. At some point, some died, and we buried them. We cry, all that. But that just goes … it goes. But it's not the same as with my parents [who were disappeared], that doesn't go.

In 2022 families are still waiting for their disappeared family members to return to their homes. Since all evidence about their family members was hidden, they do not know what happened. The lack of information, the need to know why they were abducted, what happened to them after they were taken from their homes, how were the last moments of their loved ones, and why the absurdity and chaos of the violence all contribute to the prolonged suffering of families. They still demand why their relatives' bodies were disappeared after their death, and why their families have been denied their right to truth and justice after decades.

Political violence leaves a different mark to other life-threatening events, such as disasters or accidents, due to the intentionality and directionality of the violence, the inhumanity, and the disruption of the notions of community and protection in a fair society. This scar is even deeper when this violence is directed towards children or elderly, who are supposed to be protected. This kind of violence breaks the idea of humanity, and those who survive tirelessly seek to raise their voices and seek justice:

JUANA: It has been proven; it is proven. Everything, everything. That they were innocent, they were authorities of the town. Innocent people, children and the elderly, and they were murdered, disappeared. They dumped the remains into the ravine. No, I will not be tired of telling. No, I will not be tired of talking, until the day I die.

The most salient elements of the women's situation, together with the ambiguous loss and the meaninglessness of the extreme violence, are the anger, frustration and the permanent suffering experienced in the struggle to access truth and justice. The anger is not directed at the persons who took the life of their loved ones, but at the institutions they represent, such as the Army, which were found responsible for these human rights violations. The frustration is linked to the system's inefficiency, that more than three decades after the events it has still failed to fulfil its mandate. Being denied justice is perceived as another form of discrimination in which justice is less available to rural communities. This experience of class and race discrimination is also represented in the interactions during the trials.

ISABEL: And at that time [during the trial] … those, I say 'gringas pitucas' [reference for white upper middle-class women], that's how they were. And one of them annoyed me when she did like this (derogatory gestures). That's how she looked at us, as if we were like the stinky ones, like…

BERTHA: Like the ones that haven't bathed

ISABEL: (…) I felt humiliated.

The manifestations of suffering and wellbeing are shaped by the women's own cultural expressions, leading to specific ways of dealing with the ambiguous loss in the Quechua population. They report interacting with their disappeared family members, talking to them, and being heard, dreaming about them, and asking them for advice, feeling their presence, preparing food for them, or leaving the door open for them to return.

These women share their narratives in regular meetings to mourn together, to identify healing practices, and to look for possibilities for restoration as a community.

GABRIELA: Maybe they [people] don't get it. But you can't leave it, right? When you bury someone, they say 'OK, it's already buried', right? And you have somewhere to go [a tomb]. But when you don't know anything, you are with that thought, you are always 'thinking', right? That is why we have always walked, the three of us have only walked in group.

The community space they have shaped in their group meetings allows them to normalise the unique experience of living with such a loss, and to build on their own emotional and social agencies and capabilities.

PSYCHOSOCIAL ACCOMPANIMENT: ACKNOWLEDGING THE IMPORTANCE OF THE GROUP

These experiences of "relational" coping with collective violence within informal social groups indicate potential approaches for therapeutic supports that go beyond the individualising and medicalising trends. We found psychosocial accompaniment as an appropriate method to approach this group and learn from their experiences. According to Watkins (2015), psychosocial accompaniment has its roots in Liberation Psychology and has been developed in Latin America as a practice of accompanying those who have faced adverse situations, such as prisoners, refugees, or victims of human rights violations. It involves accompanying someone on their path, walking their way, building meaningful bonds through time and commitment, but also starting to envision a different future, passing from how the situation actually is, to how it could be. Importantly, when the one who accompanies is not from the group, they need to acknowledge their own privileges, including power and social disparities, and still try to establish horizontal relationships of mutual trust and respect. We engaged in psychosocial accompaniment aiming to learn how the women-led group functions and became a source of coping with the experience of loss after the disappearance of their family members.

The group gathers many women searching for truth and justice after the human rights violations that their families were exposed to. There are approximately 25 women (between 45 and 70 years old) who meet monthly to follow up on the progress of their disappeared family members' cases. For the last three decades, they have been active in human rights demonstrations, memorialisation, commemoration activities, and in advocating for human rights and national policies for redress.

During 2018, the authors and the group members organised a series of four participatory workshops on community organisation, community participation, work team, and communication (4 hours each), plus a full-day participatory workshop with group discussions. Additionally, we developed psychosocial accompaniment activities over 16 weeks in 2018, in which we attended their monthly meetings and joined their participation in human rights activities, commemorative rituals, embroidery meetings, and social entrepreneurship activities. We conducted this psychosocial accompaniment as a practice of "walking in the company" of the women trying to establish horizontal relationships by openly talking and reflecting together on their plight, acknowledging their capabilities, and learning from the experience of each other. This also meant, as Watkins (2015) states, decolonising pre-existing structural power relations among us – "the urban professionals" – and them – "the rural victims" – into more equal bonds.

When we met this group of women, their collectivism was very salient, but we were also struck by how their work to address their marginalisation through engagement in community mobilisation activities had allowed them to transition from "victims" to "human rights activists". For us, it was relevant to learn how, even 30 years after losing their family members, they continued to engage in group activism and remained engaged in discovering the fate of their disappeared family members. Their focus did not waver from investigating where their family member was taken, how they were disappeared, where their human remains are, who was responsible, and finally to advocate for a "Never Again" movement and for human rights for all.

ESTABLISHING THE GROUP

These women felt privileged to have been able to flee from a context of extreme poverty and conflict; their flight allowed them to protect their lives and to prevent potential rape and harassment in their rural communities. Once in the capital, they gathered around religious or human rights organisations, where they found support in filing their cases for investigations. Additionally, they connected with other institutions and representative persons, such as Congressmen or other "fellow peasants", to advocate for special commissions to investigate the enforced disappearances. The launch of the TRC in 2001 was a key stage in their process. Even though most cases received by the TRC did not have enough legal evidence to become judicial cases, a few were able to begin the legal process.

These attempts to seek justice had significant impacts on victims' mental health, due to both the re-victimisation during the whole process and the failures of the legal systems in administering justice (Hamber and Lundy, 2020). Such discomfort and frustration are exemplified in the following quote: *"in the last hearing we were mistreated (…) Having all the evidence! Having everything! The relatives of those soldiers made us feel bad, so bad" (Isabel).*

In their group, they built a collective identity and enriched their sense of belonging. Moreover, since the mental health impact is not restricted to their loss but also to the daily stressors that they faced, these groups allowed them to support each other. They offered each other time and emotional, social, and instrumental support. When experiencing other life stressors, such as health issues, economic constraints or family struggles, the group was there to provide accompaniment.

In this context, the psychosocial accompaniment allowed us to understand the importance of coming together as peers to share their experiences, to provide help and support to other victims, and to embrace broader social goals of advocating for democracy and promoting non-violent cultures. In that sense, these women positioned themselves as peace builders.

DEVELOPMENT OF THE GROUP

The path to becoming a consolidated group was long. In the beginning it was mainly focused on collecting information about their cases, about the TRC, where to register family members, and where to follow up cases; but progressively, it included new demands and others. For instance, as the cases were progressing, more family members were interested in understanding the process, so there were many internal informative meetings as well as meetings with other organisations. At the same time, they were, as a group, gaining more visibility due to their community participation in human rights meetings, demonstrations, and commemorative and memorialisation activities. Their group dynamic allowed them to exchange their stories, their sufferings, but also their hopes. As was shared during the group discussions:

JULIA: It's like catching the problem that other has, Ah! I also have this problem; we can accompany each other. Of course, the neighbour's problem is different from my problem, right? But it gets to feel closer, and unity is strength, right? So, to know, to keep going (…)

PATRICIA: To know how to do too, right?

JULIA: To accompany each other

PATRICIA: Yes. How to do the paperwork? How…? Where to go? What do we want?

GABRIELA: Where are we going to go?

In the beginning, social, psychological, spiritual, and legal support was provided by church organisations and human rights NGOs, but later financial resources became harder to find.

Currently, this group of women remain in close coordination with those organisations, and they are still supported, for example with the venue for their meetings. Earlier, the women decided to officially register their group, have their own Directive Committee, and to hold monthly meetings. In each meeting, they work with an agenda led by the Directive Committee, which includes diverse topics of interest to the group. These can include: the legal progress of their cases and reparations; human rights commemoration activities; health and socioeconomic needs and initiatives to address them. The meetings are held in a "formal" environment, but once the agenda is completed, they move to informal interchanges, sharing the food they may bring, talking and joking in Quechua, and organising informal encounters. The group are also engaged in supporting other victims in coordination with human rights NGOs. They travel to other regions where human rights violations took place to contact local organisations and share experiences of handling their cases in the judicial system, and to share experiences of supporting each other within the organisation.

Through the regular meetings, women found that coming together allowed them to share ideas but also to act and to advocate for justice together. So, they started gathering around those women that seemed to be the bravest and caught their bravery and courage. They learned from each other's experiences and reported that progressively they were less afraid of stigmatisation and were more able to show themselves as who they are and where they come from. They were also less afraid of retaliations, so started talking about the disappearances of their loved ones, moving from sharing their struggles in the "safe" group meetings into publicly denouncing and claiming for justice in demonstrations. This took place in a national context framed by human rights claims and the process initiated by the TRC.

In the past, the women were more afraid of opening and trusting others, but progressively grew more certain about the value of networking and engaging in community work to demand social justice. Additionally, they have learned to act more democratically within their own organisation. They elect their Directive Committee for a set period and then they appoint other members. Even though the group members have a common focus on searching for disappeared family members, they face difficult situations and internal disagreements just as all groups do. For example, some members consider that engaging in socio-economic activities to raise money to deal with daily stressors can take the energy of the group and distract them from the main goal of searching for justice in their legal cases.

They have also gained more understanding of their own group identity, so they engage in public commemoration events and always try to honour the name of their organisation. They aim to gain visibility regarding the way they work (collectively and committed) and the way they represent themselves (for example, wearing a vest, with their embroidered banner). The messages they try to disseminate relate to advocacy for truth and justice. But also, they are sharing their cases, building a collective memory for society to know what happened and to prevent others experiencing what they lived, as well as supporting other victims of human rights abuses

Likewise, it's worth noting that their participation is contextualised. Peru is a country with a weak democracy and the division of political powers is not always evident, which means that the political forces that were responsible for human rights violations in the 80s and 90s are still powerful in 2022. In that sense, the work of these women in advocating for human rights is very relevant in the current political context at the time of writing. For instance, in the 2021 Presidential elections they participated in political demonstrations against a candidate whose father (a former president) was involved in abusing the human rights of Andean populations.

The core characteristic of the group is their resistance and determination to seek the remains of loved ones. It has been more than three decades of struggle in an exhausting, overwhelming and slow process of searching for justice in a national system that re-victimises and neglects Andean populations. In a context where it is easier to quit than to stand firm, they have learned to maintain their hope, and despite receiving adverse judicial sentences, they keep appealing to international courts. They can be absent for health or travel, but then they re-join or stay connected by social media. In contrast to a therapeutic group, what defines their participation is not a professional prescription but their own interest in searching for their disappeared. The struggles of families with disappeared family members, sadly, are not isolated experiences. In 2022, there are more than 20,000 disappeared persons in Peru. Families use the slogan "They took them alive, we want them back alive", which is also used in other Latin American countries, such as Argentina, Colombia, and Mexico.

LEARNING FROM THE GROUP'S STRENGTHS

We have seen that this community space provided the women with new meanings and with a sense of belonging and shifted their social role from victims to peace activists in a process of resistance to social injustice. In the following paragraphs we will share our reflections on what we have learned from our engagement with this group.

Moving beyond a pathologising lens

Along with strengthening their voices and finding a space for peer support, the community space was also a place for the women to share their unique ways of mourning and their experiences of permanently waiting for their disappeared family members to walk into their houses and return to family life. They also acknowledge the importance of having the space and time to share their emotions with peers, and to build a sense of carrying the suffering together in the group:

BERTHA: We tell each other the problems that have happened.

JULIA: The differences.

BERTHA: And we cry together! And how? I mean hours. No, no, it hasn't been that fast either. Now we know each other, we call each other.

GABRIELA: So close.

BERTHA: We carry the suffering, together now. We all together carry the pain now.

Sharing with their peers how they interact with their missing family members (e.g. dreaming, talking to them, cooking for them, feeling that their loved one is sitting next to them) enabled them to feel that their unique experiences of mourning were not strange but a common response, even after decades. None of them reported the need to visit a mental health professional to deal with those "symptoms". Instead, sometimes they sought mental health support for family members who did not have the chance to grieve and express their emotions towards the disappeared loved one.

Likewise, the sense of belonging and affiliation provided by the community space allowed them to be connected and prevented feelings of isolation. Indeed, when one of the members does not participate in the meetings or is not answering the phone, the group organises home visits to approach this person.

Locating their loss in a broader context

Resisting the extreme violence by enhancing leadership has located the women as active agents in the process of building collective memories and social justice. Their connectedness and engagement have put them in a special position to advocate for their goals at the national and international levels. They have taken all opportunities to share what has happened to their families and their communities. They also share their learnings and the support they have received or provided, as a way to position themselves not only as victims but also as providers of supports and knowledge.

JUANA: So, also my case, we share our cases [in those meetings with public officers]. They did not know much [about this], so we shared with other organisations and now we also know their cases. I mean, afterwards we could freely talk, go together to their trials, accompaniment, those things.

Sharing in international platforms has also allowed them to broaden their understandings regarding how extreme violence operated in Latin America as a region; how there were systematic human rights violations in other countries with similar procedures to inflict horror upon communities and to disappear human remains. These understandings strengthened the women's appreciation for democracy and awareness of strategies used by dictatorial regimes. This learning has allowed them to locate their loss in an international context of generalised human rights violations.

Collective practices of cultural continuity and wellbeing

The broader context also provided the opportunity to openly show their cultural Andean practices as an expression of cultural resistance. As Carmen states: *"This is how we are, and we like it. If this is from my hometown [then it's] good."*

They proudly demonstrate their cultural practices that bring them together and provide a holistic sense of wellbeing. For example, cooking together and sharing their traditional food, using traditional medicine, and sharing ancient recipes for relieving body aches. Moreover, sharing their dreams and building together collective interpretations, or imagining together desired situations (positive trials, the return of their family member, accessing to reparations) are also part of the traditional strategies.

The culture-specific group also provided a space for participants to express suffering in their own way. This included elaborating their own explanations of the pains and health complaints by using local understandings and languages of distress without feeling afraid of criticisms. They relate their current pains to their experience of loss or the extreme conditions that they went through due to the collective violence.

When there's no closure

In the group, they can exchange narratives; the group is experienced as a safe space to engage in storytelling and to repeat the narrations as many times as they need to, knowing that their colleagues will not censor emotional expression. Although the women were exposed to very intense and potentially traumatic events, sharing emotions, and breaking down in tears are not necessarily seen as signs of weakness or hopelessness. They have established a long-lasting peer support network that goes alongside the decades of search for loved ones.

In cases of ambiguous loss, where there is uncertainty regarding the fate of the loved one, the idea of "bringing closure" has little relevance (Boss, 2017). Instead, these women have found ways of not becoming "frozen in the past" but promoting present interactions. They have moved towards diverse endeavours such as memorialising, searching for the human remains, looking for dignification, supporting others, and advocating for democratic processes. This group mobilisation in furthering an agenda of human rights allowed them to continue living with loss, recognising that their family member may be present in different ways, and that it is not a matter of saying "It is over", but of learning to live with that experience of loss. In the group they share that this loss will not go away but nor will it hold them back and that they will continue with their new goals. By belonging to this unique group, they encourage each other with plans of reconnecting to their rural hometowns or other activities that intertwine cultural and spiritual components.

Finally, being part of the group seems to open paths for different intra-family dynamics that may need further study. For instance, some of the women reported that at home, their families find them calmer after having the chance to share with their peers, to establish new links, to support others, to receive training and to engage in future group plans.

RESPONDING TO THE CHALLENGES OF THE COMMUNITY APPROACH

The main challenge of this approach is to prevent the idealisation of peer support. Although it does address one core area of victim's experiences, the family and community sphere, it may neglect or mask others that need special attention. Thereby, it is important to keep available other mental health supports for those who may need it, including group participants or those doing the psychosocial accompaniment. Another challenge is the need to "oxygenate" from the group to prevent repetitive interactions that may saturate the group. These women found it positive to connect with other groups since this allowed them to get fresh perspectives, as well as to ease tensions and potential conflicts, and to learn from other experiences.

Working in the context of societies facing transitional justice processes is particularly challenging since those who were in power when these violations occurred are still there, meaning that no matter the strength of these women, the possibilities of finding justice may be hindered by that political influence. However, they resist and keep fighting together, as they explain:

JUANA: We have walked everywhere, with our placards, with our banner "They took them alive; we want them alive". That was our motto. In the parks, institutions, everywhere we walk, we are not afraid, we do not have [fear]. I do not have.

ISABEL: I think that fear is not, we're not going to give up because we want to get to the truth.

In this context, it is easy to feel disempowered and hopeless, due to the uncertainty of the ongoing situation. However, this situation strengthens the women in their struggle, and in their fight of "Never again"; knowing that their loved ones will probably not return, but still, they are looking for a future. They have achieved this by supporting others and taking opportunities to speak up, such as going into schools to share about the internal armed conflict or others by guiding in memory museums. It seems that the challenge is to give a new meaning to their experience and to locate it in a broader social narrative.

INSPIRATION

We are inspired by the ways in which these women reinvent themselves, and at their conviction. They have moved beyond their own cases and look further. Their strength is inspiring – how can people engage in such powerful ideals? They have come forward because of their ideals and have survived because of them; they help them to stay alive and face adversity. They are a living memory that personifies the injustices that are still present in Peru. They themselves have become an institution, a benchmark. The living memory, the evidence, the example of how diverse memories compete. In Peru there is a hegemonic memory that tries to make these struggles private, particular and invisible, but by approaching the women one is able to put a face to what is written in human rights documents. Sitting at the table with them, listening to their testimony, is inspiring.

Importantly, working with human rights victims does not mean only focusing on their sufferings. The group allowed us to share their life experiences in a holistic human way. We do not remember sad scenes with them, but their laughs, how they played and had dreams. These women who, despite having unjustly suffered, can continue living and engaging in group projects for the whole society. Their solidarity is also inspiring, feeling that they are not going to focus only on an individual case but to fight for a more collective case, for this to not happen again. Their hope. We wonder how do they have so much hope? Most of us give up whilst facing far less.

Finally, and in an opposite vein, we notice that the women themselves do not have the sense that their achievements are significant. It seems that their fight has taken place over such a long period of time, that they do not recognise the gains they have made. There is a need for social recognition, to make the achievements of these groups of women visible. However, we are also aware that cultural expectations of modesty and valuing humility may make it difficult for the women to claim this recognition.

GUIDING PRINCIPLES WHEN WORKING WITH SURVIVORS OF HUMAN RIGHTS ABUSES

Working with these groups of women has had a great impact on our work. In this final section, we reflect on what the experience has taught us about the ways in which group activities with survivors of human rights abuses can be framed in order to have positive impacts on their well-being in the broadest sense.

A key aspect of our learning is related to the diverse ways in which social suffering can be experienced, and the negative effects of pathologising and professionalising human suffering. Engagement with the women's groups made evident the importance of peer support, and the need to offer opportunities for those who have experienced human rights abuses to meet others who have experienced similar losses, rather than immediately focusing on specialised care (which frequently is not available where survivors live). For those accompanying such groups, it is paramount to respect the group's own processes and provide open and safe spaces to enable them to rely on their collective self, accepting the will of members to revisit their painful experiences.

Moreover, when addressing their suffering, it is important to also embrace their capacities and to address practical-logistic issues by motivating their own leadership and promoting self-government. If requested, providing training to strengthen their capabilities of democratic leadership and paths for community participation in society can be useful. Encourage them to find their way, to consider their own goals and values to take forward community action on the issues that impact them.

Key areas of focus for this population include cultural continuity, family dynamics, spirituality, bonding and networking, and daily stressors that often challenge their lives. It is crucial for those accompanying the groups to join their efforts to identify and denounce racialised mechanisms that hinder access to justice for indigenous populations. Finally, those working with survivors of human rights abuses are called to promote intersections between family-community and other societal spheres which allow the members to anchor themselves in a country reality, and to act upon it.

REFERENCES

Boss, P. (2017) 'Families of the missing: Psychosocial effects and therapeutic approaches'. *International Review of the Red Cross*, 99(905), pp. 519–534. doi:10.1017/S1816383118000140.

Grupo De Trabajo Sobre Las Desapariciones Forzadas O Involuntarias (2015) *Perú/Desapariciones Forzadas: 30 años después las heridas siguen abiertas*. Available at https://www.ohchr.org/EN/NewsEvents/Pages/DisplayNews.aspx?NewsID=16065&LangID=S (Accessed: 21 January 2022).

Hamber, B. and Lundy, P. (2020) 'Lessons from transitional justice? Toward a new framing of a victim-centered approach in the case of historical institutional abuse'. *Victims & Offenders*, 15(6), pp. 744–770. doi:10.1080/15564886.2020.1743803.

International Center for Transitional Justice (2013) *Hatun Willakuy. Abbreviated Version of the Final Report of the Peruvian Truth and Reconciliation Commission*. Available at: https://www.ictj.org/sites/default/files/subsites/peru-hatun-willakuy-en/ (Accessed: 21 January 2022).

International Committee of the Red Cross (2019) *Search for disappeared persons in Peru: Achievements and challenges*. Available at: https://www.icrc.org/en/document/search-disappeared-persons-peru-achievements-and-challenges (Accessed: 21 January 2022).

Jenner, F. (2018) *'Internal racism' is prevalent in Peru, survey shows*. Available at: https://perureports.com/peru-racism-survey-culture/7135/ (Accessed: 21 January 2022).

Rivera-Holguín, M., Pérez-Sales, P., Hildenbrand, A., Custidio, E., Vargas, G., Baca, N., Corveleyn, J. and De Haene, L. (2019) 'Psychosocial and community assessment to family members of victims of enforced disappearance and extreme violence in Peru: Informing International Courts of Human Rights'. *Torture Journal*, 29, pp. 16–33. doi:10.7146/torture.v29i1.114046.

Suarez, E. B. (2015) 'Surviving juntas (together): Lessons of resilience of indigenous Quechua women in the aftermath of conflict in Peru'. *Intervention*, 13(1), pp. 6–18. Available at: https://www.interventionjournal.com/sites/default/files/Surviving_juntas__together____lessons_of.3.pdf (Accessed: 21 January 2022).

TRC (2003) *Final Report*. Lima: Truth and Reconciliation Commission. Available at: https://www.cverdad.org.pe/ingles/pagina01.php (Accessed: 21 January 2022).

Watkins, M. (2015) 'Psychosocial Accompaniment'. *Journal of Social and Political Psychology*, 3(1), pp. 324–341. doi:10.5964/jspp.v3i1.103.

CHAPTER 5

WHAT IS THE USE OF TALKING WHEN I CAN'T FEED MY CHILDREN? TPO UGANDA'S INTEGRATED APPROACH TO SUPPORTING REFUGEES

Grace Obalim, Caleb Tukahiirwa, Leticia Biira Birungi and Elias Manirakiza

Mary had lived with her young son in Lobule refugee settlement in the West Nile region of Uganda for four years. Mary is South Sudanese by nationality, and before the war that rocked her country began in 2013 she was a happily married woman with one child, and pregnant with her second. Her husband was a young man whose business was doing very well. When the war became intense, Mary left with the women of her husband's family for Uganda. Her husband and her ten-year-old son stayed behind, promising to come to Uganda once Mary was settled. That was the last time Mary heard from either her husband or her son. She arrived in Uganda and was settled with many other refugees from her country in Lobule refugee settlement. A few months later she gave birth to a second son, with whom she now lives.

When she attended a community meeting facilitated by social workers from TPO Uganda, she was shy, withdrawn and gloomy. During the meeting, the social workers described to the listening community members the signs of psychological distress, and some common coping mechanisms. Mary later told the social workers that everything she heard during the meeting seemed to be a description of her life, the constant memories and dreams, sleeplessness, loss of appetite, uncontrollable anger, fear of men and remorse, coupled with the thought that life was never meant to be for her.

The social workers conducted an assessment of Mary's wellbeing, which indicated that she might benefit from the groupwork programme offered by TPO Uganda to women in that settlement. She was introduced to a group of other women, and invited to attend weekly meetings with them over the next ten weeks.

> When teacher (referring to the group facilitator) told me I was to be with these women for 10 weeks I laughed at him and said he must be crazy. No one can allow being with a person like me, who would even listen to me? I am invisible to people. Even my own child sometimes doesn't recognise me.

The initial group sessions were tough for Mary as she had to learn to manage her insecurities and constant self-talk which told her that she was unworthy. She also struggled with the fear of being judged or even accepted once her fellow-participants learned about her experiences. As the sessions progressed, Mary heard the other women in the group share stories similar to hers, and learned that they had also experienced challenges, disappointments and hurts. Alongside this realisation, the group facilitator emphasised regularly that everyone in the group was valued, their opinions and feelings mattered and there was no room for judgement but rather it was every group member's duty to make the group as safe and welcoming as possible.

During the group sessions Mary began to notice how pleasing and comforting it was to be accepted and listened to again. The group provided her with a platform where she could freely speak about her struggle to accept where life had placed her. Listening to the other women in the group also enabled her to realise that she wasn't alone, as she heard other people had been through difficult life events and were willing to try to work through them.

Over the course of the sessions, Mary saw the other group members improve over the weeks. This gave her courage to also work towards her own personal recovery. The most

DOI: 10.4324/9781003192978-7

influential point for her in the whole group process was allowing herself to learn to love her son. She said:

> Listening to one of us who had lost all her family during an attack in their village made me realise that I was blessed to still have someone I can call my own blood. Although I knew he was born from a painful moment, listening to this woman helped me realise he was innocent and just a good boy that needed his mother's love.

Once the sessions came to an end, Mary and some other group members continued to meet regularly to discuss their concerns and support each other. They were able to start up a savings group, with the support of a TPO Uganda social worker and livelihood officer. The livelihood officer provided training on business skills, and the social worker met with the group for occasional check-ins. After some time, the women were able to open a market shop that sells local greens and other food stuffs, which enabled them to support their families and reduced their financial concerns.

The group process helped Mary to face her fears and come to terms with her traumatic experiences. It enabled those who had lost family members and their sense of self-worth to work towards regaining their self-appreciation, and to find a family with which they can identify. One of the participants said:

> This group has made me feel alive again, I see these women as my sisters, daughters and mothers. I have learnt to love again and felt loved as well and through interacting with them I have realised there is more to live for.

REFUGEE CONTEXT IN UGANDA

The population of refugees and asylum-seeking people in Uganda was estimated to be almost 1.5 million at the end of 2020 (UNHCR, 2021). People seek refuge in Uganda primarily from South Sudan and The Democratic Republic of the Congo (DRC), with smaller numbers arriving from other countries, such as Burundi. More than 12 districts in Uganda host refugees either in settlements or integrated within the host communities. According to the UNHCR 2019–2020 response plan, refugees continue to face numerous protection challenges due to the magnitude of displacement and growing vulnerabilities, compounded by diminishing resources and strained social services in the refugee-hosting districts. A protection needs assessment conducted by UNHCR to inform the 2019–2020 response plan revealed that 40% of refugees reported that a family member was in psychological distress and unable to access care.

Refugees in Uganda have experienced numerous stressful events because of political or religious oppression, war, migration and resettlement. Potentially traumatic events often preceded the war-related events that caused them to flee, including imprisonment, torture, loss of property, malnutrition, physical assault, extreme fear and loss of livelihood. The process of fleeing can last days, months or years during which refugees may be separated from family members, robbed, forced to inflict pain or kill, witness torture or killing, go through the loss of close family members and have to endure extremely harsh environments. Perhaps the most significant of all the experiences is the sense of betrayal, either by their own people, by the enemy forces or by the custodians of the country's democracy. Having the cynical actions of others become the controlling factor of one's life can have significant effects on mental health and hinder the development of the healthy interpersonal relationships critical to resettlement and healing. These refugees are dealing with untold levels of pain from the events of their near pasts. Mentally, they are still running away from their captors and this can become a barrier to healing.

When refugees arrive in Uganda, they are often hosted in places that are not of their choosing. They must adapt to a new place and language, living amongst strangers under uncertain circumstances with uncertain futures. Re-establishing a home and identity, while trying to juggle the tasks of daily living, is yet another significant challenge that the refugee must undertake. Post-migration stress significantly influences the emotional wellbeing of refugees and often provides a risk similar to, or greater than, war-related trauma.

TPO UGANDA

TPO Uganda is a rights-based non-governmental organisation that works in partnership with communities, civil society, the private sector and government to empower communities to improve mental health and socio-economic wellbeing in a sustainable way. The goal is to leave behind communities capable of resolving their own problems. The organisation has operated in post-conflict and non-conflict areas of Uganda for over 25 years, and works with both refugee populations and host communities.

The main thematic focus of TPO Uganda is food security and livelihoods along with mental health and psychosocial support (MHPSS), but other thematic areas include child protection, prevention of HIV and AIDS, and prevention and response to gender-based violence. Key MHPSS interventions include psychoeducation, group therapies, case management, Psychological First Aid (World Health Organization, War Trauma Foundation and World Vision International, 2011), Problem Management Plus (PM+) (World Health Organization, 2018) and capacity building for different community support structures (e.g. village health teams, community-based counsellors, volunteer psychosocial assistants, probation and child protection officers, refugee leadership structures and community influencers such as youth groups, women groups, religious leaders and cultural leaders).

TPO Uganda has over the years been a source of employment to many young Ugandans. It prides itself on recruiting people who share its values and are passionate about humanitarian work. Although specialities differ depending on the project, TPO Uganda ensures that as many staff as possible are indigenous to the community of operation, or share an ethnic background with the communities they serve. This enables the organisation to both build capacity within the local communities and establish a sustainability process for when the projects end.

INTEGRATING GROUP THERAPY WITH LIVELIHOODS SUPPORT

TPO Uganda integrates livelihood or income generation activities (IGAs) into MHPSS programming. The rationale for this is based on evidence for the strong relationship between livelihood opportunities and the psychological wellbeing of individuals (e.g. Nuwagaba, Najjingo and Arinaitwe, 2019; Schininá et al., 2016). Some TPO Uganda clients are unable to engage in any productive activity due to the distress they experience. Therefore, TPO Uganda aims to address multiple aspects of refugees' lives in an integrated way, in order to contribute to positive and sustainable change in wellbeing.

Before beginning work in a new location, TPO Uganda conducts assessments to determine the specific MHPSS needs of the community. This is usually followed by awareness-raising initiatives to increase community understanding of the available MHPSS services. This commonly stimulates community interest and referrals for MHPSS support from either community members, community structures or self-referrals. The awareness packages are tailored to specific communities; for example, there are differences between the sessions for refugee and host communities. Sessions with host communities often focus on depression and the mental health consequences of sexual and gender-based violence, whilst those with refugee communities place more emphasis on post-traumatic stress disorder (PTSD) and anxiety resulting from the extreme experiences and changes in their lives.

Once an individual is referred to TPO Uganda's MHPSS team, standardised mental health screening tools are used to assess whether they are likely to benefit from the services provided. Individuals whose scores indicate moderate or severe distress are invited to join one of the group therapy intervention programmes, such as Group Cognitive Behavioural Therapy for Trauma. This consists of ten weekly sessions for groups of around 10–15 members, who work through sessions focusing on stabilisation, trauma narration and processing, integration and consolidation. The pre-intervention assessment is followed by an assessment around session five in order to determine the level of recovery. This mid-term assessment also includes a socio-economic assessment, to understand the client's needs and economic status, and their opinions on the type of livelihood opportunities they would like to be engaged in. This information is used to plan a comprehensive training on different business opportunities. The group members continue with the group therapy sessions until they graduate following session ten. At this stage, the recovery rate tends to be high with around 80% reporting low PTSD and depression-related symptoms and improved social functioning; they are also able to make informed decisions regarding the types of livelihood activities that they would like to engage in both individually and as a group.

We have observed that the risk of relapse among individuals who complete the group therapy is much higher amongst those with limited livelihood opportunities compared to those who access both MHPSS services and livelihood opportunities. Therefore, for MHPSS achievements to be consolidated and sustained, TPO Uganda facilitates linkages and referrals of graduated clients to other service providers who offer IGAs or Village Savings and Loans Associations (VSLA). VSLAs are an instrument introduced by the government of Uganda to enhance women's socio-economic empowerment, and are now used by many partners. It involves a group, usually single-sex and primarily women, who save together and take small loans from the savings collected by the members. The members of each group normally share a common interest, have common livelihood needs and financial strength. The VSLAs are self-managed and self-capitalised savings groups in which members' savings are lent to each member in turn. This platform provides members with a means to cope with emergencies, to manage their household cash-flow, build a capital base and, crucially, rebuild social networks, solidarity and trust.

TPO Uganda provides women's VSLA groups, consisting of graduates of the group therapy programme, with livelihood capital after they participate in a basic training on savings and record-taking. The group is supported to elect leaders (chairperson, secretary and treasurer), and the TPO Uganda social worker who facilitated the psychosocial therapy groups makes bi-weekly visits to each group to ensure that any issues are resolved and the group is functioning effectively. A TPO Uganda livelihood officer makes monthly visits to support with any difficulties in their saving operations. The groups are also encouraged to engage in more income-generating activities like selling simple items in the community markets. In addition, they carry out activities such as community sensitisations (speaking to communities about topics like mental illness, its effects and the services available), planting vegetables around their homes for daily consumption, and most of all practising positive coping mechanisms they have learned together in order to develop as a team. This not only reduces the potential risk of relapse but also increases bonding amongst group members.

I (Grace) have facilitated cognitive-behavioural therapy (CBT) sessions with three groups who had high levels of distress. Once they completed the CBT programme, TPO Uganda supported each group with funds to start a VSLA group and a small business venture. One group of women from Kiryandongo refugee settlement opened a small shop and were able to save alongside this. With their accumulated profits and savings, they bought tailoring machines and started learning how to use them. At the community church where these machines were kept, adolescent girls who had not benefited from the therapy group and were not members of the saving group were also able to learn how to use them. When the COVID-19 pandemic began, this group of women were contracted by UNHCR to make reusable masks for the community, which empowered them economically whilst also supporting the community with easy-to-access and affordable masks.

As a second example, a group of adolescents who benefited from the TPO Uganda group intervention and livelihood programme formed themselves into a sports team after graduating, and held sports activities at a Child Friendly Space (a space created to provide play and learning areas for children in a safe environment). The group was given a pair of goats, and over time the goats bred so that every member had at least one or two goats in their homes. The adolescents became change agents in the settlement. Some contributed to TPO Uganda awareness-raising sessions on mental health; some became youth leaders and have inspired and supported their peers.

RATIONALE FOR SOCIAL ECONOMIC APPROACH

We don't heal in isolation, but in community.

At TPO Uganda, we know that realistically, the biggest contributor to psychological distress in the refugee settlements is poverty. Trauma is usually a secondary thought for most of these survivors. Their children provide refugees with a reason to live another day, in order to support and protect them. The inherent need to survive obscures and buffers trauma; survival mode takes over.

The combination of therapy with livelihood activities enables some of the factors contributing to distress to be addressed, as well as the feelings of distress themselves. When a group has been enrolled for therapy, we often ask the group members what they want from the process. Often the answer will be: *"I want not to feel like this anymore. I want to be able to wake up every day and be happy even with the little I have."*

However, frequently the answer will refer to their material wellbeing: *"I don't want to be poor anymore; I need some sort of business that can help my family. I am tired of being poor."* Our clients' needs for money, medicine, food and other basic provisions are more salient to them than their need to address their traumatic experiences. We have had clients who have told us:

> What good does talking about my problems do me, when I can't even feed my children? What good is healing my mind going to do for the hunger pangs I feel every day?

The combination of group therapy and livelihood opportunities, which are also implemented in a group format rather than individually, builds on the community-based approach which is crucial to effectiveness in this context. Most African cultures have strong foundations in family and community. The essence of the support is to empower the client to be self-reliant but also be in a position to contribute to the growth and development of their community. This can only be achieved by working with individuals within their value system. Groupwork has been found to provide the members with a sense of belonging similar to a family context, which enables them to work through underlying difficulties.

The group approach is effective in this context for other reasons as well. One important factor is the recognition of shared experiences and feelings among group members. The universality of the problems discussed serves to remove an individual's sense of isolation, validates their experiences, and raises self-esteem. Secondly, the group becomes a place where members can help each other. The experience of being able to give something to another person can lift the member's sense of self-efficacy and help them to develop more adaptive coping styles and inter-personal skills. Thirdly, the group setting instils hope and encourages healing and perseverance. In a mixed group that has members at various stages of development or recovery, members are often inspired and encouraged by another who has overcome the problems with which they are still struggling, and this goes a long way in healing and growth for the members who have just joined. They are mentored and encouraged by those further along in their healing journey.

The group setting also provides a safe and supportive environment for members to take risks by strengthening their social skills through, for example, sharing personal feelings, showing concern, and supporting others. The groups have also promoted cohesiveness. Humans have an instinctive need to belong to groups, and a cohesive group is a place in which all members can feel a sense of belonging, acceptance, and validation.

The group also promotes catharsis. When members tell their story to a supportive audience, they can obtain relief from chronic feelings of shame and guilt but they can also learn from the group that one has to take responsibility for one's own life and the consequences of decisions. The group members can achieve a greater level of self-awareness through the process of inter-acting with others in the group, giving feedback on other members' behaviour and its impact on others. They can also achieve greater levels of insight into the genesis of their own problems.

Recovery is an undulating and tumultuous process but, overall, the groups do relatively well. Most are able to feed their families and re-enrol their children in school. They have become functioning members of the community by engaging in community activities, such as joining the choir in church.

CHALLENGES

As effective as group therapy has been in this setting, there have also been challenges. Some of our staff came together to discuss what makes it a beautiful process and what can make it quite difficult.

> When dealing with a group of people, it is common as a therapist to mostly concentrate on what bonds them rather than their individuality.

It is rather common to look at the group as a whole rather than as individuals. It may be diffi-cult to go through each person's issues, understand their motivations, setbacks, emotions, what drives them and their thought structures. In a group of twelve, facilitators have to work extra hard to make sure they understand each group member as an individual, as well as how they fit within their group.

> Some people may stay silent about their problem from start to finish of therapy, while others may monopolise sessions as if they are the only ones going through something.

> Not all groups cohere well. There have been those where cohesiveness isn't easily attained or not at all. They may instead breed conflict.

> Some clients are more interested in what they are getting out of the group rather than recovery. They come in every session; say the right words just for an opportunity at livelihood.

> No shows are common, in a group of twelve; full attendance may only happen a handful of times, with almost half the members absent on some occasions.

In such incidences, the session is usually postponed to the next meeting day, when the majority of the clients can be available. Despite some of these challenges, we have managed over time to learn and unlearn what we think we know about trauma, about the way life is supposed to flow and we have challenged ourselves to make sure the group members get the most out of the therapeutic process.

OUR LEARNING FROM THE GROUPWORK EXPERIENCE

As facilitators of the groups, we have been privileged to accompany the participants and learn from them, as they learn from each other. Over the years we have witnessed groups of clients who have received MHPSS support from TPO Uganda who go on to embrace the changes in life and become influential not only in their families, but also in their communities at large. Some of the groups have continued meeting months and years after their group therapy sessions have ended. TPO Uganda has also continued to provide follow-up sessions through community structures and field social workers, with support from a clinical psychologist.

Through its livelihood officers TPO Uganda has provided one-time cash grants to some graduated client groups, and successes have been noted within these groups and communities. This support always follows the VSLA guidelines to enable group members to support each other as they work on their recovery journey (both psychological and economical) together. TPO Uganda also continuously provides refresher livelihood trainings for these groups. Inevitably, there are cases where the funds are misused, with members borrowing and failing to repay the loan, or failing to keep up with the membership contributions. However, this does not overshadow the many persons who have managed to improve their economic livelihood through these one-time cash grants provided by TPO Uganda.

In this final section, we share our own reflections on our experience of being involved with the TPO Uganda therapeutic activities with refugees in the settlements.

> The most amazing thing for me about groupwork is how in the first place you have to drag these people to come together; each has their own struggles and fears of being known or heard, their faces are always filled with worthlessness, hopelessness and helplessness. So you get them together and as weeks pass by a ray of hope seemingly shines upon them and slowly you see them brighten up and dream again about a better tomorrow together.
>
> (Caleb Tukahiirwa, Clinical Psychologist with TPO Uganda)

> It is very satisfying to see individuals from two tribes that have been rivals for years coming together in a group, sharing traumatic experiences they have gone through as a result of violence in their country. Coming together in MHPSS/Livelihood support groups has not only enabled the individuals from these tribes to support each other to recover from trauma, but has also been an avenue of forgiving one another and promoting peaceful coexistence among the communities. To me, forgiveness is part and parcel of healing, and an enabler of achieving the peace and wellbeing (mentally, physically, spiritually, emotionally) which all humanitarian workers advocate for. Working with these groups has allowed me to understand the different sorts of problems that come from being displaced, and witnessing participants overcoming these adversities is an inspiration. At every graduation ceremony of these groups, I feel like a proud mother watching success.
>
> (Elias Manirakiza, Regional Coordinator with TPO Uganda)

Grace Obalim (Clinical Psychologist, MHPSS Advisor with TPO Uganda) reflects on the groupwork from the perspective of her experience as a clinical psychologist in a hospital setting:

Coming from my work in a private mental health hospital, adjusting to humanitarian community-based MHPSS implementation was one of the greatest professional challenges I have faced. As a trained mental health practitioner in a structured hospital setting, a normal day would involve me seeing four clients, holding one family session and then sitting in a well set-up office to record and file my session notes. Learning to conduct assessments under a tree, just a few metres away from many other hundreds of clients lined up waiting to be assessed, and holding community mental health awareness sessions in my local Uganda language was a challenge. It led to a realisation that a complete attitude change was required. Through engaging with the refugee community, I learnt that the greatest strength of those affected by adversity is the resilience that can be built through close social networks. Shared suffering becomes a community suffering, hence no one is stigmatised and everyone becomes a keeper of the other.

As a manager, my frequent field visits and participation in some of the graduation ceremonies of the groups has always left me humbled by the impacts our field team are creating in the lives of others, and how resilient they are, living in tents and riding motorbikes close to 50 kilometres each day. I have experienced the power of close coordination with other service providers, to ensure that individuals receiving TPO Uganda MHPSS services can be referred to others for complementary forms of support, such as livelihoods, enabling a more holistic approach.

I am challenged to advocate for a community-based approach towards addressing the mental health and psychosocial needs of the general public beyond humanitarian settings. I have seen how it can reduce stigma about mental health disorders, improves awareness of mental health issues and leaves long lasting evidence of its effectiveness in terms of persons who have recovered from severe forms of distress and are able to function effectively and develop the strong social connections that will support their wellbeing in the long term.

REFERENCES

Nuwagaba, D., Najjingo, D. and Arinaitwe, F. (2019) *Prevalence of SGBV and Impact of TPO Psychosocial Support Model and Livelihoods Interventions on Mental Health Recovery of SGBV Survivors in Emergency in the West Nile Region.* Kampala: TPO Uganda and UN Women. Available at: https://www.alnap.org/help-library/prevalence-of-sgbv-and-impact-of-tpo-psychosocial-support-model-and-livelihoods (Accessed: 20 January 2022).

Schininá, G., Babcock, E., Nadelman, R., Walsh, J.S., Willhoite, A. and Willman, A. (2016) 'The integration of livelihood support and mental health and psychosocial wellbeing for populations who have been subject to severe stressors'. *Intervention*, 14(3), pp. 211–222. Available at: https://www.interventionjournal.com/content/integration-livelihood-support-and-mental-health-and-psychosocial-wellbeing-populations-who (Accessed: 20 January 2022).

UNHCR (2021) *UNHCR Global Focus: Uganda.* Available at: https://reporting.unhcr.org/uganda (Accessed: 30 July 2021).

World Health Organization (2018) *Problem Management Plus (PM+): Individual psychological help for adults impaired by distress in communities exposed to adversity. (Generic field-trial version 1.1).* Geneva: WHO. Available at: https://apps.who.int/iris/rest/bitstreams/915902/retrieve (Accessed: 20 January 2022).

World Health Organization, War Trauma Foundation and World Vision International (2011) *Psychological First Aid: Guide for Field Workers.* Geneva: WHO. Available at: https://apps.who.int/iris/rest/bitstreams/53113/retrieve (Accessed: 20 January 2022).

CHAPTER 6

HOME AWAY FROM HOME

Healing among Congolese refugees in Rwanda through community-based sociotherapy

Theophile Sewimfura, Emmanuel Sarabwe and Annemiek Richters

FROM MISERY TO EMPOWERMENT

Mutesi is a 31-year-old Congolese woman living in a camp for Congolese refugees in Rwanda. She had fled the armed conflict raging in her place of residence in Congo on a motorbike, holding three of her children in her arms and the fourth one tied on her back. When in the camp, she accidently got pregnant by a man other than her husband. She felt guilty and ashamed, even though her husband had left her long ago and she had not heard from him since. Still caring for her children, Mutesi tried to torture herself to death through starvation for two months to no avail. When her in-laws, considering her behaviour leading to her extra-marital pregnancy unacceptable, took her children away from her, Mutesi felt that her life was finished, and she thought of committing suicide. Luckily her children, expressing their need to see their mother, were returned to her.

Back in the camp with her children Mutesi lived in despair. She was unable or unwilling to speak or be in eye contact with anyone, cried unceasingly day and night, and suffered from recurrent headaches. One morning, still pregnant, Mutesi went to a river nearby to drown herself. However, the thought of her children being left without someone to care for them made her return home. Soon after, Mutesi was invited to join a sociotherapy group that was about to start. She accepted the invitation with the intention to only listen and not speak about her troublesome life. During the first weekly sessions that is what she did. Eventually, however, Mutesi gained the courage to talk and tell her life story. She had become aware of the care that group members gave her, by even visiting her at her home. Also, the life stories two women had shared in the group made Mutesi realise that her plight was less serious than that of others; that she had never been physically injured and that none of her loved ones had been killed.

Empowered by the group, Mutesi started to take care of herself and her children again. She realised the value of being supported and now supports others. When she meets someone who is lonely, she tries to comfort that person and advises the person to join a sociotherapy group. Mutesi goes again to church to worship with other people. She socialises with others and no longer blames herself for what happened.

INTRODUCTION

The story of Mutesi is an excerpt from one of eight accounts of the ways in which the lives of Congolese refugees living in a camp in Rwanda changed through their participation in a community-based sociotherapy programme. The eight stories were written by Congolese refugees trained as sociotherapists, who were asked to describe the most significant changes they had observed in the lives of those who had taken part in the programme.

DOI: 10.4324/9781003192978-8

Sociotherapists, also called group facilitators, live among the people they bring together in groups for the 15-week community-based sociotherapy journey. Rwandan sociotherapy participants named the journey *mvura-nkuvure*, which can be translated as 'you heal me, I heal you' in Kinyarwanda, the national language of Rwanda. This chapter is based on the eight stories and our experience in community-based sociotherapy in Rwanda and surrounding countries since 2005. In the following section we present some background information about Congolese refugees in Rwanda and their lived experiences of distress that create a need for the support provided by community-based sociotherapy (below shortened to sociotherapy). The names used are pseudonyms.

LIVED EXPERIENCES OF DISTRESS AMONG CONGOLESE REFUGEES

In 2021, Rwanda hosted nearly 75,000 Congolese refugees (UNHCR Rwanda, 2021). Most of them live in one of the five Congolese refugee camps spread over the country. They include refugees who fled their home country in the 1990s as well as more recent arrivals who fled during 2012–2013 due to renewed hostilities in the eastern part of the Democratic Republic of Congo (DRC), a country neighbouring Rwanda. Congolese Tutsi were the most hated, hunted and killed. Extreme violence related to ethnic conflicts, or the threat of this violence, caused many to flee, leaving behind their properties and often their family and community. These experiences, together with the pressures of trying to integrate into a new living environment, were factors that contributed to a high level of distress among many of the refugees. As Leonard, a 28-year-old man married with two children, shared:

> When I arrived in the camp, I was not aware of where I was coming from nor where I was going. This was caused by psychological trauma I developed due to the bad things I had experienced during the wars that took place ever since I was young and lastly due to soldiers having taken away all the money we got from selling our properties. Life in the camp was very difficult. The camp was overpopulated, people shared latrines and bathrooms. In a nutshell, life was without any freedom. These problems were common among camp dwellers, but they did not hurt me too much.

Leonard fled Congo out of fear that his Hutu relatives would kill him because of his interactions with Tutsi. Within the camp he suffered most from being insulted and discriminated against by Tutsi youngsters. "*My heart was about to burst as it were. I did not want to talk to anyone in the camp. I was dumb for two months. … I intended to take revenge one day.*"

Most of the other sociotherapy participants whose stories were collected emphasised their social and psychological suffering as exceeding the distress caused by poor living conditions in the camp. Therese shared: "*I hated my life in the camp because I had no one to live for.*" Therese's children and husband had been killed in an army attack, whilst she was seriously injured and barely survived. "*I hated myself and could not accept the death of my children. I isolated myself and I spent a lot of sleepless nights. … The thoughts of wanting to commit suicide did not leave me.*" The storytellers spoke of the violence they had been exposed to or witnessed; abandonment; loss of loved ones; communal and family bonds being shattered; high levels of mistrust, fear, and social tension; hatred and revenge; shame and guilt; lost self-confidence and low self-esteem; lack of taste for life; suicidal ideation and behaviour (Ingabire and Richters, 2020); social isolation; sleeplessness and mood disturbances; headaches; and an orientation towards the future being disrupted. There is no sign of hope for refugees from the DRC of returning to their homelands as long as political tensions with persisting insecurities continue to reign in their zones of origin.

While various humanitarian organisations have responded to the concerns of refugees by providing tangible support – food, water, livelihood development – with some effect, the scarce mental health and psychosocial support available is usually not very effective because it is mostly individual oriented and not adapted to local realities. This is confirmed by refugees who have benefitted from participation in sociotherapy, as for instance by Kwihangana.

Kwihangana is a 33-year-old man with a wife whom the community refers to as "*a mad woman*". Kwihangana takes care of her and their four children. He tried many options to get help for his wife, even bringing her to Congo for treatment. However, all in vain. He had a grudge against the family that, according to his wife, had poisoned her. He felt like "*dried leaves of banana trees*" due to the hardship and not seeing a way out. Being beaten by his wife made him feel ashamed and afraid to meet other people. He did not speak to other people and did not listen to anyone, including his wife. He was ready to do just anything to find a solution for his problems. The psychiatrist he consulted could not help him. Eventually Kwihangana participated in *mvura-nkuvure* which he experienced as "*a place you step in dirty and tired and you get out clean and relaxed.*"

How Kwihangana and our other seven storytellers were helped by their participation in sociotherapy to find a home again away from their original home in the DRC, is what we will explore in the following sections.

THE PATHWAY TO THE DEVELOPMENT OF COMMUNITY-BASED SOCIOTHERAPY IN RWANDA

Sociotherapy was brought to Rwanda by Cora Dekker, a Dutch sociotherapist who had years of experience with practising sociotherapy among traumatised refugees in support of their psychiatric treatment in clinical settings in the Netherlands. Sociotherapy in the Netherlands evolved from the therapeutic community model developed in military hospitals in the United Kingdom during the Second World War for the treatment of the many psychiatric casualties of that war (Whiteley, 2004).

The idea behind healing and health promotion within the context of therapeutic communities is that the methods to support recovery from overwhelming experiences should be environmental and not solely dependent on expensive individual forms of treatment (Bloom and Norton, 2004). The social anthropologist Robert Rapoport, who observed one of England's therapeutic communities after the war, considers the social rehabilitation unit he studied to be an experiment in milieu therapy. He wrote about his observations in his book *Community as doctor* (1960). The psychiatrist Maxwell Jones, one of the pioneers of the therapeutic community movement in the UK, ends his Introduction to this book as follows:

> By studying the individual in the social setting of both hospital and home it forces us to reconsider what are the relevant social factors that affect the course of patients' lives and how they can be used in a therapeutic way. Thus, the concept of a therapeutic community as a somewhat artificial hospital social milieu gives way to the wider concept of socio-cultural therapy in all relevant environments in which a patient must function as a social being.
>
> (Jones, 1960, p. 6)

The therapeutic community model became known as sociotherapy in the Netherlands, where since the 1970s it has been part of the mental health care provision.

In 2004 during a visit by Cora Dekker and Annemiek Richters to the Byumba Diocese of the Anglican church in Rwanda, the main pastor of this Diocese, Emmanuel Ngendahayo, became interested in the sociotherapy approach. He stressed the limited success of one-to-one pastoral and trauma counselling in helping people to recover from the complex wounds of genocide and the preceding war (1990–1994) and asked his visitors to bring sociotherapy to his Diocese. A year later the first steps in the implementation of sociotherapy in the Byumba Diocese were made (Richters et al., 2008). Since psychiatric clinical care was extremely scarce in Rwanda and given the enormous needs among the Rwandan population for the type of care that a sociotherapy intervention can offer, it was decided to transform the clinic-based sociotherapy as practised in the Netherlands into a community-based approach through experimenting and learning by doing. It was assumed that practising sociotherapy at a community level would meet the needs of many more people than an individualistic approach could do; would do so within a relatively short period of time; and would be cost-effective.

The widespread recognition of the positive impact of sociotherapy on people's lives resulted in sociotherapy travelling from the Byumba Diocese to communities, prisons, and refugee camps spread over Rwanda; the neighbouring countries DRC, Burundi and Uganda; and, further away, Liberia (Dekker, 2018). Each new environment asked for adaptation of sociotherapy to the socio-cultural, historical, and political specificities of that environment. *Due to those specificities, in Rwanda sociotherapy developed from a mental health and psychosocial support intervention to a psychosocial peacebuilding intervention, contributing to reconciliation between genocide survivors and* perpetrators and between their respective descendants (Ingabire et al., 2017; see also cbsrwanda.org). However, the values underpinning the approach and the core of the 15-week sociotherapy journey remained intact. Regarding sociotherapy for Congolese refugees in Rwanda, very little adaptation was necessary, since these refugees have much in common with Rwandans, such as language, culture, and a high level of human rights abuses.

THE VALUES THAT UNDERPIN SOCIOTHERAPY'S GROUP APPROACH

The main values that underpin the sociotherapy approach include the principles of interest, equality, democracy, participation, responsibility, and learning-by-doing using actual and current situations, to be applied throughout the sociotherapy journey (Richters et al., 2008). The principle of interest is what distinguishes sociotherapy from mental health and psychosocial support interventions that have an individual-oriented approach. The concept of interest was taken from Hannah Arendt (1958). It refers to the "subjective in-between reality" or "the web of human relationships", indicating its somewhat intangible quality. Jackson, with reference to Hannah Arendt, observed in his anthropological research on the impact of mass violence on people: "Because violence […] occurs in the contested space of intersubjectivity, its most devastating effects are not on individuals *per se* but on the fields of interrelationships that constitute their life-worlds" (2002, p. 39). Therefore, in the aftermath of the mass violence experienced in Rwanda, the DRC, and other countries around the world, one of the major challenges is the re-invention of shattered social worlds, of the web of human relationships. Particularly in places where people affected by mass violence must live together in conditions of proximity and depend on each other in day-to-day life, a renewed form of social cohesion is essential for survival and a dignified life.

Dekker used to explain the principle of interest to future sociotherapists by saying that people who are interested in each other can ask questions like 'how are you?', 'what do you mean?', 'how do you do things?', 'how do you see things?', 'how do you experience things?'. In this way a dialogue starts. That dialogue, together with other activities – such as games, songs, and cultural activities – carried out in sociotherapy groups, make people arise from social death, from "a disempowering descent into passivity and privacy, solitude and silence" (Jackson, 2002, p. 44).

The idea behind sociotherapy is that through active group participation, people practically re-engage with everyday life (cf. Summerfield, 2002). Its emphasis on the here-and-now distinguishes sociotherapy from trauma therapy that focuses specifically on the processing of traumatic memories of a painful past. Speaking about traumatic memories in sociotherapy cannot be avoided. However, this speaking is not encouraged at the start of the intervention. Sociotherapists are trained to contain it to prevent people from becoming too overwhelmed by emotions. The focus in the sociotherapy journey is first on actual daily life problems. However, once an atmosphere in the group of trust and mutual respect has been established, painful memories of the past can be shared.

Values other than the six principles include: the meeting of groups in the direct living environment of the participants and not in training centres; the facilitation of groups by sociotherapists who live in the same environment as those participating in the groups they facilitate; the inclusion of all people – regardless of education, gender, age, religion, profession, ethnicity, etc.; speaking the local language throughout the group sessions; no provision of drinks, meals, or money. The latter was much debated among staff and sociotherapists at the start of the programme in 2005. The then bishop of the Byumba Diocese, Onesphore Rwaje, who was asked for advice on this controversial issue, said very simply, "Providing food or money is the end of this programme." The underlying thought was that meeting requests for material support would not help in breaking through the state of victimisation and dependency many of the sociotherapy participants are in. Material support would bypass the goal of sociotherapy, which first is to restore people's dignity and create connectedness. Nevertheless, before people fully understand what sociotherapy is about, many of them, being familiar with the NGO culture of providing material 'compensation' for participating in meetings, do expect some material benefits from participating. As Leonard said:

> I joined the group with much curiosity. To tell you the truth, I thought I would get material support (money), especially because I had heard other members of the group whisper that they would get something out of this project.

However, during the first session Leonard, like many other participants, realised that he got something else that proved to be worthwhile.

THE GROUP PROCESS

Sociotherapy uses the group as a therapeutic medium to establish trust, create an open environment for discussion and manage together daily psychosocial problems. Sociotherapy groups are composed of an average of 10 to 15 people. They meet weekly for approximately three hours over a period of 15 weeks in a place located in people's direct living environment that group members experience as safe. The location can be a school, a church, an office, a private sitting room, a place under a tree, or the grass in the open air. Each group is facilitated by two sociotherapists. These sociotherapists were selected from community members based on criteria such as knowing their community well, trustworthiness, availability, having at least finished primary school, but preferably having an education higher than that, not necessarily in psychology, social work, or the clinical domain. Throughout their work they are supported in various ways by programme staff.

Sociotherapists invite people who they think are likely to benefit from the sociotherapy process to participate in a group during one or more visits to their home. No diagnosis is made beforehand. They explain to potential participants what the process is like and what to expect. As Kwihangana said: "*Subjects such as confidentiality, caring for one another, building confidence and peace of mind for everyone would be covered. Moreover, I was told that everyone would be there to help his or her neighbour."* Some people had doubts that they would gain anything from sociotherapy and were reluctant to join. However, most of them were so desperate that they are willing to try anything that may help them. They then often join with the intention to keep silent and not participate in the discussions, as was Mutesi's intention.

People receive a warm welcome from the sociotherapists and are invited to sit with them and the other participants in a circle, which is a new experience for most. Leonard, who came expecting to get material support, said:

> But on the first day, when I found myself sitting with other people, something that I could not explain was happening in me. I felt taken from one level to another because it was my first time to sit in a group forming a circle. Even though I had attended different meetings like church services, it was my first time I sat with others while facing one another and not behind others.

Sitting in the circle symbolises the principles of interest and equality that guides the group process. Sociotherapists explain again what participants can expect from the group sessions and how the group will work. For instance, as Aimé understood it, *"sociotherapy is about receiving and giving ideas or sharing testimonies to help anyone who faces a problem. No one is forced to talk about themselves. Everything is to be done out of one's own will."* Therese remembered that it was explained that:

> … group members help someone understand what happens to him or her and what causes that to happen, link the causes to the psychological wounds suffered in life before giving someone advice, help others by sharing testimonies of the progress they have made thanks to the socio-therapy program.

During the 15 sessions, the two sociotherapists guide the group through the sociotherapy phases of safety, trust, care, respect, new life orientations, and memories. Throughout the journey the six principles are applied. It is the dynamic complexity of principles and phases that makes sociotherapy work effectively. As sociotherapists observed, both the phases and the principles encourage participants to take care of each other and help one another to cope with the problems or situations troubling them, which enables them to think about the future in a constructive way (Richters et al., 2010). When a person experiences that they are safe and can trust the other group participants, that person starts to have contact with others, is able to listen to them and gets ready to share their troubles with the group. A demanding challenge for sociotherapists is to guide the group in building that safety, so that, as trust builds, people open up and gradually present their problems in some detail before any suggestions are given for potential actions or solutions.

Following the last group session, participants, whether or not with the help of sociotherapists, organise a conviviality meeting to celebrate what they achieved and share their testimonies with family members, friends, neighbours, and local authorities. The majority of sociotherapy groups in communities in Rwanda continue to meet after the 15 sessions have ended. This continuing contact can involve supporting each other through discussions about daily life or forming associations to generate an income together, or a combination of the two. In refugee settings groups also continue to meet. However, it is seldom that they engage in income generating activities as refugees have limited access to financial resources they could invest in associations (Ingabire and Richters, 2020).

THE IMPACT OF GROUP PARTICIPATION ON PEOPLE'S LIVES

A sociotherapy group can be considered as a 'transitional space' in which participants gradually experience the value of listening, sympathising with others, speaking with others about one's problems, making decisions together, and empowering each other. The group provides a safe space where they can practice new behaviours based on these values, behaviours which they subsequently introduce in their daily life outside the group, in their families and communities. The story of Mutesi illustrates this behavioural change. Leonard's story provides another illustration. Leonard realised that the peace of mind he got thanks to *mvura-nkuvure* had positive impacts also on his wife and their way of relating to each other. "*In the unhappy days of my life, she was sad, too. Nothing went well at home. Can you imagine that I spent two months lying in bed without going out to seek work! That affected my family obviously.*" Leonard started to listen to his wife, which changed her way of behaving. The fact that the group visited his wife was much appreciated by her. She stopped wandering around and beating Leonard and again took up household chores.

One very frequently hears those who have completed the 15-week sociotherapy journey testify that they discovered in the group that they are not the only one suffering or the only one who has been exposed to injustice. This often results in relativising one's own suffering and problems, as again the story of Mutesi illustrates. In such cases, the proverbial saying 'a burden shared is a burden halved' applies. However, with the support of the group that burden may even be reduced further, as was the experience of Claudine, a 50-year-old mother of seven children. When Claudine joined *mvure-nkuvura* her heart was broken. She cried unceasingly. She refused to be comforted and overcome the injustice perpetrated against her and her family. In one of the sociotherapy sessions, somebody gave a testimony interrupted by sobs and tears. Claudine also burst into tears. The group let her cry and she went back home feeling released. A participant visited her and asked her how she was feeling. Claudine said,

> You know, that day, when I heard the testimony from the other woman who was left by her husband and whose children were all poisoned, and seeing her crying, I started to cry too. I thought about her plight and mine and I felt released. I was like a person who got released from a heavy stone on his/her shoulders.

The group helps people to raise their self-esteem and confidence and helps them to re-engage in everyday life again. This happened to Aimé, a 34-year-old man. Criminals had attacked Aimé and injured his legs with machetes. Eventually his legs were amputated. His wife had left him taking their children with her. Aimé felt alone, worthless, hopeless, and afraid of other people. He had no self-confidence. He shared this story in the group and the group helped him to understand that he still had value. They tried to convince him that even though his limbs were disabled, his brain worked properly. They showed him that he could find other talents in himself which he could develop and that he could be of value for himself and for others. A visit by the group, which is a naturally occurring part of the group process once participants have been encouraged to care for each other, was particularly important as Aimé began to rebuild confidence in himself, to see that he had value and could contribute to helping other group members who had problems.

A final example of the impact of participation in a sociotherapy group on people's lives relates to the reconciliation of people in conflict. This can be reconciliation between family members, between people who relate to each other as survivor and perpetrator of mass violence, or between people with a different ethnic identity who see each other as representatives of parties in violent conflict but not necessarily relate to each other as victim and perpetrator. Unlike Rwandan communities where genocide victims and perpetrators often live side by side and may participate together in a sociotherapy group, camps for Congolese refugee accommodate mainly people with the same ethnic identity who lived through the violence as victims. The latter explains why in sociotherapy groups in the camps direct victim–perpetrator encounters, if they are there at all, are an exception. Nevertheless, tensions related to ethnicity do occasionally arise within a group. Therese shared with the group that she did not have any peace of mind and had a grudge against anyone of Hutu ethnicity. The group helped her to realise that not all Hutu are killers. Leonard often felt hurt whenever he heard Tutsi neighbours pointing at Hutu like him in the camp who had taken refuge with them. Leonard was so troubled when Tutsi youngsters harassed and insulted him that he seriously considered taking refuge again, returning to the DRC and joining some armed groups there far from his former place of residence. Referring to the members of the sociotherapy group he had joined, he testified:

> I have trust in them, and I really feel safe in the camp thanks to those people! I am not afraid of those who have not changed yet because the group would not let me suffer any form of injustice from those people. I am at peace with the world now.

LESSONS LEARNED

The implementation of sociotherapy is a process of continuous learning, for staff as well as sociotherapists. Below we present some of the many lessons we learned over the years.

Organisational capacity

We found that the approach depends heavily on the involvement of an organisation – for instance, a church or civil society organisation – which is interested in the approach, has staff available with the capacity to implement it, and can establish a good working relationship with local authorities throughout the implementation of sociotherapy. Starting a new programme in a new setting benefits from the engagement of people with experience in different aspects of sociotherapy. For instance, we always make sure that experienced trainers partner with an organisation starting a sociotherapy programme in a new setting to deliver the first trainings, until the organisational staff can continue alone.

Sociotherapists as key pillars

The work of facilitating groups requires an understanding of the sociotherapy approach, good facilitation skills, love of the work and a desire to support people who are experiencing problems, commitment, high moral values, and being trusted by community members. It can prove difficult to identify people in the community who possess all these qualities, which requires creativity from sociotherapy staff and trainers to create a pool of qualified sociotherapists who complement each other in their group facilitation. A continuous challenge is to guide people used to preaching and/or teaching into becoming 'real facilitators' in the sense that group members start to realise that their own wisdom, individually and as a group, is important for handling problems and that they build self-confidence. Similarly, programme staff do not interact with sociotherapists as leaders, telling them what to do, but act in partnership with them. The philosophy is that sociotherapists should have space to be innovative and find out what works best in a specific context and in the particular group they are facilitating.

Another challenge is that many sociotherapists are wounded healers. A principle of sociotherapy is that group facilitators are from the same living environment as participants. This is helpful as those group facilitators understand the problems and culture of group participants. On the other hand, facilitators themselves have usually experienced the same challenges and adversities as participants and are similarly affected. Therefore, during the training, trainees are facilitated to engage in their own healing process. However, as healing is a long process, sociotherapists may be severely emotionally affected by the life stories shared by group participants or reminded by these stories of their own suffering and problems in life. For that reason, socio-therapists need sufficient support by programme staff. In addition, peer support and psycholog-ical supervision proved to be helpful. The latter also applies to programme staff.

Ongoing adaptation to the local context

It is our experience that sociotherapy is intrinsically adaptable to different contexts. For us, the outcomes of various monitoring and evaluation activities as well as participatory action research facilitated an ongoing adaptation during programme implementation. For instance, there is no general rule for the formation of groups; it will depend on the context in which sociotherapy is applied, the needs of the people to be served, and the specific objectives of the sociotherapy programme to be implemented. These objectives may include healing of wounds, solving family conflicts, or reconciliation between people of former rival groups. If, for instance, in a certain area family violence is perceived to be rampant, then programme staff and sociotherapists may decide to take that into account in their recruitment of group participants.

Emergency settings, like refugee camps, raise specific challenges in terms of adaptation. In these settings sociotherapy participants live in an unstable environment where situations con-stantly change due to, for instance, insecurity and relocation. It is challenging for sociotherapists in such situations to assist participants in developing at least some peace of mind. Relocation is beyond the control of programme staff. What staff can do is negotiate with decision makers to bring sociotherapy to the area where refugees are relocated.

Financial expectations among group participants and local leaders

Time and again we confronted challenges in resisting the NGO culture of providing mate-rial incentives. Sociotherapy is provided to people in post-conflict or emergency settings, such as refugee settings. Participants, people with mental health and psychosocial problems, are in many cases the most vulnerable people in terms of material needs. They are more aware of their material basic needs than of psychosocial needs. When they attend sociotherapy sessions these people expect to receive material support. Understandably, once they realise that this support is not provided, some are reluctant to participate, especially at the beginning before realising that sociotherapy has something relevant to offer them. This happens in particular in communities where sociotherapy is newly introduced and people have not yet had a chance to observe the results of participation in sociotherapy among their community members. Our experience is that once psychosocial stability has been reached, people individually or in a group often initiate economic development activities and may subsequently benefit effectively from additional material support. Without this stability, people may misuse that support by, for instance, spending money on alcohol and drugs instead of investing it in business or farm-ing activities. This behaviour may increase family conflict instead of mitigating it. Also, local leaders are in many cases unaware of psychosocial problems, both their own and those of the population they serve, whilst they do see physical and material needs. Consequently, they only value projects providing material support or infrastructures. It is only after they have seen positive changes in behaviour and attitudes among people in their constituency as a result of psychosocial support that they become aware of the psychosocial needs of the population and the relevance of psychosocial support. Their support as local leaders of economic development activities graduates of sociotherapy then starts developing. This awareness increases their sup-port of a programme like sociotherapy and facilitates their support of the income generation activities of sociotherapy graduates.

Follow-up of groups after the completion of the 15 sociotherapy sessions

Sociotherapy graduates frequently testify that they will remain guided by what they learned in sociotherapy in dealing with daily stressors in future life. Graduate groups frequently take the initiative to continue to meet to share daily life issues and/or to form an income-generating association. However, most of the sociotherapy participants are vulnerable and may need continuous support. Once they have completed 15 sessions with a positive result, they may relapse. It has been challenging to find a structure that can provide follow-up psychosocial and economic support to sustain their growth.

CONCLUSION

What one can learn from those who experienced the sociotherapy approach is the power of the group in helping people speak about their problems, often for the first time; in enabling people to support each other as well as care for themselves; in empowering people to use new coping strategies; and in having new friends to socialise with. As we often hear sociotherapy graduates testify, they have found a new family. Group participants share similar life conditions, which helps them to understand each other. They advise each other based on experiences in their ordinary life. Participants learn together and they continue to evaluate the implementation of what they learned in their life together.

As some of the excerpts of the refugee stories presented in this chapter illustrate, the positive changes in group participants often have spin-off effects on their family members and community members. The credo among sociotherapists is, if one person is 'healed', on average five other people benefit from that.

For us, each context in which sociotherapy is implemented and each story we hear has its uniqueness. We always find something new to learn. This, added to the many benefits programme staff, graduates, sociotherapists and their respective families and communities gain from the process, continue to inspire us to engage in a further development of community-based sociotherapy.

REFERENCES

Arendt, H. (1958) *The Human Condition*. Chicago: University of Chicago Press.

Bloom, S.L. and Norton, K. (2004) 'Introduction', *Psychiatric Quarterly*, 75(3), pp. 229–231. doi:10.1023/B:PSAQ.0000031793.86933.30

Dekker, C. (2018) *Handbook Training in Community Based Sociotherapy: Experiences in Rwanda, East Congo and Liberia*. Leiden: African Studies Centre Leiden. Available at: https://scholarlypublications. universiteitleiden.nl/handle/1887/68342 (Accessed: 6 June 2020).

Ingabire, M.C., Kagoyire, M.G., Karangwa, D., Ingabire, I., Habarugira, N., Jansen, A., and Richters, A. (2017) 'Trauma informed restorative justice through community based sociotherapy in Rwanda', *Intervention: Journal of Mental Health and Psychosocial Support in Conflict Affected Areas*, 15(3), pp. 241–253. Available at: https://www.interventionjournal.com/sites/default/files/Trauma_ informed_restorative_justice_through.6.pdf (Accessed 6 June 2022)

Ingabire, M.C. and Richters, A. (2020) 'Suicidal ideation and behavior among Congolese Refugees in Rwanda: Contributing factors, consequences, and support mechanisms in the context of culture', *Frontiers in Psychiatry*, 11, 299. doi:10.3389/fpsyt.2020.00299.

Jackson, M. (2002) *The Politics of Storytelling: Violence, Transgression and Intersubjectivity*. Copenhagen: Museum Tusculanum Press.

Jones, M. (1960) 'Introduction', in Rapoport, R.N. *Community As Doctor: New Perspectives on a Therapeutic Community*. London: Tavistock, pp. 1–6.

Rapoport, R.N. (1960) *Community As Doctor: New Perspectives on a Therapeutic Community*. London: Tavistock.

Richters, A., Dekker, C., and Scholte, W.F. (2008) 'Community based sociotherapy in Byumba, Rwanda', *Intervention: Journal of Mental Health and Psychosocial Support in Conflict Affected Areas*, 6(2), pp. 100–116. Available at: https://www.interventionjournal.com/sites/default/files/6.2_02_%20 Richters.pdf (Accessed 6 June 2022)

Richters, A., Rutayisire, T., and Dekker, C. (2010) 'Care as a turning point in sociotherapy: Remaking the moral world in post-genocide Rwanda', *Medische Antropologie: Tijdschrift over Gezondheid en Cultuur*, 22(1), pp. 93–108. Available at: http://tma.socsci.uva.nl/22_1/richters.pdf (Accessed 6 June 2022)

Summerfield, D. (2002) 'Effects of war: Moral knowledge, revenge, reconciliation, and medicalised concepts of "recovery"', *BMJ Clinical Research*, 325(7372), pp. 1105–1107. doi:10.1136/ bmj.325.7372.1105

UNHCR (2021) *Operational portal refugee situations: Rwanda*. Available at: https://data.unhcr.org/en/ country/rwa (Accessed 20 January 2022)

Whiteley, S. (2004) 'The evolution of the therapeutic community', *Psychiatric Quarterly*, 75(3), pp. 233–248. doi:10.1023/B:PSAQ.0000031794.82674.e8.

CHAPTER 7

WOMEN AND GIRLS SAFE SPACES

The power of feminist social groupwork in humanitarian settings

Melanie Megevand, Micah Williams and Laura Marchesini

INTRODUCTION

On any given day, in different corners of the world, women and adolescent girls living in humanitarian and emergency contexts are making time to visit Women and Girls Safe Spaces (WGSS). They visit to seek respite from their daily challenges; and the emotional, social and practical support that enables them to face those challenges again when they leave. They may be greeted by the sounds of singing or drums, or a nurse sharing information on family planning or breastfeeding. Whilst in the WGSS they may participate in a knitting or literacy class; decorate their feet with henna; spend time with friends or make new friends; share information on safety risks in their community; learn about new services available, or discreetly and safely seek help from a gender-based violence (GBV) caseworker after surviving an incident of violence.

Women and Girls Safe Spaces are dynamic centres that have become features of communities in diverse humanitarian settings, including natural disasters and conflict situations. They can be found in all phases of an emergency, from the initial onset, through the relief and recovery phases, and in protracted emergencies which merge into development contexts. A Women and Girls Safe Space can be defined (Megevand and Marchesini, 2020) as a structured place where women's and adolescent girls' physical and emotional safety is respected and where they are supported through processes of empowerment to seek, obtain and share information, access services, express themselves, enhance psychosocial wellbeing, and more fully realise their rights. WGSS create opportunities for feminist social groupwork and the transformational power of co-creation.

We, the co-authors of this chapter, have spent more than ten years working with women and girls in humanitarian settings and have recognised the transformative potential of groupwork in WGSS. With the support of a team of GBV advisors, we developed a 'Women and Girls Safe Spaces Toolkit' (Megevand and Marchesini, 2020), in collaboration with more than 20 WGSS and more than 50 staff in Cameroon, Ethiopia, Lebanon and Thailand. The International Rescue Committee and International Medical Corps led the development of the Toolkit, which introduces technical standards and provides guidance for teams implementing WGSS.

Unintentionally, and yet quite appropriately, our experience developing the WGSS Toolkit mirrored women's experiences of taking part in groupwork delivered in WGSS: it was powerful and empowering. Applying feminist-informed principles and approaches to capture practice-based learning and experiences, we were able to learn from and amplify the voices of a broad network of mentors, peers, female field staff, women, adolescent girls and community members in diverse humanitarian settings. We drew on this synergy of voices to develop this chapter, which will demonstrate how the group-based support available through WGSS can be transformative.

WHY ARE WGSS NEEDED IN EMERGENCIES?

Conflict and disaster-related displacement magnifies gender inequality and intersecting forms of discrimination, compounding internally displaced and refugee women's and girls' experiences of isolation, exclusion, disempowerment and violence. One in five displaced women in

DOI: 10.4324/9781003192978-9

complex humanitarian settings has experienced non-partner sexual violence (Raising Voices, 2008), and even more experience intimate partner violence (UNFPA, 2019). Internally displaced and refugee women and girls are at particular risk of violence, and experience higher levels of distress, due to factors brought on by humanitarian crises and displacement, including: loss of social network; limited power and participation; limited access to services and opportunities (including educational, income-generative and recreational); reduced mobility; and a reduced sense of freedom and independence (Bradshaw and Fordham, 2013; International Rescue Committee, 2014; Women Refugee Commission, 2019).

> Everyone harasses us now because of this conflict. People see us girls as being cheap. Everyone harasses and abuses the girls.
>
> (Adolescent Syrian refugee girl)

In many emergency contexts, women and girls describe experiences of needing permission from the men in their families to leave their homes. Mobility is particularly limited where security threats are perceived as high or where expectations related to traditional gender roles are strong. Leaving home, for some, is perceived as inappropriate or undignified and could be met with social sanctions, as a displaced Iraqi woman shared:

> You feel that women and girls are under pressure. They do not have support from the brother, husband or father. The woman doesn't own herself. She does not own herself. They are under pressure. If a woman goes outside her house, people gossip about her.

Women and girls are further limited by the tremendous responsibilities they carry, particularly in emergencies. They are often preoccupied with securing basic needs for their families.

> We are strong because we get up early in the morning and we prepare food for the children, because we go to the market, we get the water and we go collect firewood. Women are strong because we support the family when the husband is not around.
>
> (Displaced South Sudanese woman)

The WGSS approach is responsive to the multiple constraints faced by women and girls. WGSS are designed for safety and acceptance, with attention to maximising access. They are also designed as hubs where women and girls, without time or ability to visit multiple service centres or participate freely in public affairs, can receive information on a range of services and participate in a range of activities. When women and girls are able to leave their homes, they commonly identify WGSS as the first or only space they can visit. WGSS provide a vital link to other people and services, and even a lifeline for women and girls to meet their survival needs.

Skilful and relational facilitation of group interaction invites women and adolescent girls to co-create, hold and own the space dedicated to them. In contexts where conflict and displacement have eroded social trust and polarised communities, groupwork safely, yet boldly, encourages diverse groups of women and girls to come together through shared experiences, understandings and interests to form supportive relationships. WGSS create a space to question power imbalances and opportunities for women and girls to explore and express their power, a sense of belonging, safety, equality and solidarity.

Although WGSS have been a feature of humanitarian emergencies for some time, the spaces have not received sufficient recognition for their contributions and potential to serve women and girls. The GBV prevention and response programmes that typically support WGSS are undervalued and underfunded in emergency settings, with less than 1% of humanitarian funding invested in GBV prevention and response (International Rescue Committee, 2019). Often, even within GBV programmes, WGSS-based interventions have been considered less essential, technical and substantive than casework, where survivors of violence receive one-on-one support from trained caseworkers.

WGSS MEET THE DIVERSE NEEDS OF WOMEN AND GIRLS: ONE SIZE DOES NOT FIT ALL

The person-in-environment perspective is integral to feminist and social work practices that GBV programmes apply in humanitarian contexts. While all WGSS should share a common framework, no WGSS is the same. Each WGSS uniquely reflects participating women's and girls' experiences, abilities, priorities, needs and interests. But also, because groupwork supports women and girls through empowerment, each WGSS evolves as women and girls gain knowledge, confidence and skills and exercise their leadership and power to take collective action.

Despite the diversity of WGSS, three factors are common to all:

- Context-tailored: Tailoring relates to the humanitarian context as well as the physical layout of the WGSS, available resources, programming environment and selected implementation approaches. For example, in an urban setting, a WGSS may be set up in a rented apartment building, while in a camp setting, the WGSS is likely a tent or container. In Northern Thailand, a WGSS is rectangular and constructed from bamboo, while in specific areas of Cameroon and Ethiopia, WGSS are circular and constructed from mud blocks.
- Women and girl-led: From the outset, women and girls must be involved in decisions related to design, implementation and monitoring of the WGSS. Women's and girls' ownership of WGSS, and leadership of activities organised in WGSS, should increase over time.
- Community-informed: Key stakeholders in the community, including community leaders and male community members, are engaged from the outset of WGSS planning. Doing so secures support for the WGSS and creates greater and safer access for women and adolescent girls.

WGSS should be accessible for all women and girls in humanitarian settings, with the understanding that not all women and girls experience emergencies in the same ways. Intersecting forms of oppression and discrimination related to factors such as race, age, disability, sexual orientation, gender identity, nationality, class, ethnicity, citizenship and religion can heighten risks and experiences of violence and isolation for specific groups of women and girls. It is therefore important for WGSS to recognise diversity among women and girls, including older women; adolescent girls; women and girls belonging to national or ethnic, religious and linguistic minorities or indigenous groups; women and girls with disabilities; and women and girls from sexual minorities. Additionally, WGSS may recognise specific needs among women and girls living with HIV/AIDS, women engaged in sex work, and any other group which is socially excluded, discriminated against and at heightened risk of experiencing violence in a community. Ideally, WGSS staff and volunteers will reflect the diversity of women and girls in the community, and programmes must be attentive to principles of diversity and inclusion at all stages of establishing and running a WGSS.

OBJECTIVES OF WGSS AND THE FOCUS OF SOCIAL GROUPWORK

Empowerment is central to WGSS. The WGSS Toolkit identifies four dimensions of empowerment, with different activities contributing to each.

Cognitive empowerment relates to the saying 'knowledge is power' and encompasses activities and opportunities that allow women and girls to learn new skills and gain new knowledge to make choices and take control of their lives. Cognitive empowerment includes women's and girls' awareness and understanding of their rights, services available, how to access them, and reporting complaints and safeguarding concerns.

Psychosocial empowerment includes activities and services that recognise women's and girls' strengths, encourage expression, strengthen coping mechanisms and support networks and foster mutual support.

Personal empowerment refers to 'power within' and encompasses activities that develop self-confidence, self-awareness, self-respect, ability to assert rights and make choices. In some programmes, personal empowerment embraces a component of economic development, in which income generation activities are instrumental to women's and girls' access to and control over the use of resources and reduce their dependence and vulnerability to exploitative and abusive situations.

Socio-civic empowerment encompasses activities and services focused on participation in public life and opportunities to mobilise and organise for social change.

We identified five standard objectives that all WGSS should meet to effectively support women's and girls' empowerment in humanitarian settings. The objectives were identified through formative research carried out in the four pilot countries (Cameroon, Ethiopia, Lebanon and Thailand) during the initial stage of the WGSS toolkit development. The specific objectives were endorsed by global GBV advisors, WGSS frontline staff, GBV programme managers/ coordinators and GBV sub-cluster co-leads.

WGSS activities vary across contexts as well as time, and a wide range of activities might contribute to each objective. Under each objective below, we highlight illustrative activities, dimensions of empowerment linked to the objective, and women's related experiences (Table 7.1).

WGSS CORE CONCEPTS: FEMINIST SOCIAL GROUPWORK IN PRACTICE

Due to the highly relational, fluid and constantly unfolding nature of WGSS, methods to best hold the space for women and girls and support them through processes of empowerment will vary over time and between spaces. Nonetheless, WGSS should share common principles, key approaches, objectives and standards. This section focuses on crucial concepts rooted in feminist social groupwork, which distinguish WGSS from other spaces.

> Working in a woman safe space is not like working in an office. You really need to have a team that finds the balance between sharing and confidentiality; having a certain level of trust in the supervision; being able to interact with the other stakeholders to have smooth referral pathways. Once you remove a piece and you change it, it can have dramatic consequences for the whole running of the safe space.
>
> (Senior staff, Lebanon)

Multi-faceted power of co-creation: Feminist social groupwork

WGSS promote both feminist and social groupwork practice. WGSS are means of creating safety, social connections and support for women's empowerment. WGSS also represent the result of the groupwork, as spaces co-created by women and held by women's relationships. Eventually the WGSS contributes to the goal of transforming power as women and girls take

Table 7.1 Standard Objectives of WGSS

Objectives	Sample Activities Contributing to Objective	Quotes and Notes
1. To facilitate access for all women and adolescent girls to knowledge, skills and a range of relevant services.	Hosting information sessions on relevant topics and available services, inviting experts and service providers (e.g. legal, nutrition, sexual reproductive health). Life skills sessions for groups of adolescent girls. Skills-building groups or hosted skills training (e.g. vocational or livelihood service providers).	"Before the WGSS I was stressed, especially with my children and our difficult situation. Now I am more patient. I have more information on my children, on myself as a woman, and I feel like I am part of a support group. Now I spread the word about the centre and always bring along new women." WGSS member, Ethiopia.
2. To support women's and adolescent girls' psychosocial wellbeing and creation of social networks.	Arts-based activities (e.g. music, dancing, theatre, drawing). Exercise and sport (e.g. yoga, volleyball, football). Leisure and relaxation activities (e.g. coffee or tea ceremonies, meditation, storytelling, movies). Craft-making (e.g. soap making, tailoring, beading, basket making). Community development initiatives (e.g. gardening, rehabilitation of community spaces). Positive support groups (young mother support groups, community development groups). Communal income-generating activities to support the WGSS.	"I love it – I feel like I have freedom here. I'm learning and growing. I decided to come to the WGSS to be more sociable – to meet others. I feel comfortable in this space and now I see these same women on the street and we talk, we visit each other. I feel like I am part of a group." Adolescent WGSS member, Iraq. "I initially heard about the WGSS through word of mouth from neighbours. About two years ago when I arrived here I decided I would check it out. I walked several kilometres to meet the bus. The WGSS changed me. There, I get emotional support. The kind of support I have not found anywhere else. I talk often about my stresses and problems and the other women help me, like I help them. And I take what I learn – how to manage what is going on in my life – and I pass that education on to others. My sister calls me all the time and asks me about the sessions. There is no place like this where she lives, and she encourages me to go and come back and share with her everything I've learned." Adult WGSS member, Lebanon.
3. To serve as a place where women and adolescent girls can organise and access information and resources to reduce risk of violence.	Facilitated discussions to understand concerns and safety risks. Awareness sessions on risks to GBV, including sexual exploitation and abuse by humanitarian workers. Awareness sessions on feedback and reporting mechanisms. Community mapping and safety planning exercises. Hosted information sessions from safety/ security actors (e.g. peacekeepers, police, community watch groups). Direct or hosted distribution of dignity kits, cash or voucher assistance.	"We had two girls with us who told us that the boys used to annoy them. (…) [The WGSS staff member] used to ask them about the available roads. 'Is there another road to use?' […] We used to draw it and discuss of which roads we were afraid. For example, I am afraid of this road, so I put a red dot on it. I am scared of this shop, so I put a red dot. Then we would agree on several plans, so we could feel more safe but also well prepared in case anything happened". Adolescent WGSS member, Jordan.

4. To serve as a key entry point for specialised services for GBV survivors.	Hosted GBV case management and individual psychosocial support services for survivors. Confidential referrals from WGSS to other service points for health, psychosocial and other GBV response services.	*By upholding survivor-centred approaches and ensuring spaces are only for women and girls, WGSS create an environment to support the safety and healing of survivors.* *In fact, WGSS are often the first place survivors choose to disclose their experience of violence, and many WGSS host case management services, where survivors can meet with a caseworker discreetly without raising suspicion from the wider community. WGSS members across all four pilot countries listed WGSS as an essential service for survivors. Among WGSS members surveyed during the development of the WGSS Toolkit, 93.5% reported knowing where someone can get support if they're experiencing violence, and 87.0% were able to identify safe methods of reporting sexual abuse and exploitation.*
5. To provide a place where women and adolescent girls are safe and encouraged to use their voice and collectively raise attention to their rights and needs.	Facilitated discussions to understand women's and girls' perspectives and needs. Women's forum meetings and advocacy planning. Mentorship, peer facilitation and side-by-side support from active members. Meetings of women and girl-led initiatives (e.g. associations, savings and loans groups). Leadership and advocacy training.	*"I am a woman but I am a leader. I am a centre point for the community. Women and men come to me for guidance, advice and information, and I work hard to make sure everyone knows about the needs women and girls share with me and that the community upholds and respects women's rights."* Adult WGSS member and community volunteer, Lebanon. *"Before, women were [...] not allowed to meet, not allowed to speak… We had no say, no voice, as if we were no one. But look at us now. We gather, we meet, we work, we help others, we teach others. We rose up and taught people here what women can do. We are a force."* Adult woman, Democratic Republic of Congo.

an active role and harness their collective power so that the WGSS becomes an expression of women claiming space.

Participation and co-creation of WGSS offers women and girls the opportunity to reclaim their personal and collective agency in a supportive environment focused on the relational, personal and collective.

Exclusively women

The rationale for women-only safe spaces begins with the importance of reducing risks and preventing further harm in humanitarian settings. These spaces provide women and adolescent girls with a place to access critical information, in a context in which women and girls are often excluded from public spaces and networks, and the spaces also offer a safe entry point for a range of services. WGSS further offer women and girls opportunities to engage with each other, exchange information, rebuild support networks and increase social assets.

WGSS relieve women and adolescent girls from commonly felt pressures and prejudices of men. Women and girls across contexts express that the absence of men in WGSS makes the environment more relaxed, less judgmental and safer. This allows them to more freely express themselves, explore their potential, make decisions affecting their lives, and learn and practice skills. One WGSS participant from Ethiopia shared "*The [WGSS] place is safe, and we can freely chat as men and boys are not allowed to come to the centre.*"

Maintaining an exclusive space for women and girls also promotes access to WGSS. In many humanitarian settings, community norms would not deem it safe or acceptable for women, or particularly adolescent girls, to spend time in social spaces shared with men and boys. These norms do not allow women and adolescent girls to express themselves or partici-pate freely and equally in the presence of men. In developing the WGSS Toolkit, we surveyed hundreds of women and girls, as well as male community members and leaders, across 18 com-munities in humanitarian settings. We asked which factors enabled women's and girls' access to and participation in WGSS. Without prompting, "keeping the space female only" was the first factor raised by almost all respondents.

All about power

Agency (the ability of women and girls to consider options and meaningfully choose between them) and opportunity (the context that influences women's ability to transform choice into action) together influence the degree of an individual's empowerment. WGSS aim to both increase opportunity and strengthen women's and girls' abilities to make effective choices in their lives. This involves breaking down barriers between service providers and beneficiaries and ensuring that implementation informs, consults, involves, collaborates and empowers women and girls as co-creators of the WGSS. It is the collective process between women and girls who choose to gather and contribute as beneficiaries, members, facilitators, mentors, service providers, agents of change or any other role, which creates the relevant space for women's and girl's empowerment.

> To do this kind of job you need to be very open to listen to people, understand, not being judgmental, which is also sometimes difficult because in some places you have very entrenched cultural and religious ideas that may actually lead you to judgement. It is important to find objectivity, neutrality.
>
> (GBV Working Group Lead)

Through dialogue on expressions of power, WGSS can create a space for women and adoles-cent girls to question power imbalances and offer opportunities for women and adolescent girls to explore, express and celebrate their own power. Using everyday language, different forms of power are named and distinguished: power over, power within, power to and power with (Drumm, 2006).

Gender-based violence is based on imbalance of power. Not all types of power drive GBV; it is mainly the 'power over' that perpetuates inequality and injustice. This type of power may apply to patriarchal relationships, as well as other types of relationship where power is used to control and dominate. WGSS staff need to be mindful of their power as service providers (e.g. through control of resources and decision-making in the safe space) over women and girls seeking WGSS services.

> I was in a bad place until I met an outreach volunteer for the WGSS. I decided to go with her one day to help her lead a session with girls on creating handicrafts. The women and staff they treat us like our sisters. There is no difference between staff and us.
>
> (WGSS member, Ethiopia)

The remaining three types of power may drive different types of empowerment and, interchangeably, may support the personal and social development of group members. Starting from the individual level, the 'power within' is critical in WGSS programming. The 'power within' supports women and girls in understanding that their lives matter and that they have the right to have control over strategic life choices despite the systematic oppression, the strict gender roles, and the impact of displacement and violence on their ability to exercise their rights.

> Everything I have gone through has made me strong and confident. I discovered this by coming to the WGSS. I know now I am strong on the inside. I'm not afraid to stand up for myself when no one else will. I've had to do it so many times in my past and I will do it in my future.
>
> (Adolescent WGSS member, Syria)

WGSS do not promote empowerment to achieve only personal goals but seek common objectives and positive social change. Group activities and initiatives that work at the level of 'power to' give women and adolescent girls opportunities to exercise their leadership skills, socio-civic engagement and ability to engage in social change efforts.

> I am strong and powerful because of the experience I've had. My words are important and this I learned here at the WGSS. My words and my beliefs drive me forward and are my weapons in helping other women. This is my message to the world.
>
> (Adult WGSS member, Lebanon)

Finally, the 'Power with' refers to the unity arising from everyday experiences, interests and beliefs between individuals and groups demonstrated by collective support and action. This is the power of the group. Based on solidarity, trust, mutual respect and cohesion, 'power with' forges collective efforts for social change and multiplies the power of individuals and their networks.

> I feel like we are one family here, that our differences don't matter. You are from here, I am from elsewhere. You are Christian, I am Muslim. You can read and write, I am illiterate. It doesn't matter, we are all women, as individuals we are equal, as a group it is only our strengths which add up to the benefit of each of us.
>
> (Adult WGSS member, Turkey)

WGSS provides a space for women and girls to establish meaningful relations, mutual support and (re)establish support networks while also forming strategic relationships with local women's community-based organisations and women's movements based on shared values and a commitment to support existing efforts.

At the WGSS, I knew there were many women from different backgrounds. I wanted to be part of that. We are one community made up of women from all over. It is an important place where we can reduce our stress, talk about our issues and share our stories and overcome whatever we decide to take on as a group.

(Adult WGSS member, Syria)

BENEFITS AND CHALLENGES OF THE WGSS APPROACH FOR THE WELLBEING OF WOMEN AND GIRLS

I am happy that someone is hearing us. I feel like the problems we face are those faced by all, which helps me - that it is not just me. I feel like I can handle these problems now. All these women are strong - so I must be strong. She has suffered the same thing and made it through - so I can as well.

(Adolescent WGSS member, Lebanon)

For women and girls who have experienced the dispossession of displacement, female-only spaces create conditions for women and adolescent girls to support each other and create social networks.

I used to think it was useless to leave the house, to go where? to do what? But now I come here to the centre, I meet new people, I have someone to talk to, the staff, the other women. I feel safer. I'm very happy.

(Adult WGSS member, Thailand)

During the development of the WGSS Toolkit, 96.8% of women and girls surveyed reported that WGSS increased social support networks to which they can turn and 65% reported an increased sense of empowerment. *"Now that I've been coming to the centre. I feel more empowered. I feel like I have time to myself - to take care of myself. I feel like I can breathe" (Adult WGSS member, Lebanon)*.

Social groupwork theory (Drumm, 2006) has evidenced that members of groups can experience a common identity that fosters a sense of belonging, which in turn can reduce anxiety, increase self-expression and willingness to try new ideas and boost self-esteem. The WGSS effectively increase women's and girls' social connectedness, confidence and access to confidential response services such as psychosocial support and case management. Skills-building activities, training of women in leadership and other women-led empowerment activities yield positive outcomes in terms of women's and girls' agency, self-esteem and social connectedness, even while bigger-picture constraints of gender inequality and militarisation continue to limit women's and girls' voices and freedom.

During the development of the toolkit, we identified common challenges among WGSS frontline staff and programme managers who feel discouraged at times by the persisting challenges women and girls face, the continued need for GBV services, and the perceived indifference of some who hold power. Given our shared experience, with empathy and in solidarity, we offer perspectives on several challenges common to WGSS interventions:

Backlash and resistance are inevitable responses to social change. When patterns of inequality and injustice shift, individuals and groups, particularly those advantaged by the status quo, resist. In a sense, the backlash is a sign of progress and success of interventions, whereby changes to women's status seem possible or are underway. A significant amount of evidence underscores the importance and benefit of spaces only for women and adolescent girls in humanitarian settings. And yet, during humanitarian response, donors, humanitarian coordinators and even senior staff from organisations implementing WGSS still raise questions about the need for such a space. While we may not be able to avoid this resistance, we can anticipate it. WGSS staff should carefully consider all the stakeholders who might contribute to supporting or constraining WGSS from achieving its objectives and engage them accordingly to minimise setbacks.

Engaging in an equal, transparent exchange of information with women and girls from the onset of an emergency, before trust is established, can be challenging. Ensuring women and adolescent girls are key decision-makers who guide the design of the WGSS is difficult when they are not yet familiar with the benefits of such spaces, and often because of common gender norms, where women and girls may not be encouraged, used to or comfortable with making decisions and providing feedback. Key to managing this challenge is valuing process rather than a specific result. When staff recognise their relative power as humanitarian workers, they can choose to use their power with, rather than over, women and girls. This may start with discussions where women and girls are less responsive, or share few ideas, but the process of engagement itself is foundational to the significance of a WGSS.

In contexts where community dynamics are tense or discriminatory due to conflict or other factors, these dynamics can affect the inclusiveness of WGSS. It can be challenging to build an environment of trust and supportive groupwork when communities of women are suspicious of one another. Impressions can also take hold within a community that WGSS are only welcoming of women who occupy a specific space in society. While addressing larger issues of community dynamics is beyond the ability or scope of the staff implementing WGSS, they can apply sensitive strategies that neither replicate nor endorse discrimination or abuse of power within the WGSS. Staff can engage women and girls in gender and power analyses to understand intersecting forms of discrimination and how these affect women and potentially undermine the WGSS.

The motivational value of a group's work is subjected to the beliefs, attitudes and power balance of its members. While WGSS can be most valuable in very patriarchal and hierarchical societies, attention is required to not replicate such power dynamics within the space and within groups. For example, women and girls commonly reflect that they do not feel comfortable sharing opinions in front of leaders or powerful women. One WGSS staff member summarised this challenge in her environment: "In the refugee camp there are clear differentiations among social classes. Women from the lower social class sometimes interpret the WGSS as a space for rich and educated women, not for them." The idea of WGSS is to create a space of equals where women can celebrate their own empowerment, as well as achievements of other women. Regular attentiveness to the dynamic of a space is required to spread a sense of support that can foster groupwork and empowerment.

WGSS: AN INTERVENTION FOR TRANSFORMATIVE CHANGE

Despite significant evidence of how emergencies disproportionately affect women and girls, few interventions are truly tailored to women's and girls' needs and rights. Where humanitarian programmes are specifically attentive to women, it is almost always from an instrumentalist perspective where women are recognised as caretakers and guardians of children, communal utilities or communities. WGSS assert a different, and often radical, perspective that women themselves matter, and that women and girls deserve literal and figurative space dedicated to serving their needs and interests. We have been fortunate to observe the benefits of WGSS in many parts of the world and we have ourselves benefited greatly from the shared community of WGSS. Grounded in feminist social groupwork, WGSS provide opportunity for transformative changes in women's and girls' lives, and they demonstrate that even in the most adverse contexts, women and girls can, together, find and create space for security, respite, healing, solidarity and hope.

REFERENCES

Bradshaw, S. and Fordham, M. (2013) *Women, girls and disasters – A Review for DFID*. Available at: https://assets.publishing.service.gov.uk/government/uploads/system/uploads/attachment_data/file/844489/withdrawn-women-girls-disasters.pdf (Accessed: 20 January 2022).

Drumm, K. (2006) 'The essential power of group work'. *Social Work with Groups*, 29(2–3), pp. 17–31. doi:10.1300/J009v29n02_02.

International Rescue Committee (2014) *Are We Listening? Acting on Our Commitments to Women and Girls Affected by the Syrian Conflict*. New York: International Rescue Committee. Available at: https://www.rescue.org/sites/default/files/document/1144/ircwomeninsyriareportweb.pdf (Accessed: 20 January 2022).

International Rescue Committee (2019) *Where's the Money? How the Humanitarian System is Failing to Fund an End of Violence Against Women and Girls*. New York: International Rescue Committee. Available at: https://www.rescue.org/sites/default/files/document/3854/whereisthemoneyfinalfinal.pdf (Accessed: 20 January 2022).

Megevand, M. and Marchesini, L. (2020) *Women and Girls Safe Spaces: A Toolkit for Advancing Women's and Girls Empowerment in Humanitarian Settings*. Available at: https://gbvresponders.org/wp-content/uploads/2020/02/IRC-WGSS-English-2020.pdf (Accessed: 20 January 2022).

Raising Voices (2008) *SASA! Start module*. Available at: https://raisingvoices.org/resources/sasa-activist-kit-start-phase/ (Accessed: 20 January 2022).

UNFPA (2019) *Interagency Minimum Standards for Gender Based Violence in Emergency Programming*. Geneva: UNFPA. Available at: https://www.unfpa.org/minimum-standards (Accessed: 20 January 2022).

Women Refugee Commission (2019) *Where Do We Go from Here? Moving Forward with the Gender Equality Objective of the Call to Action Road Map*. New York: Women's Refugee Commission. Available at: https://reliefweb.int/attachments/759fadbf-8b30-3a3f-b7da-6c9325fa0c36/GenderEqualityReport-Final--Screen.pdf (Accessed: 20 January 2022).

CHAPTER 8

A THERAPEUTIC COMMUNITY FOR SURVIVORS OF TORTURE AND HUMAN RIGHTS ABUSES

Room to Heal

Room to Heal is a registered charity and therapeutic community based in London, England. We support people seeking asylum and refugees who have experienced torture and human rights abuses to rebuild their lives in exile. Room to Heal takes a holistic approach to post-torture recovery and the harm enacted by the UK immigration system.

Cultivating our therapeutic community lies at the heart of Room to Heal's approach. Our programme is composed of individual and group therapy, socio-legal casework, community gardening and residential retreats. We refer to the people we support at Room to Heal as 'Members', conferring a sense of agency and belonging.

This chapter begins by offering an understanding of Room to Heal's community approach. It goes on to outline how this works in practice and then situates the work in its wider socio-political context. In exploring what makes our community approach effective, we look at the values underpinning the work and we hear Members' experiences of being in a community. The chapter concludes with reflections on the challenges and learning since 2007 when we were founded.

ROOM TO HEAL AS THE PRACTICE OF COMMUNITY

Room to Heal is a community of survivors, most of whom have experienced torture, human rights abuses and other harm in their home country, and of staff and volunteers working in the community. The majority of survivors in the community suffer from (complex) post-traumatic stress disorder (PTSD) and/or depression. They have suffered multiple losses: home, family, friendship, culture and community. When people first come to Room to Heal they are often a shell of their former selves and suffer from debilitating PTSD symptoms, unable to sleep at night, experiencing regular panic attacks and flashbacks. Many Members feel a lack of self-worth, suffer periods of low mood, loneliness, hopelessness and suicidal ideation. Intrusive memories and memory loss are common. Alongside the psychological symptoms, physical health issues that often relate to torture and trauma manifest, including headaches and somatic pain in different parts of the body. Feelings of shame, relating to the experience of torture and seeking asylum, mean that forming meaningful relationships can be difficult.

The daily struggles of living in exile and experiencing hostile environment policies first-hand exacerbate Members' poor mental health. Some describe their experience of living in the UK as a 'second torture'. Many people seeking asylum in the UK endure a protracted asylum legal process and years of living in destitution. Asylum-seeking people are excluded from living a normal life and are expected to live in long-term isolation, unable to work or support themselves.

Our work takes place against this backdrop of dehumanisation, enforced isolation and widespread anti-migrant sentiment and violence. The deliberate nurturance of community and connection is in direct opposition to this. Room to Heal is a space where our shared humanity underlies everything. Scott Peck writes that humans only thrive within the context of a true community characterised by empathy and open communication: "Community is a safe place precisely because no-one is attempting to heal or convert you, to fix you, to change you" (1987, p. 68). We create the 'room to heal' rather than seeking to heal.

DOI: 10.4324/9781003192978-10

HOW IT ALL STARTED

Room to Heal began with the premise that human rights abuses injure communities as a whole and that, in the aftermath, community becomes a resource for healing. These were the views of Ugandan colleagues, with whom the founder of Room to Heal, Mark Fish, worked during the civil war in Northern Uganda in the early 2000s. This led to a model that embraces group therapy as part of a wider community approach. Room to Heal was born in 2007 when Mark asked five individual clients as a group what they needed – they said somewhere to come together and to grow food. A relationship with a local community garden was established and Room to Heal came into being when these clients and Mark began to meet there weekly to tend the garden and to talk around an open fire.

Relating in this way, outside of the traditional therapy room, went against the grain of what is viewed as therapeutic best practice in the West, particularly the rigid demarcation in the client–therapist relationship between what happens inside and outside of the therapy room. In contrast, at Room to Heal therapists and Members share space outside of the group therapy sessions, for example, in the garden or having lunch together. While boundaries play a central role in the way we work, our approach brings different levels and spheres of relating that go beyond the therapy room and into the wider community spaces.

The Rogerian person-centred approach has been a strong influence – in particular, the primacy of 'authentic' human relationships in the therapeutic encounter, the corresponding importance of an 'empowering' environment in which the 'client' can be trusted to find their own solutions and truths, and the necessity of addressing the power differential in the relationship. Scott Peck's notion that community is fundamentally a process was also present, a process that required constant vigilance and maintenance to stay vibrant and relevant.

WHAT WE DO

Room to Heal's way of working is always in motion and continually negotiated within our community. This approach did not come about didactically and cannot be taught. Rather, experiential learning is required by all – Members, staff and volunteers.

A therapeutic community

Everything we engage in, from the overtly therapeutic group therapy sessions to the cooking and informal chats in the corridor, is orientated towards offering a safe space for reconnection. There is an unspoken and perhaps even unconscious intention towards rediscovery of self, of meaningful relationships and of the world around us. Just as a flower leans towards the Sun, to be in the community at Room to Heal indicates hope and a desire to grow.

Our community approach applies to staff, volunteers and Members alike and needs to be enacted, embodied and practised intentionally. Everyone is part of its creation and evolution.

This relates to Rogers' therapeutic condition of congruence. Members will not benefit from and internalise the feeling of belonging to a community if only part of that community is authentically participating. One therapist referred to this as 'practising what you preach': Room to Heal *is* the practice of community.

Our Community Charter outlines our aims, values, rules and responsibilities. It was developed with Members, and is a living document that is reviewed and revised with input from the community. We go through it with each new Member to help facilitate and ensure common understanding of what we mean by community.

Individual therapy

When a person joins Room to Heal, their journey starts with short-term one-to-one therapy. The aim of these sessions is to support the individual's entry into group therapy. For many, group therapy will be a new experience, so these sessions can build a sense of what groups are about. They are also important for the individual to begin to form an attachment with the therapist and the organisation. Our experience is that many individuals need practical input at this stage, including support on how to manage panic attacks and sleeplessness. On occasion, we will provide urgent casework, for example finding an immigration solicitor or advising on a housing or asylum support problem.

Group therapy

Our weekly therapy groups lie at the heart of the community. The primary focus of the groups is on the relationships within it, and the highlighting of shared experience by the therapist plays a central role. For example, Araniya, a group member misses a group one week; some of the group members notice her absence and ask the therapists if she is okay. When Araniya comes to the group the following week, the therapist relays that group members were asking about her. This may seem inconsequential, but can be very powerful for somebody who holds a belief that their existence does not have an impact on others. This relational group therapy approach enables people to develop the confidence to support themselves and their peers and to rebuild self-worth. The emphasis on peer-led healing nurtures a sense of belonging and personal value. One Member describes what it's like in a Room to Heal group:

> The main help I've got has been from Members themselves and not the therapists – they just run the group. Sometimes we have sessions where the therapists don't talk at all. Everyone brings in their feelings. When people can't speak, we encourage them to speak. You see after a few sessions that people begin to speak. The atmosphere of the groups give safety and comfort to open up and to speak.

Through shared experiences of struggle, a sense of belonging is established:

> Group therapy is unique in being the only therapy that offers clients the opportunity to be of benefit to others. … Members of groups can speak to one another with a powerful authenticity that comes from their first-hand experience in ways that therapists may not be able to do.
>
> (Yalom and Leszcz, 2005, pp. 8, 13)

A member expresses this movingly: *"One time, I remember, one of the others said exactly what I wanted to say. That was comforting whilst also sad; knowing that you are not alone"*.

Our therapists describe how a 'Room to Heal approach' has evolved, underpinned by an integrative way of working that places Members' own experiences at the core of the therapy:

> They [the Members] are the experts, they are the ones who know how their experiences of seeking asylum here impacted them and how they are still impacted in their day-to-day living – not us, the therapists; we have no idea, to be honest. But what we can do is to make space where people can share with each other and listen to each other so that they can help each other. This is so valuable.

In 2022, Room to Heal is running three therapy groups. Two are open-ended and one is a time-limited group that runs for 12 months. Each group is co-facilitated by two therapists. Group membership varies but is generally limited to 10 to 12 people.

Open-ended groups are a response to the lack of long-term therapeutic support available that takes account of the ongoing trauma and protracted asylum system that people endure on arrival in the UK. Open-ended groups also enable Members to have more agency in working with therapists to decide when they leave the group. More recently, we have set up a time-limited 12-month group to expand our service to more people; this was a pragmatic step due to short-term funding. However, we have witnessed benefits to having a time-limited group. It has enabled Members to start and end the group and build relationships together at the same time. Members seem to be making the most of the group, knowing time is precious. This, in turn, emboldens them to join in community activities sooner compared to a more tentative approach of open-ended group Members, who sometimes focus more on their group than the wider community.

Casework

Casework is an integral part of our work. We recognise the therapeutic value of non-clinical interventions such as casework in fostering a Member's healing potential (Sigalas, 2019). Clearly, offering therapy to someone who has no food, money or place to sleep will have a limited impact. Similarly, precarious material circumstances inflict a considerable psychological toll. Casework support is therefore critical for a Member to be able to engage effectively in the emotionally intensive practice of group therapy.

A distinctive feature of Room to Heal's work is that therapists and caseworkers work closely together. A fortnightly caseworker–therapist meeting brings a therapeutic input into the casework and ensures that therapy is informed by casework.

We continually look for a 'middle ground' at Room to Heal, where Members are experts of their own experience, but where therapists and caseworkers also bring their training and expertise to work together to cultivate the most therapeutic outcomes. To illustrate, housing is a central theme in casework. Through a therapeutic lens, we learn that housing goes beyond physical walls and structures, and involves underlying feelings around missing family and acute loneliness. The therapist, caseworker and Member can work together to address actual material needs as well as their associated psychological and emotional needs.

Our small casework team helps Members resolve practical issues that they face: for example, accessing suitable legal representation, housing and medical care. Caseworkers support Members to develop their potential by preparing for employment, education and training in line with their own interests. Our approach to casework supports and equips Members to advocate for themselves by building confidence and agency.

Gardening

Room to Heal focuses on a person's engagement with space and nature as well as their relationships with others. Room to Heal began in a garden, born out of the need for connectedness to nature and to each other. The community still gathers at Culpeper garden, a little oasis in the city, every Friday to garden, cook and eat together.

Here, Members can reconnect with nature. Cultivating the land, planting seeds, tending to seedlings and watching them grow can have a profound therapeutic impact. Nurturing plants with patience and care has parallels with Members' own healing journeys.

The smaller garden next to our therapy rooms is an additional accessible space where gardening sessions take place after group therapy. This is also used as a resource for therapists and Members during one-to-one therapy. If a Member becomes dissociated, the therapist may take them into the garden and use sensations of sight, smell, sound, touch and taste, for example, picking and smelling some lavender, to bring them back to the here-and-now.

Therapeutic retreats

Residential retreats for Room to Heal Members and staff take place twice a year in a rural location that becomes the 'home' of the group for five days. Everyone participates in communal living, from cooking and cleaning to making outdoor evening fires. This helps level out power differentials and encourages people to relate with each other beyond their roles. Retreats are integral to strengthening and deepening understanding and relationships within the community. On retreats we witness a shift – the quality of sharing often changes and people become more open and trusting. Being removed from their usual environment in London, which is often associated with stress, can create psychological space for Members; it allows people to think and talk in a way that may not be possible in the thick of their usual situation and helps them to 'meet' each other more fully.

> It was a great opportunity to be together in one place, sharing cooking and helping each other like one team, we got space to learn and communicate to each other. I learnt a lot about every friend in the group – their culture, music, food, and lifestyles. I got new good friends. I can now have confidence to speak and express myself more openly.
>
> (Member)

We notice that the group therapy sessions on retreats tend to go deeper. Sharing the time and space intimately for five days allows stronger trust. Members are more able to share explicitly the experiences of torture, war atrocity, imprisonment and witnessing death that made them seek protection in the UK. In these daily group therapy sessions on retreat Members often also speak about separation from family and losses.

The retreats create an intensity of emotion and an authenticity that is often the catalyst for profound and sustained healing.

Community activities

We have a programme of activities for Members:

- Weekly community gardening (see above) and cooking
- Recreational, creative or advocacy groups: e.g. exercise, drama, reading, photography, anti-racism
- Occasional trips to the seaside, theatre, gardens and sporting events

All our activities have a therapeutic orientation and most have a therapist present so that any issues arising can be mindfully addressed in the moment and where appropriate taken into a different space, often back to the group.

A specific example of how this works comes from a community visit to the Palm House at Kew Gardens in London. A Member suddenly became quiet and withdrew from the rest of the group. A therapist observed this and was able to provide support in that moment. The Member shared that seeing tropical plants brought back memories of their childhood and they then spoke about the grief of losing their family. With the support of a therapist, they were able to share more in the group the following week and received generous support from other Members who could relate to the feelings of grief.

The spaces between

So much unfolds at Room to Heal in the 'spaces between', in the kitchen, making coffee or chopping vegetables for a meal. These spaces often feel more accessible to Members and offer non-verbal ways to connect. A level of intimacy can arise from collaborating on a practical task. These in-between spaces can also dismantle power dynamics. Therapists come to experience the Members they know from the therapy groups in a different way; similarly, Members get to experience their therapist as just another human being carrying out everyday tasks. Therapists and wider staff alike often talk about real moments of connection which take place in these spaces.

Bringing it all together

While the therapy groups are central, we recognise the limitations of talking therapy alone as a means for healing trauma. The activities surrounding our therapy groups are equally important, and this is reflected in how we allocate our time, care and resources. All activities and services combine to enhance the connection, communication and authenticity that are core to healing. We are striving continuously to cultivate a balance between intensity and depth of relating, and lighter and more playful, everyday ways of being together. Tuesday is when two of our group therapy sessions take place and Friday is when we gather to garden, cook and be in nature. As one member summarised: "*On Tuesdays we cry and on Fridays we laugh*". This 'balance' is not a final destination, a place we can arrive at fully, but a practice of ongoing reflection and modification.

> It's a nice experience on a Friday evening, we experience different cooking, different cultures, it's nice. For me it's a good release, it's good fun. When you're stressed, you go to Culpeper [Community Garden] and everyone comes together and makes jokes, shares their problems; it's good therapy.
>
> (Member)

HOW DOES THE COMMUNITY SUPPORT HEALING?

This section explores what makes our approach effective in helping torture survivors begin to heal.

The power of shared experience and human connection

> We can get courage when we see other people's problems. When we are alone, we feel like it's just me who is suffering and these things are only happening to me. When we see everyone in the community from different communities, we see that they also have so many problems. When we see these, we feel like our own problems are very small. And so we get courage, then we can face our problems and understand and solve them.
>
> (Member)

The people we support have experienced violence at the hands of others in their country of origin. Many Members have been raped, tortured, indefinitely detained and seen their families killed. After torture and forced exile, it is common for people to feel isolated and as if no-one else can understand what they have been through.

The shared experience of survival has a profound impact on Members. Seeing other people getting past seemingly insurmountable shame, loss and barriers engenders hope in other Members.

Herman highlights the power of survivor groups in the recovery process (1992). This also applies to the processes of community. At Room to Heal, community is fundamentally about being human together: "It is only by regaining a sense of being 'a human among humans' … that we have any hope of emerging from the unbearably lonely exile of trauma" (Brothers, 2009, p. 56).

Members are often isolated. The solidarity of human contact, where each person experiences the reciprocity of giving and receiving, is therefore fundamental to our work. The community approach creates spaces for everyday relating and this is often where therapeutic benefits can be felt.

A place to feel held

> They [Room to Heal] are there to walk with you on that path; that path that is so dark that you don't even know how to come out of it.
>
> (Member)

Witnessing and being witnessed in a group provides a much-needed experience of being held in mind. Being part of the community also means you are not alone with your day-to-day struggles. It is notable that the word most used by Members to describe Room to Heal is 'family': "*Having Room to Heal as a family and community gives positive senses of care and support which definitely had positive influence on my mental health*".

The therapists find that discussions in the groups are internalised and held by Members once the group is finished. Being able to hold each other in this way is fundamental. Care is at the heart of our groups, how people listen to one another and remember things about each other.

One Member who is required to report to a government reporting centre regularly, with a risk of being detained indefinitely, explained how the group supports him in these difficult moments: "*I went alone, but I knew I wasn't alone. The group was with me*".

A safe place to reconnect with a sense of self and others

One of our therapists likened being in the community to the experience of being surrounded by mirrors, reflecting yourself back at you from all 360 degrees, making it "harder for you to miss yourself". In a group setting, through subtle interactions, observation and direct feedback, we are frequently confronted with our responses and the impact that we have on others, and how others respond to and impact us.

The community approach helps to equip a person to the challenges of life outside the community, whether living in limbo in the UK's asylum process, or as someone with newly acquired refugee status. Our approach offers people a safe space in which to 'practice' ways of 'doing' and 'being' with their peers. In a context where refugees are rendered invisible by the state, this helps Members to take steps towards becoming more visible:

> Before I became part of Room to Heal, it was almost impossible for me to speak openly to other people. I was very negative, sad and depressed. Just after one year at the group, I felt a lot changing. I started to speak and express how I feel. I became less negative and started having a good time. The community at Room to Heal gave me confidence and the feeling of being part of a community where I was not rejected.
>
> (Member)

The fact that our groups are usually open-ended and are embedded in a community makes it possible to practice new ways of being, at a pace that is right for each individual. Each new

Member will approach this differently, depending on their unique history and character. Participation is often tentative at first and time is required to gain confidence and trust. Gradually and sometimes seemingly against all the odds, changes that occur in the therapeutic community are replicated in a Member's life outside of Room to Heal.

Conflicts and tensions in the groups and wider community are an inevitable part of forming meaningful relationships. Often, these are moments when past experiences affect the way current issues are being perceived. We recognise these moments as potential precursors to growth. We promote a non-shaming approach in working through these difficulties together. Our Community Charter is a useful tool to manage conflicts and tensions and to uphold the values that ensure our community remains a safe and welcoming space for all.

Agency and empowerment within the community

The community offers Members agency in a context where, for most people seeking asylum, this has been taken away. Recent research supports the importance of approaches that further agency and empowerment. Morgan *et al.* indicate that psychological interventions, such as cognitive behavioural therapy, are compromised by the powerlessness of individuals to alter their situation (2017). Our approach fosters agency both at individual and interpersonal levels, cultivating interconnectedness. A Member explains this when talking about the garden: "*The garden is our space, our place to go there, to feel joy. It's special. It's not for everyone, it's for us. It brings joy to go there, to share cooking and every week is different.*"

The staff team explicitly encourages self-help and mutual help. For example, our approach to casework strengthens the capacity of Members to advocate for themselves. If excessive praise or reliance is directed towards therapists and caseworkers, they remind Members of their own efforts and role in the healing process, and those of the wider group and community.

Despite this clear intention to facilitate empowerment and agency, Members can still idealise Room to Heal as omnipotent, with the power to change the wider, hostile system. In moments of crisis, such as when someone is experiencing homelessness, this idealisation can be broken, as Members recognise Room to Heal's limits.

It is often in these difficult moments that Members give each other most support. There is a recognition that when there is no 'solution', having a community of people who understand, support and empathise, with the authenticity of lived experience, is enough to get through and build strength through collective resilience.

We do not ignore, however, the ongoing risk and pull for our work to morph into a helper/helped (doer/done to) relationship. The role of staff supervision is key to ensure this dynamic of dependency does not play out. Clinical supervision supports therapists to gain greater insight about their work with Members. Therapists take their processing back to the group and emphasise the role of the support that Members receive from each other in allowing for change and transformation.

Members are regularly reminded in groups, 1:1s and community activities of their essential place in the community through encouragement to take on roles within it. Members do this in many ways, for example, facilitating a reading group, participating in an advocacy group, being lead chef or supporting each other in community gatherings. Members are encouraged to participate in decision-making through community forums, where organisational plans are considered; they take part in day-to-day decision-making in community activities, such as meal plans and deciding what is grown in the garden; and they are involved in the recruitment process of new staff. One Member described their participation at Room to Heal:

I was able to give my opinion about any matters been going, also help to be part of the decisions that taking place within the community. It gave me more feeling and confidence that I'm really part of the community, not only as a Member who is receiving help and support, instead it make me feel like part of a family.

CHALLENGES TO OUR COMMUNITY APPROACH

Our community approach presents opportunities for healing and growth, but also challenges, some of which are explored below. This potentially creative tension indicates the importance when working in this way of reflective practice and learning through experience. Rogers describes this powerfully: "Experience is, for me, the highest authority. The touchstone of validity is my own experience. No other person's ideas, and none of my own ideas, are as authoritative as my experience" (1961, pp. 22–23).

As a staff team, in supervision and in community meetings we reflect on our interactions with each other in order to learn from our experience, and we adapt our ways of working accordingly.

Unequal power, privilege and responsibility

It is important that we recognise key differences between community members and staff in power, privilege and responsibility. Members have experienced torture and other serious human rights breaches; they do not have a permanent form of immigration status and live in a hostile environment with constant uncertainty. Most Members are black or people of colour. In 2022, approximately 60% of Room to Heal's paid staff are white, and the majority have secure citizenship and have not had the experiences described above. Staff are paid for participating in the community, whereas Members join for mental health support.

We recognise that it is common for organisations comprising helping professionals to be permeated by white culture. Ryde reminds us that although white professionals are aware of practicing without discrimination, they often do not see the impact of their own cultural identity in a multicultural workplace (2009).

Working within the wider social and historical backdrop of racism and inequality, it is inevitable that transcultural issues arise, both consciously and unconsciously, within our community. It is critical that our staff team recognises, values and represents cultural differences in our community, and that staff are aware of the impact of their own cultural identity. The power of people with lived experience supporting each other is at the core of our work and we recognise that no amount of learning and training can replace lived experience. We actively encourage people with relevant lived experience to apply to join our staff team and board of trustees.

Recognising our limitations

We are a therapeutic organisation working with refugees and people seeking asylum, primarily torture survivors, and this is where our expertise lies. However, we strive to understand the intersectionality of the identities and experiences of our Members in relation to such areas as race, sexual orientation, gender, disability, addiction and trafficking.

For example, some of our Members have fled persecution based on their sexual orientation, and a significant proportion of Room to Heal staff are LGBTQI+. We are aware that, in our therapeutic groups and wider community, issues related to sexual orientation often remain an undercurrent. In our experience, respecting a Member's choice, pace and readiness has shown to be beneficial to the long-term process of healing. There is much to explore on this topic that space does not allow for here, for example, an exploration of taking a more overt LGBTQI+ affirmative approach that also recognises the influences of race and culture.

Initially, Room to Heal had separate men's and women's groups and it was our view that this provided the safest space for everyone. With time and experience, Room to Heal moved to running two mixed-gender groups. This decision was made consciously to allow for more opportunities for women, and some men who had also survived sexual violence, to work with fears and mistrust, to experience safety with men.

We recognise that this focus has its limitations. There are people who would not find mixed-gender and/or mixed-racial groups a safe space to begin to unravel gender-based violence that they have experienced. Some people who have been persecuted based on their sexual identity will benefit more from being in a group of people who have had similar experiences. During our assessment process we endeavour to identify where this is the case and refer to relevant specialist organisations that have a more in-depth understanding of the intersecting issues that are identified.

We also recognise that our work so far has operated within the limitations of the gender binary – issues around gender identity and trans inclusion have not yet been fully explored.

Power dynamics within our therapeutic groups and wider community

Inevitably, some of the tensions, inequalities and hierarchies in wider society are played out within our community. For example, within our therapeutic groups, we note the role that seniority can play, with some long-standing Members sometimes dominating. The distinction between 'asylum-seeker' and refugee status, and the differences in power and privilege, can set Members apart from each other.

Given the diversity of our community, cultural difference and how we engage with it is another ever-present consideration. While it is natural for sub-groups to form (for example, between French or Farsi-speaking Members), as a community we need to be alive to the risk of one group dominating and excluding others.

Awareness of power dynamics within the groups and wider community is vital. It starts with setting up a therapeutic group and giving consideration to balance in terms of, for example, gender, age, race, sexuality, nationality and religion. Within the community as a whole, it means being vigilant to and sensitively addressing imbalances in who takes part in particular community activities so that we offer an inclusive and safe environment for all our Members.

Linguistic challenges

All activities, including group therapy, are in English, without the use of interpreters. Some therapists have observed that, where not a first language, talking about experiences of torture in English can give Members emotional safety and distance. There are also limitations: Favero and Ross show that where the therapist does not speak a person's first language, "important details may be lost or hidden" (2003, p. 287), and this may reduce the quality of a therapist's response.

Although using a common language helps build a unified community, we recognise the complexities. Fortier (2017) describes the colonial legacies of language, with English having been forced on populations throughout the British Empire, and the ongoing hostile use of it, for example as an assimilationist tool in the language requirement on immigration applications. We strive to remain aware of these issues of language at Room to Heal.

BEGINNINGS AND ENDINGS

Beginnings and endings are ever present in our community, with Members, staff and volunteers joining and leaving. All Members have suffered extreme loss and trusting people after torture can take a long time. Once trust is formed it can be difficult to separate. One Member recently described a therapist they were close to leaving:

> To be honest, I don't like it when therapists change. I know it is difficult but I feel like when I'm seeing someone in therapy for a long time, it's so difficult and uncomfortable when a new therapist comes. I know it can't be changed but I just want to be honest.

To alleviate some of this difficulty and ensure that Members have some agency in the comings and goings in the team, they are invited to be part of the recruitment of therapists and have influence over these decisions.

We give long notice of any changes to enable Members to prepare, often in direct contrast to past experiences of loss. Time is given in therapy groups to share thoughts, feelings and concerns that Members may have about changes. We also give time to appreciate the benefits of change and see this as an important part of the healing process: "*I had lost hope. I didn't trust anyone. I was nearly a different person. Room to Heal brought me back to life. Now I see myself, I can trust myself and some others, and more trust will come.*"

In concluding, perhaps it is helpful to go back to the essence of what Room to Heal is. A Member puts this best: "*The meaning of Room to Heal is in its name; it's really for healing.*"

There is a saying that 'what you feel, you can heal' (Gray, 1984). Through the practice of community in its multiplicity of forms, be that in therapy, cooking together, tending to the garden, Room to Heal offers Members, more than anything, safe and supportive space to feel. We know that healing is not linear and often isn't neat. It's important to re-emphasise then, how Room to Heal is the practice of community, with an emphasis on 'practicing' – testing, exploring, reflecting and always adapting. The power of community in its entirety can offer hope and transformation. A Member who recently received his immigration status reflects: "*When I joined, I was someone else and when I progressed, I became someone else – someone better, much better.*"

REFERENCES

Brothers, D. (2009) 'Trauma-centered psychoanalysis: Transforming experiences of unbearable uncertainty', *Annals of the New York Academy of Sciences*, 1159(1), pp. 51–62. doi:10.1111/j.1749-6632.2009.04350.x.

Favero, M. and Ross, D. R. (2003) 'Words and transitional phenomena in psychotherapy', *American Journal of Psychotherapy*, 57(3), pp. 287–299. doi:10.1176/appi.psychotherapy.2003.57.3.287.

Fortier, A.-M. (2017) 'On (not) speaking English: Colonial legacies in language requirements for British citizenship', *Society*, 52(6), pp. 1254–1269. doi:10.1177/0038038517742854.

Gray, J. (1984) *What You Feel You Can Heal*. Norwich: Heart Publishing.

Herman, J.L. (1992) *Trauma and Recovery*. New York: Basic Books, Hachette Book Group.

Morgan, G., Melluish, S. and Welham, A. (2017) 'Exploring the relationship between postmigratory stressors and mental health for asylum seekers and refused asylum seekers in the UK', *Transcultural Psychiatry*, 54(5–6), pp. 653–674. doi:10.1177/1363461517737188.

Rogers, C. (1961) *On Becoming a Person*. London: Constable.

Ryde, J. (2009) *Being White in the Helping Professions*. London and New York: Jessica Kingsley Publishers.

Scott Peck, M. (1987) *The Different Drum: Community Making and Peace*. New York: Simon & Schuster.

Sigalas, A. (2019) 'Inferiorisation: Approaching a stigmatising reality in therapy', in Baffour, A. and Littlewood, R. (eds.) *Intercultural Therapy Challenges, Insights and Development*. London: Routledge.

Yalom, I. D. and Leszcz, M. (2005) *Theory and Practice of Group Psychotherapy*. New York: Basic Books.

CHAPTER 9

THE USE OF *GROUPES DE PAROLE* AS A MEDIUM FOR CHANGE IN THE TUNISIAN PENAL SYSTEM

Confronting institutional violence in a context of democratic transition

Mark Fish and Rim Ben Ismail

During the last fifty years of autocratic regime and dictatorship, the Tunisian institutional apparatus had been functionally inclined to violence and had regularly used torture. In the transition to democracy, since January 2011, it needed external support to engage in a self-reflective process about the impact of such violence on its employees and on future generations. The prison system, as one of the purveyors of violence in Tunisia, was an obvious place to begin to analyse work practices, as it became clear that this particular institution was open to change.

This chapter describes the development of a model that combined the experience of Room to Heal, a London-based organisation that provides group-based therapeutic support to torture survivors (see Chapter 8), Organisation Mondiale Contre la Torture Tunisie (OMCT), an international NGO operating in Tunisia since 2011 and having established the first comprehensive assistance programme for victims of torture in Tunisia, and Psychologues du Monde Tunisie (PDMT), a Tunisian organisation, knowledgeable about the context of psychological practice in Tunisia and the psychological impact of institutional violence. We wanted to provide a safe arena in which people could talk about the violence of the past and its consequences, such that change could happen and reparation be made.

Our challenge was to develop a system of psychological support that would allow for structural change. To this end, we designed a pyramidal support system that was able to work within environments where violence was endemic. We started with the hypothesis that violence in a closed environment would generate significant stress in the workplace. Our aim was to reduce this violence in the system, not by confronting it directly, but by working on the psychological impact violence had on its agents. We focused, therefore, not on the detained individual, usually serving a short sentence, but on the prison staff, who often worked in the prison for life.

To support the process, we decided to use a therapeutic groupwork approach. We wanted to create an environment in which the prison staff could talk about the realities of their work and its impact on them. We surmised that through sharing their practices as well as their emotions in the group, participants would realise the commonalities of their feelings and experiences and build a mutually reinforcing environment of support. We aimed:

- To work with the institution: engaging with and alongside the prison system, generally regarded as part of 'the oppressor' regime, listening to and being empathetic to those people who worked at the core of it and who might have witnessed or perpetrated violence. No one knows the institution and its problems better than the people who work there.

- To provide groupes de parole for prison staff to share and reflect on their experiences[1]: a safe reflective space would allow prison staff to consider the impact of their work on their physical and mental health, share their emotions, connect to their own suffering and create an impetus for change. This needed to be done with significant empathy and without judgement.

DOI: 10.4324/9781003192978-11

A CONTEXT CONDUCIVE TO CHANGE

We came to this work with the prisons in 2017, six years into Tunisia's transition from dictatorship to democracy, at a moment when the environment was alive with change. We were already engaged in the care of victims of torture in Tunisia through OMCT, when the Conseil Général des Prisons et de la Réhabilitation (CGPR) decided to open its doors to the PDMT programme. In the freedom of this moment, the CGPR understood both that PDMT reflected the potential for change and that it wanted to support the institution, rather than threaten it. This is how PDMT psychologists and groupes de parole entered the 'omerta' of the prison. And being in 'the silence' with the prison staff, PDMT was able to confront the power and the entrenched violence of the system, without stigmatising those people, the prison staff, who perpetuated it and who like the prisoners themselves were also victims of it.

The prison staff wanted change just like anyone else. When presented with the opportunity, they wanted to talk. They realised that if they didn't take it, the chance might not come again. Indeed, whether prison psychologists (the first cohort of prison staff to be involved in the programme) or educators or social workers or even prison guards (subsequent cohorts of prison staff involved in the programme), each cohort saw itself as somehow closer and more important to the prisoner, more impacted by their work, and more in need of help and support than the others. Crucially, however, when each group accepted and understood that the PDMT psychologists' fundamental role was to be there as group facilitators, neither to upbraid nor denigrate, nor to take the weight of the situation from them, they then talked about the immense and often-terrible impact of their work on themselves and their families. In this way, each cohort and each group came to realise that they had to work both on themselves and together for any real, lasting change to materialise.

FROM INDIVIDUAL TO GROUP TO INSTITUTION

It was clear that there were simply too many victims affected by the endemic violence of the regime to provide individual care and support, and that an individual approach could neither impact the structural violence inherent in the system nor generate the necessary changes in practices to stop future acts of torture. Prior experience of providing individual therapeutic support to torture survivors in Tunisia had already revealed the challenge of working in an environment where people were simply not used to talking openly, or indeed where such activity was prohibited by the dictatorship. Resistance to change had been inculcated at a deep level over many years.

We therefore decided to use groupes de parole as the medium by which we would provide psychological support to the prison environment. Over a period spanning 18 months, our intention was to provide support to all the psychologists working in prisons throughout Tunisia.

Being in a group would give the prison staff the experience of no longer being alone with their suffering. Instead, they would be together with their peers and able to position themselves as enablers of change. Unlike in the individual setting, the victim no longer has to face an expert; rather they find themselves in front of a group of people who, like them, need strengthening, and who are able to seek a solution together. The group can restore a feeling of belonging and a renewed sense of what it is to be human.

The approach we have adopted in this project is fundamentally experimental because we think that the solutions to the difficult and often-intractable issues of the prison cannot be manufactured outside the system. Indeed, we think that the solutions can only be realised by those professionals (the prison staff) who work in the prison environment. Such thinking reflects a 'theory of action', as defined by Argyris and Schön (1974, p. 21): "They make sense of their environment by constructing meanings to which they attend, and these constructions in turn guide action. In monitoring the effectiveness of action, they also monitor the suitability of their construction of the environment."

We developed the groupes de parole as places for sharing, exchanging and listening, such that participants could reflect on their professional activity and its impact on them personally and professionally. We sought to encourage them to find answers to questions such as: Why am I doing this job and what are my unconscious motivations? What are the differences between the realities of this job and the ideas I had about it beforehand? How do I manage my personality and emotions in a professional environment? How can I better know what I should and shouldn't do in my work situation? How can I establish more robust boundaries for myself so that I am more able to manage conflicts? How can I acquire the necessary skills and self-understanding to allow me to communicate more effectively in professional situations?

In setting up such a framework we anticipated three challenges:

Tunisian psychologists had little experience of therapeutic groupwork or group supervision

Working with a large cohort of PDMT psychologists significantly increased the potential impact and reach of the project and allowed us to work with all the psychologists working in Tunisian prisons. But how could the PDMT psychologists facilitate these groupes de parole with the prison psychologists, when they too had little experience of group supervision or therapeutic groupwork?

Confronting the 'omerta' of the system

Offering these groupes de parole to psychologists working in prisons meant giving them a space in which they could finally break the shackles of the silence of the system and speak openly. But would they be able to express their difficulties to their colleagues? Would they be able to talk about their work environment and its impact on them? It was apparent that they were extremely frustrated by the role they were forced to play in the prisons, having to act as 'guards' rather than psychologists. Their aspiration to engage in meaningful work as psychologists was often thwarted and they despaired of this reality.

Keeping the focus on the detainee

Our pyramidal model meant that our focus was firstly on the PDMT psychologists (via the PDMT psychologists' clinical supervision group, facilitated by us) and secondly on the prison psychologists (via the groupes de parole, facilitated by the PDMT psychologists). However, we had to keep in mind that the ultimate beneficiary of this work was the prison detainee. What we ultimately hoped for was an improvement in the detainee's conditions of detention and potential for rehabilitation.

OUR WORK WITH THE PDMT PSYCHOLOGISTS

In order to overcome the first challenge, we provided training in therapeutic groupwork and clinical group supervision to the PDMT psychologists. We ran these at intervals of three months, typically over a two-and-a-half-day intensive period. The intensive format provided a richness and depth to the supervision for the PDMT psychologists, and sufficient time for the PDMT psychologists to conduct two or three monthly groupes de parole with the prison psychologists during the periods between the supervision sessions.

Our fundamental aim in these training sessions was to provide a framework for supervision for the PDMT psychologists and a framework for the supervision of the groupes de parole with the prison psychologists. It was also to create a 'safe space' for the PDMT psychologists to learn through experimentation.

To begin with, it was apparent that although the first cohort of PDMT psychologists had significant clinical experience working with individuals in Tunisian public institutions, they had little experience of working conjointly with colleagues and, as we had thought, little experience of either therapeutic groupwork or clinical group supervision. Initially, this left them in a rather ambivalent position; on the one hand, they had years of clinical experience and considered that they had excellent skills and knowledge; on the other hand, however, they were fearful about working with a group of colleagues (the prison psychologists) who had significant experience in the prison field which they lacked.

The first sessions with the PDMT psychologists concentrated on their identity as psychologists and the impact of their work on them. As the sessions progressed, we built up a model that was very similar to the analysis of professional practice generally used in clinical supervision.

It was first necessary to create a sufficiently safe space for the participants to express their difficulties, concerns and emotions, both about their day-to-day work as psychologists and in relation to the forthcoming groupes de parole with the prison psychologists. Experimenting with the expression of emotions was at the heart of our work – facilitating the psychologists to explore their feelings and the impact of emotional repression allowed them to open their practice to this type of approach with the prison psychologists.

An example of this is the emotional scale, which is one of the tools developed during the sessions. This is a physical scale from 1 to 10, represented on the floor. Participants are asked to identify the impact of the work on them and to identify the emotion that is linked to this impact. Then each participant in turn stands up and moves along the scale and stops at the level they think represents the degree of intensity of the impact on them. We invite them to express themselves if they wish, and then invite people who have felt a similar emotion to move up the scale. Finally, we ask them to re-evaluate their position on the scale after talking about it (often we observed a decrease in the intensity of the emotion felt by the participant). Thus, this exercise allows participants to appreciate the intensity of the impact of an emotion and to feel it in the body through the movement on the scale. But there is also in this exercise, a sharing of the emotion, an awareness of the degree of collective impact on all the group members and an appreciation of the sense of wellbeing derived from expressing and sharing deep emotions together. We have also seen that the exercise has been taken up by the PDMT psychologists in their respective groupes de parole with the prison psychologists and that each has adapted it to their individual preference and sensitivity.

In order for the sessions with the PDMT psychologists to be effective in preparing them to work with the prison psychologists, they needed to be able to take on the exercises for themselves and creatively adapt them in their groups. Thus we wanted the psychologists to leave the session with an embodied experience, a feeling with which they could build their practice.

The PDMT psychologists facilitated their groupe de parole with the prison psychologists in pairs. This was something that we initiated from the outset, both as a support system to the individual psychologists within the pair and to showcase a model of open, emotionally literate communication to the prison psychologists.

Co-facilitation of the groups meant that the individuals in the pairs had to constantly negotiate the group space together, both before the groupes de parole in terms of planning and strategizing, and afterwards in terms of debriefing, including an analysis and reflection on their functioning as individuals and as a pair during the session. This was central to our supervision of the group process in the PDMT psychologists' group, where the participants were able to observe that there was a direct link between the quality of the relationship between the pair of PDMT psychologists and the quality of relationships between the prison psychologists in the groupe de parole. In short, a healthy, functioning, emotionally expressive pair of PDMT psychologists engendered a healthy functioning groupe de parole; and conversely, if dysfunction existed in the pair of PDMT psychologists, then it was quickly translated to the groupe de parole.

Moreover, co-facilitation ensured that the PDMT psychologists had to talk to one another about themselves, to share what it was like to be in their respective groupes de parole, not just as a psychologist but as a human being, and they had to do this in front of their peers in the PDMT psychologists' group. It was precisely this sharing of doubts that allowed the PDMT psychologists to go further into reflection together, and the group as a whole to cohere at a deeper level. In parallel, as vulnerabilities were shared, the pairs opened the door more fully to their creativity. In talking about their sessions in their groupes de parole and reflecting on all the processes with their partner, they came to realise how important it was to prepare for their groups beforehand, practically and emotionally, such that they could be in unison in front of the group. The depth of sharing between the individuals in the pairs, between pairs, and finally altogether in the PDMT psychologists group provided an emotional template for their work with the prison psychologists. As the PDMT psychologists explored and experienced their own emotional vulnerabilities and the creativity that naturally ensued from the encounter, they were able to carry this 'embodied' experience into their work with the prison psychologists and support them in doing something similar.

THE GROUPES DE PAROLE WITH THE PRISON PSYCHOLOGISTS

The groupes de paroles with the prison psychologists were at the heart of the project. The learning garnered in the PDMT psychologists' group about therapeutic groupwork needed to be used in the groupes de paroles so as to encourage communication and the expression of emotions. The hidden suffering within the prison had to be expressed for the benefit of everyone in the prison system.

The groupes de parole took place on a monthly basis. Each group had a membership of approximately 10. We chose to locate the sessions in a hotel rather than within the confines of the prisons, so that the prison psychologists could enjoy a 'safe space' outside of their normal working environment. We ensured that those psychologists who worked in the same prison were distributed within different groups and that where possible the groups were mixed-gender. The ratio of male to female psychologists in the prisons was 70% to 30%.

The PDMT psychologists were apprehensive about working with the prison psychologists. The latter were often older, had many more years of work experience, and were used to working within the challenging prison environment. The tension in the initial sessions was palpable, as the prison psychologists gave voice to this asymmetry, maintaining: *"[T]hat's all very well, but you don't know what prison is like"*, and *"[W]e invite you to come and spend a day in prison, it would help you to understand us better"*. The PDMT psychologists had already explored their own expectations and fears about facilitating the groupes de parole within the PDMT psychologists' group and anticipated some of these challenges. Moreover, the therapeutic work on their emotions ensured that the PDMT psychologists were able to support the prison psychologists' expression of their emotions when articulating their most pressing issues. In addition, the preparation of session objectives, the 'ownership' of group exercises and interventions, and the knowledge that they would have ongoing clinical supervision of their work were all elements that enabled the PDMT psychologists to make progress.

Another issue that surfaced at the beginning of the groupes de parole was that some of the group members were no longer practicing as psychologists and were now in managerial positions within the CGPR. After elaborating the problem in supervision, the PDMT psychologists decided to keep the managers in the groups. This required particular attention so that matters of hierarchy did not hinder free speech in the groups, and above all it allowed a collective awareness of the degree of the impact of the work on all the prison staff and the need to confront those impacts. These sessions enabled the prison staff in the groupes de parole to distance themselves from their daily work-lives and to envisage changes within their institutions. Little by little, it helped them to become actors in the system again, with the power to change things, and to be able to continue working in the prison without being destroyed by the system.

Whatever the issues in these initial sessions, each pair of PDMT psychologists conducted their groupe de parole in a more or less similar manner, according to the training and supervision undergone in the PDMT psychologists' group. However, it was clear that each groupe de parole followed its own distinct trajectory, each taking its own time to get to a place where individual members could share their concerns and emotions in depth. Despite this, we observed that the life and process of the various groupes de parole shared a common turning point; the same turning point as had been evident in the PDMT psychologists' group. That is to say, it was during the session that focused on 'family' and the impact of the psychologist's work on their own family, that the members of the group opened to their withheld emotions and became closer to one another. It was at this point that the group began to work on itself, where defence mechanisms weakened and group members became more able to communicate openly, where, according to Tuckman's model of group development (1965), the group shifted from 'forming and storming' to 'norming and performing'.

THE IMPACT ON THE PRISON ENVIRONMENT

It has been difficult to measure the impact of our work on the prison detainees, as we have not been working with them directly. We can only therefore assess the impact on the prison environment as a whole. The impact of violence on the prison psychologists revealed the nature of institutional violence and the violence involved in working with prisoners. In the early sessions, the prison psychologists submitted that it was the prison environment itself that had rendered them complicit in institutional violence and that because of this they felt as if they had lost their humanity.

The groupes de parole provided a space for them to express the reality of their difficulties in their relations both with the detainees and their families. They were able to voice their frustrations with the working conditions in the prison and the lack of consideration by the authorities for the impact of their work on their physical and mental health. They came to realise the importance of having 'a therapeutic space' in which they could talk with one another about their work and its attendant problems, and the lack of such a space within the typical ambit of the prison.

The groupes de parole, and their emphasis on providing a space for the expression of emotions, helped the prison psychologists to understand the degree to which they suffered from vicarious trauma as a result of more or less constant immersion in violence. In sharing the emotional impact of their work, their weaknesses and their vulnerabilities the prison psychologists were able to realise how much humanity they had lost and the extent to which they had come to dehumanise the detainees.

Over time, the groupes de parole and the work on emotions helped the prison psychologists to change the paradigm in the prison, restoring humanity to the institution, both their own humanity and humanity towards the detainees. *"As for the prison environment, the* [prison staff] *changed their perception of the inmates and have a better attitude. [The] conditions of detention … are more human and respectful"* (Project Evaluation, PDMT psychologists, 09/2021). This could happen only because the focus was on the prison psychologist and the whole body of prison psychologists. Typically overlooked, in this project they found themselves at the heart of the endeavour, allowing them to think of themselves first and foremost as human beings with feelings. The restoration of their own emotions helped the prison psychologists to recognize the importance and place of emotions in the prison environment more generally.

This project has helped the prison psychologists to restore a sense of purpose and dignity in their work. It has allowed them to once again recognise the importance of what they are trying to do as psychologists. They work in the prison system with a marginalised, traumatised and largely rejected population, people who will eventually return to society. Despite their frustrations about the difficulty of changing the environment, the prison psychologists have been vocal about the importance of the groupes de parole. The programme was subsequently extended to other departments in the prisons, with the result that in 2021, four years on from starting the project, more than 250 prison staff, including social workers, chefs du pavillon and educators in juvenile detention centres had participated in groupes de parole facilitated by the same PDMT psychologists.

PERPETRATORS AND VICTIMS

Sironi (2017), who has worked with perpetrators of collective violence, insists on taking the collective dimension into account. It is not that one is born a perpetrator of collective violence, but one becomes a perpetrator. It is the environment and the surroundings that transform the person and lead them to either witness acts of violence 'silently' or to commit acts of violence. Through this work, we have observed that individuals do not consider themselves as violent or agents of violence, but rather they recognise themselves as working in an environment where violence is rife. They thus consider themselves to be victims of this violence too. The analysis of practice carried out with the prison staff enabled us to work on institutional violence by creating a distance from it, by providing the opportunity for them to articulate and elaborate difficult experiences. This work enabled the participants to become aware that they themselves were victims of vicarious trauma.

The prison staff isolate themselves in much the same way as victims of torture. But here, they isolate themselves through the routine of violence, engaging in the inexpressible, and through the routine of their status as 'persecutor'. They live this situation in isolation, never permitting themselves to talk about its reality. However, by working as a group on the impact their work environment has on them, on the image they have of themselves, on the image the prison milieu reflects back to them, they have the opportunity to build resilience together. Resilience is made possible through the realisation that they have the expertise to change things, rather than importing solutions via external 'experts'. Only they know the difficulties they face in such an environment. It is only the prison staff who can progressively become channels for change.

EVALUATION

Security protocols in the prisons meant that we were not able to evaluate the impact of the project on the prison staff directly, so we sent anonymised evaluation questionnaires to the 20 PDMT psychologists who were involved in the project over the whole period. Of these 20 participants, 12 replied (4 PDMT psychologists had left the project during the period and 4 others did not reply). We asked 15 questions about the impact of the groupes de paroles on: themselves, the prison staff, the detainees and the prison environment as a whole.

Bearing in mind the goal of our project, to impact the structural violence in the institution by working closely with the prison staff, we concentrate here on the evaluation findings in relation to the prison staff, the detainees and the prison environment.

100% of respondents thought that the groupes de parole had given prison staff something positive on both personal and professional levels; 83.3% thought that the groupes de parole had a positive impact on the prison environment as a whole, whilst 8.3% were unsure and a further 8.3% thought that they would not have a positive impact; 83.3% thought that the groupes de parole had a positive impact on the detainees, 8.3% were unsure of the impact and a further 8.3% didn't think that it would have a positive impact. From the verbatim remarks made by the PDMT psychologists we noticed particular themes:

- *"Exteriorising emotions"*

  The psychologists pointed out that this work allowed the prison staff *"to have the possibility of sharing the suffering … and the fact they feel secure, listened to, not judged, free. The groupe de parole is a renaissance for the prison staff"*, and *"to share their negative experiences and release the emotions that come from them, in a secure environment where they felt understood and not judged, allowed to minimise the negative impact of some stressful experiences lived at work"*. By the fact that they built a safe environment together, *"[the prison staff] became capable of exteriorising their emotions and putting words on them"*, which was difficult given the prison culture.

  According to the PDMT psychologists, as the sessions progressed, they noticed *"[a] better understanding and management of emotions, more empathy and self-respect"* and that *"[the prison staff] were able to speak about their difficulties to find alternatives"*. They wanted to find solutions for themselves and also for their family lives. They maintained that *"the [groupe de parole] allows the release of negative emotions and to prevent psychological disorders such as burn-out and or depression"*, but equally *"the work that each has done on themselves must have an impact on the family lives of the group members"*.

- *"Re-humanising"*

  According to the PDMT psychologists, the groupes de parole created a space where *"a real work on oneself and a reflection on the way [prison staff] approach the professional life in the prison environment"* was made possible. Through *"a more concrete look on their practice"*, they could develop *"a different way of approaching problems at work"* and *"a reflection on the possibilities to change the working conditions"*.

  In the prison environment, opportunities to share good practice between prisons are rare. The psychologists noticed that *"the [prison staff] understanding of the prison environment is a lot more positive which can allow a change in the perception of their tasks and their mission as part of a team"*. It appears that this also allowed them to *"benefit from the experiences of their colleagues to learn new strategies of problem solving"*. As the sessions progressed, *"the staff became more and more open to communication which itself [created] a new atmosphere at work"*.

  Another important aspect which was noted by the PDMT psychologists relates to the impact of work on the prison staff themselves and on their relationships with their colleagues. As the project progressed, they noticed that the prison staff were beginning to *"help each other"*, creating more significant connections with one another and becoming *"more empathetic with their colleagues"*. This was a significant change. Some of the psychologists even spoke of the *"humanisation of the relationships between prison staff and inmates"*. Such a re-humanisation of relationships (whether between staff themselves and/or staff and detainees) developed as a result of the prison staff learning to appreciate the sensitivities and emotions of one another in relation to their work: *"an approach which looks at and affects the whole system, not just the inmates"*.

- *"A door is partially open on rehabilitation"*

    Since the aim of the project was to work indirectly on institutional violence, it was difficult to measure its direct impact. However, through the evaluation questionnaire, the PDMT psychologists shared their own views about the impact of the project and the views expressed by the prison staff on the impact of their work on the detainees. The most important gains related to improvement in the quality of communication: *"As for the prison environment, the* [prison staff] *changed their perception of the inmates and have a better attitude.* [This] *can therefore allow better communication and a reciprocal change."* The project has led to *"an improvement in the relationship with the detainees"*, and *"[a] lot less violence"*. They described *"less relational problems and a good management of conflict"* and that the emotional changes allowed *"*[the prison staff] *to become more empathetic towards the detainees and understand better how they function"*. The psychologists described how *"it has allowed the staff engaged in this work to feel less stressed at work and more available psychologically to work with the inmates, and to provide help when needed"*. Most importantly, they point to the broader impact of the work: *"Some conditions of detention that are more human and respectful; a ground favourable to change"*, *"A door is partially open on rehabilitation"*, and *"The wellbeing of the staff, the professionalism to reach, one hopes, a better rehabilitation of the inmate"*.

- *The enduring impact*

    Whilst the majority of the respondents reported positive impacts of the groupes de parole on detainees and the prison environment as a whole, it was apparent that a small number of respondents were unsure of the impact on either the prison environment as a whole and/or on the detainees: *"[I]n the absence of follow up, there is a risk that new gains won't last … quite quickly old habits take over."*

    Some psychologists expressed the notion that for the prison staff to carry on working together in a spirit of sharing and positive exchange it would necessitate *"a sincere willingness"* at governance level to continue the project. They have also expressed doubts about this happening: *"I don't have any certainty at this level"*.

    For some other psychologists it would have been useful to have *"more frequent sessions on a continuous basis"* or *"to work with another group such as* new [staff] *recruits,* [because] *they are more affected by the system and they're not yet trained"*.

CONCLUSION

The transition to democracy in Tunisia has brought with it the need to address the legacy of state violence and torture. The Tunisian prison system has been one of the purveyors of this endemic violence. Fortunately, in the context of this transition, the prison system has been open to change. Our project, in collaboration with the CGPR, has sought to reduce the structural violence within the institution by focusing on the impact of this violence on the prison staff, those people that often spend a lifetime within the system, the system functionaries who often have themselves become aggressors. To facilitate the process, we sought to create groupes de parole, safe reflective spaces, in which prison staff could consider the impact of their work on their physical and mental health, acknowledge and share their own suffering and create a potential for change.

In basic terms, the project has been successful. Since inception, it has not only provided groupes de parole for all the prison psychologists in Tunisia but, following positive feedback from the CGPR, has subsequently been extended to other departments in the prisons, such that more than 250 prison staff, including social workers, educators, chefs du pavillon and educators in juvenile detention centres have engaged in groupes de parole.

The evaluation with the PDMT psychologists has highlighted the importance of the groupes de parole in providing a 'safe space' for prison staff to share and reflect together on the realities of their work. This has helped staff to register the physical and psychological impacts of their work and to understand and feel the ways in which they have suffered vicarious trauma. It has enabled prison staff to acknowledge and address both their own dehumanisation within the institution and the dehumanisation of the detainees who are in their charge. The groupes de parole have shone a light on the structural violence endemic in the prison system. This had led to improvements in the physical and psychological well being of the prison staff, and as a corollary, to positive changes in their relationship to their work and to their relationships with detainees.

The project has shown the necessity of self-care for frontline workers who in many contexts do not have it, revealing the importance of not only talking about the subject but 'feeling' it directly in relation to the impact of vicarious trauma on the body and the emotions. The virtue of a groupe de parole is that the group begins to take self-care seriously. This can lead to a benign shift in institutional thinking about the importance of self-care in the workforce.

The extension of the project to other professional groups working in Tunisian prisons has shown that the dynamics within the various groupes de parole have followed a similar process. We have noticed consistent dynamics in subsequent non-Tunisian projects in hugely different contexts (e.g. frontline psychologists and community counsellors working in refugee camps, city slums and with victims of torture and violence). This demonstrates the scope for using the groupes de parole approach in diverse settings as a transformative and community-building approach in the aftermath of human rights violations and endemic political violence.

NOTE

1   We use the French concept 'groupe de parole' rather than 'support group' or 'therapy group' because it connotes the dual function of providing a space to share views and emotions on the one hand and a space to analyse work practices on the other, and it was a term that was amenable to the Tunisian prison psychologists.

REFERENCES

Argyris, C. and Schön, D. (1974) *Theory in Practice: Increasing Professional Effectiveness*. San Francisco: Jossey-Bass Publishers.

Sironi, F. (2017) *Comment Devient-on Tortionnaire: Psychologie des Criminels Contre l'humanité*. Paris: La Découverte.

Tuckman, B. W. (1965) 'Developmental sequence in small groups', *Psychological Bulletin*, 63(6), pp. 384–399. doi:10.1037/h0022100.

CHAPTER 10

AUTHOR DISCUSSION
Building communities

Five of the authors who contributed to the 'Building Communities' section of the book took part in this discussion, representing three of the chapters: Jilna Shah; Miryam Rivera-Holguín; Emmanuel Sarabwe and Sewimfura Theophile. The discussion was facilitated by Rebecca Horn.

REBECCA: Welcome, Jilna and Miryam, it's good to have you here for this discussion! I hope others will join us as we go on, but let's make a start with the first question, which is "what is the core message that you'd want readers to take from your chapter?"

JILNA: At Room to Heal we run groups alongside casework, because we understand that people's material needs and psycho-emotional needs are so linked, along with things like body work and therapeutic gardening as kind of a holistic framework for healing. While the therapy groups are at the core of our work, we recognise the limitations of talking therapy alone as a means for healing trauma. So the activities surrounding our therapy are equally important.

I guess the main thing for us is the power of shared experience in human connection and the power of having a safe space where we can reconnect fully with others as a way of restoring that sense of humaneness in a system that essentially dehumanises people. We place our work in the context of UK's notorious hostile environment for migrants.

MIRYAM: In our chapter, we highlight the importance of being together to share experiences and support each other. Another core message is how the women I worked with in Peru, whose family members disappeared during the conflict, have learned through the group to locate their loss in a broader context. They take active roles in their own communities, so move from the experience of being passive to active citizens. They engage in collective activities within their society, their community, and in advocating for human rights.

Another key point is how they use traditional or cultural practices to support each other and to create a sense of cultural continuity that impacts on their wellbeing.

REBECCA: As I'm listening to you both, I'm seeing some differences between the two groups that you're writing about, but also some overlap. So one difference I've noticed is the group that Miryam's working with have a similar culture, similar experiences to draw on; whereas, Jilna, your participants are from a whole variety of different backgrounds. But both groups are displaced, so they have that in common.

JILNA: I think if we zoom out to less about the specifics of everyone's situation, because they are obviously very different, there are common experiences in being isolated, displaced, uprooted, and people having similar challenges to surmount. For example, we see when one person gets their immigration status, that becomes a really powerful symbol of hope that they finally did it. So we do find that despite those differences there is enough shared experience, or enough content that feels relatable. And there's something about being unified in the face of hostility, because the vast majority will be experiencing racism and discrimination that comes with being visibly people of colour who are migrants in England.

DOI: 10.4324/9781003192978-12

REBECCA: This experience of living in a context of hostility, I guess that's also part of what the women you're working with experience, Miryam?

MIRYAM: Yes. Peru is a very diverse country with a legacy of colonial relations that are still part of the way people relate to each other. So when people from Andean rural areas fled to the city they experienced otherness, discrimination and exclusion. They did not speak their own language, to prevent being harassed and excluded due to their cultural background. So in this case, the group that the women formed really helps them to reframe their own identity and their own social networks. I think what's also powerful in the group is the building of a sense of community and belongingness.

REBECCA: Yes. Does any of that resonate with you, Jilna, thinking about the people you work with?

JILNA: Yes, it's interesting because I think people do take a lot from the identity of being a member of Room to Heal. We refer to people as members, and that does seem to have some meaning and currency. People often refer to Room to Heal as their family, and have a sense that this is their space with a lot of pride. So I think that sense of belonging in itself is very therapeutic. Although we recognise that we have paid staff, and a lot of our staff members are white, so that's a different dynamic. We're not saying, oh, it's great, and everything is led by members. It's not necessarily like that. That's the ideal and at the same time it's something we're always reflecting on and trying to address.

REBECCA: We've been joined by Emmanuel and Theophile from the sociotherapy team in Rwanda. We're happy you can join us. We have been talking about Jilna's and Miryam's work, and the chapters they have written for the book. Could you summarise for us, Emmanuel, what core message you want readers to take away from your chapter?

EMMANUEL: Yes, thank you. The core message I want to convey is the power of the group to help people who have gone through stressful life or traumatic experiences. In a group, people meet others who share similar life experiences, and are heard, understood, and cared for without any judgement. Sometimes people who have a bad life experience blame themselves or they blame life in general. Hearing the suffering of others, and others hearing their suffering, helps them to grow psychologically.

REBECCA: It is clear from what all of you have said that this sense of belonging, family, community, being part of something, is really a key element of the process for the people that you work with. And I wondered whether you might be able to say something about what it is about the groupwork that you're involved with that contributes to building that sense of community and belonging?

JILNA: Compared to some other organisations we provide something that's quite long term, and I think that can really allow for trust to build, for relationships to grow. These things really do take time. So with our National Health Service in the UK you can wait ages for therapy, and often it's very, very short, time-limited, so it's difficult to start really meaningfully addressing trauma healing.

Prior to COVID we used to run residential retreats twice a year and that was really precious where people live in community together, cook together, go out to the countryside, really spend time together. And that meant that a lot of things that would maybe stay on the surface, there was space for that to come out.

And I think as an organisation as well, Room to Heal is very organic. So things are always changing and we're adapting and discarding things, or having a plan and then changing that plan because the reality has changed, and I think that that allows us to mirror where people are actually at. I guess the balance between having some structures in place, like our weekly gatherings, the therapy groups, and space for more informal relating to occur, creates that space for relationships to build.

REBECCA: So actually spending time together is a key part of building relationships, and also the flexibility to adapt to changes as they occur.

JILNA: Definitely.

MIRYAM: Adding to what Jilna said, I think it's very important also to acknowledge that the people we are working with have strong personalities, and this not only includes their inner personal strength but also the way they relate to each other, to the institutions, to the organisation. This is connected to the need they have to be part of something. In the case of the women I work with they really attach to each other after being isolated. So this joy of being together, this time for activities, also what Jilna said about these retreats or activities that take them out of their reality for a time and allow them to connect with the things they have as a group, that's something important. Also by being in the group they start having small routines that they feel make the time they are together special, and they have the opportunity to introduce a spontaneous activity, like jokes, artistic things or singing together, which also connects with the cultural continuity that I mentioned before.

As well as that, as a consequence of migration and displacement, the women experience poverty and daily stressors, so allowing time to address these everyday needs, and to share and to think about what they can do together to address their situation, that's also very important in this group.

SEWIMFURA: As far as a sense of belonging is concerned, in the contexts in which we have been operating people have experienced violence. They went through wars, and many have lost their family members or become separated from family members. This leads them to live in a situation of loneliness. So when the groups of sociotherapy were organised, that provided a space where these people could meet and speak about their problems. For many of them it was the first time to share about their experiences. Through discussions, the group members were able to support one another, to care for one another, even to care for themselves. It also enabled them to find new strategies of navigating in a life full of problems. Often, when listening to people who graduated from those groups, we heard them say "this has been my new family". Remember that the wars and violence destroyed their primary family. The groups were able to provide ways to build that new family.

EMMANUEL: Many people approached experts using an individual approach to help them. But they were not helped effectively because in their community they still did not have any person to relate to, to socialise with, or to talk to. In contrast, when they are supported by the group approach of sociotherapy, they are able to remain connected, embedded in a team. They live together in the same community. So to me, this is the strength of community approaches, it contributes to this sense of belonging and community.

REBECCA: Thank you very much. Let's have a look at our second question, which is, has writing the chapter changed your approach to groupwork in any way?

JILNA: Yes, it's made us look a lot more critically at what we do and to look at issues around power and privilege and hierarchy and how that actually plays out. So we're thinking, OK, this is the ideal and what we're trying to do and what's the actual reality? Where are the areas where we're not being so inclusive or where people aren't actually that empowered? And so I think it's given us a bit of space just to step back and identify areas we would like to focus on a bit more.

MIRYAM: I was very happy writing the first part of the chapter, because that's about the power of coming together, but then when coming to the end it makes me realise the challenges of this approach. Because we like to work with groups, there's a risk of idealising our group, our approach. It's like we think that's the best way to do it but we need to acknowledge that groups exercise power over individual members. It's very important for us to also think about the limits of this kind of groupwork, and when some people may really benefit from an individual clinical approach. It can be that the group is so strong that members feel like they better stay in the group instead of stepping out to search for specific support. Those were the things that were on top of my mind as I was writing the chapter.

EMMANUEL: What I have learned from writing this book chapter is that what is lost in people who went through traumatic experiences is not only loved ones they lost or material things they lost, but it is also humanness they lost. It's a loss of a sense of belonging, they don't experience themselves as humans anymore. In our chapter that experience is represented by the fact that you see many people unwilling to join a group, or, even if they do join, being hesitant to share anything related to their suffering. To me, what I learned from this chapter is that this is a representation of a loss of humanness. "I lost dignity, I'm no longer human, so I don't belong to any community". But by participating in this community-based intervention with its group approach, people regain this sense of belonging, this sense of humanness, and they are capable of building a new family together.

REBECCA: As we come to the end of our time, I'd like to give you the opportunity to share your thoughts on the final question, which is "what statements or messages can we as a group together come up with to encourage more groupwork opportunities"?

MIRYAM: One important point is that when we as professionals are working with victims of human rights abuses, there's always a gap, a social gap. Human rights abuses isolate people and take them out of their group. So I think collective approaches are a way to restore the social relations that were fractured due to the victimisation.

JILNA: Just a simple but I think quite important thing is that when we are working with groups we can really enact this kind of "solidarity not charity" idea, where we all practice giving and receiving. So it's not just like there are these experts who are giving this thing. It's this very much, "none of us are free until all of us are free" kind of approach.

SECTION 2

'BODY AND SOUL'

CHAPTER 11

ADVERSITY, THERAPEUTIC WITNESSING AND THE ARTS

Enda Moclair

Creativity is a vital and powerful enabler of healing, learning and development. In this time of collective global crisis there is an unprecedented need for responsive creative healing processes. Trauma can stunt our creative potential and this chapter explores interventions designed to restore it. Therapeutic interventions focusing on imagination ask us to reconceptualise the past, envisage a brighter future and illuminate our internal world, helping to break down barriers that prevent us from seeing new possibilities and feeling new sensations. In this chapter, I describe how connecting to our innate creative instinct, via creative expression and exploration, especially in groups, is a powerful, non-pathologising and very accessible means of individual and collective healing. I draw on 20 years of experience working as a facilitator and integrated arts therapist with a range of different groups: survivors of torture, prisoners, refugees, those living with and fleeing from conflict. In this chapter I share my experience of how connecting to our innate creativity can promote healing, development and learning from adversity.

Drawing on case examples from groupwork in Cambodia, Vietnam, Iraq, Syria, Yemen, South Sudan and Sierra Leone, I will illustrate how the creative approach is fundamental to witnessing, healing and reconnecting to personal and collective resiliencies that may have been lost or damaged. These are essential for adversity-activated growth and the restoration of a sense of safety and wellbeing for people who have survived torture, loss of home, disasters and human rights violations. This type of groupwork is culturally attuned and follows an iterative process where 'choice' and 'discovery' are fundamental.

My work has also involved working with humanitarian psychosocial staff so that they have an experiential parallel journey to those they are working with. This enables them to better trust the creative process and be confident and competent in facilitating such groupwork themselves. Being vulnerable and open to a personal healing journey is very important for support staff and can be immensely challenging, especially when their own backgrounds involve conflict and upheaval.

My practice is rooted in the traditions of systemic theory, and recognises the importance of the therapeutic relationship and community as central to resilience and healing. I believe the best way to support healing within a living system is to strengthen connections within that system, and the most powerful way to enable this is through relationship with others. Coming from Northern Ireland, the Irish proverb *"Ar scaith a cheil na mhaireaan na daoine"* – *"it is in the shadow of others that we find life"* – is one that has resonated loudly down the years. Whilst different groups will have different needs and cultural considerations, a strong, safe working co-alliance and focus on creativity aligns with Jung's (1983) contention, which is at the heart of resilience studies, that *"therapy is less a matter of treatment than of developing the latent creative possibilities within the self"* (p. 306).

THE IMPORTANCE OF CREATIVITY

The awareness that creative expression can make a powerful contribution to the healing process has been embraced in many different cultures. Throughout recorded history, people have used pictures, stories, dances, and chants as healing rituals.

DOI: 10.4324/9781003192978-14

> When I reflect, and saw how we moved and danced, I felt the journey (of the group) was like the journey of life, we face new lives through the seasons, people come and people go, while we dance accordingly.
>
> (Syrian woman, 2014)

The inner and outer fragmentation that people can experience from adversity, in living with and through conflict, of leaving and losing home, being displaced, of enduring mental, physical and social violation cannot easily be captured, reflected or honoured by conscious rational thoughts and words alone. I have been privileged to witness the restorative qualities of creative approaches in enabling people to cope with extensive adversities. They stimulate our imaginations, which informs our ability to hope. For people who have lived with and through extreme stressors in conflict contexts, this is often an aspect of their humanity that is deliberately targeted for denigration and destruction.

Adversity and trauma can have many long-lasting impacts on a person. Impacts are varied, from flashbacks to depression, debilitating grief, withdrawal, isolation, relationship breakdown, addictions, and risky behaviours. The field of neuroscience demonstrates how trauma can affect the part of the brain associated with memory (Van Der Kolk, 2014). The creative expression of images and symbols can be very powerful in supporting people to understand and express what happened, and what may still be happening to them, especially in working with memories that are not always accessible to consciousness. Furthermore, working with individual and group images and metaphors can enable multiple levels of safety, communication and deeper dialoguing with oneself and other group members. This form of expression can help externalise inner feelings, thoughts, confusions, fears, unconscious needs and witness them from different angles and perspectives. An extra quality of safety is enabled through the indirect and oblique nature of image and metaphor work. Physical and embodied exercises that promote regulation of inner states is enabled more easily through the collective effort of practicing together activities that make us open to being vulnerable. Whilst vulnerability is important for curiosity and learning, it can be necessary to disconnect from this aspect of ourselves in order to survive. Furthermore, to have our inner symbols and language heard, embodied, mirrored and witnessed by others is another powerful amplification of the therapeutic power a group can provide. This is where art, music, drama and movement therapy enable a more collective and embodied means of connecting with the unconscious than the problem/solution orientation of some other talk/goal-centred therapies.

> When I joined the group I felt it a very safe place where I could sit down and think about what happened in the past and could share with others. I felt very happy to feel trust and share and have the belief again in myself and feel more trust outwards towards others. Because for the first time in my life I feel heard, people listened to me. I really enjoyed to play so much – I haven't done like this since I was young.
>
> (Cambodian woman, 2007)

The creative arts, drama, dance, movement, songs, poems also have physical components and thus provide opportunities for the release of tensions and body memories. A line from a song or poem, an image from a painting can be enacted and inhabited. Flexing the imagination enables participants to step outside of themselves and travel back and forwards in time, to engage and dialogue with people alive or departed, to co-create preferred visions for their futures. Creating art, embodiment, poetry, music and drama are therefore integral to "restore continuity and facilitate integration of dissociated states and splits in experience by reuniting affect, cognition, and perception turned asunder by traumatic experience" (Richman, 2014, p. 95).

Creative expression can enable groups in all cultures to contain and capture the complexity of their experiences, particularly non-literate groups or where emotional literacy has not been taught. Mental health and wellbeing is so often a taboo subject; talking about such issues directly is uncommon in many countries, particularly for men.

> We have a saying, "If you are not wolf the wolf will eat you." So if you are not strong or you show weakness you will not be able to protect yourself or your family.
>
> (Syrian PSS worker 2015)

Experiential and multi-modal work is especially relevant in contexts with high power differentials and where childhood experiences of learning tend to focus on rote educational approaches. In such contexts, critical thinking and creativity are rarely promoted. Being able to explore different artistic modalities that promote connection, communication and relationship, within self and with others, is particularly important and powerful for those who have experienced disempowerment in so many realms. An essential aspect of the groupwork described here is for participants to be at the centre of their own healing and learning processes, creating multiple ways to notice and express, capture and affirm the often incremental steps of insight and restorative connections.

PROMOTING COLLECTIVE LEARNING AND HEALING

The bedrock of trauma-informed therapeutic and community-based psychosocial work, as with the person-centred approach advocated by therapists such as Carl Rogers, is the recognition of the affected individual and community's capacity for recovery, resilience, healing and development.

In my work with groups, I employ a diverse palette of creative methods informed by psychotherapy, theatre and the arts which connect members to more of their own story (through self-awareness); to others (through enabling relationships); to their innate creativity; to their self-power (and the choices this brings) and the power in others; and to their own adversity-activated developments (strengths gained from exposure to adversity) (Papadopoulos, 2007). It is hard to describe this non-linear process as it's very intuitive and often I fumble at the beginning to get the lens focused and attuned to the diverse needs within a group. It's a process-led structure that requires an array of facilitation skills to both tune into and respond to the needs of the group. It requires one to be comfortable with the unknown, flexible, adaptive and responsive. Skills of attunement and communication are required to be able to co-create and shape the experience together with the group rather than govern with a pre-determined agenda.

Three central stepping stones of this process framework are Connection–Communication–Relationship. Each session begins with a co-created ritual, and threaded through each session is the empowering, attuning weave of story. I began work in the humanitarian world during the Rwandan genocide response and always remember a T-shirt one person in the camps had that read "*You cannot hate someone whose story you know*". As Ben Okri (1996, p.21) states: "*Stories are the secret reservoir of values. Change the stories individuals and nations live by and tell themselves, and you change the individuals and nations.*" Stories take us to the heart of lived experiences; taking the story to action allows us to enter, to be an active participant and witness.

I've also learned that a story can only be told when it's ready, and for people who have experienced inner and outer violations the first requisite of being ready is safety. Only then are we potentially open to connection to lost or exiled parts of self; connection to strengths; hopes and dreams; connections with others. Centring, through meditative and physical exercises, aims to help participants quieten their minds and begin to develop inner and external awareness before action. Spatial awareness and movement, from inner to outer, self to others, needs to be a regular practice as it can often cause anxiety for those who have learned that to be safe requires them to avoid vulnerability. Connection to each other is also safely experienced and promoted through this practice, building gradually to using exercises that promote safe expansion of physical and emotional ranges.

WHERE TO BEGIN

For sustained groupwork, inviting participants to create a baseline of internal and external strengths, challenges and hopes to describe their current situation can be particularly empowering in enabling witnessing of adversity-activated growths. This baseline can be expressed through a combination of images, objects and words to represent key aspects of functioning – body, mind, heart, relationships, strengths, power, behaviours and dreams. The baseline informs the practice of reflection and participants return to it during and at the end of the groupwork to witness their own incremental growth over time.

The process of mapping baselines with image and materials of choice is also a very helpful and invitational way to introduce a range of artistic modalities. It encourages participants as a collective to try out a range of natural materials: beads, beans, stones, wood, sand, metal, clay, cloth. It promotes curiosity and gentle risk taking, again encouraged by the collective work going on around them.

I call the next phase 'Tilling the Soil' as it is a preparatory, but vital step for seeds to grow and towards what follows. Tilling the soil supports participants to consider and concretise commitments they may need in the work ahead, to consider challenges, concerns and supports they can draw on when the seas get choppy. Tilling the soil also involves, for psychosocial support staff, dialoguing with their line managers and organisational directors to co-create a shared vision of what impacts are realistic and what forms of support are needed. This entails exploring what blocks and resistances might be encountered and what the organisation can do to support their staff's learning and ensure adequate resourcing for the groupwork. At a minimum, this will include the provision of a safe space and materials, and providing supervision for support staff.

As the pioneer of psychodrama, Jacob L. Moreno understood a core feature of such groupwork is the nurturing of the creative discovery instinct within people, and that the best way to promote this is via spontaneous action-orientated activities. When we are spontaneous we are in the moment, free-flowing, authentic and not censoring or being blocked by inhibition or judgements, so how we play is how we are. When members reflect on how they are in such moments, it enables a powerful self-assessment of their current functioning, one devoid of shame or rebuke. Psychodramatic action methods enable group members to experience authentic expression, something previously out of bounds for many, and to reflect on personal issues, and give themselves permission to try out new roles in safe and non-judgemental ways. The necessary ingredients for spontaneous behaviour include: safety and trust, receptivity to images, intuitions, feelings and playfulness, and movement towards risk taking, exploration and novelty.

Creating the conditions which facilitate spontaneity begins with the 'warm-up' phase of the groupwork; exercises that get people moving, interacting and improvising. The quality of the warm up will influence the depth and authenticity of what emerges through the action later. A common initial reaction from group members to creative expression as a therapeutic methodology is that they are not creative, often assuming only 'artists' are. I often draw on Picasso's adage that *"we are all born creative, then we go to school and learn not to be"*. Active improvisation requires 'warm up' as a process that warms physical, mental, social and emotional expression and promotes spontaneity. Much of Moreno's work may be understood as being methods and ideas for promoting spontaneity in the service of creativity as healing (Blatner, 1996). An effective warm up is not a one off game but a series of calibrated exercises that promote spontaneity and then bridge into the main content/action phase, and bridge out again afterwards through grounding that encourages participants back to the here and now and present in their bodies.

> Being in this group helped me to have creative ideas that I can use. I feel that I have not used this part of me for such a long time so the knife is not so sharp but it is improving already.
> (Vietnamese woman, 2011)

Receiving feedback from other members as part of the post-enactment sharing is a form of 'therapeutic witnessing' that is vital for group cohesiveness and compassion. Developing feedback strengths is an important part of the process, since this is very often a new way to interact that takes time to be valued. Few bring experience of receiving and giving feedback as intended to contribute to healing, learning and development. Many have experienced it as rebuke, competition and control, involving degrees of shame, coercion and loss of face. The giving and receiving of feedback, therefore, is a primary muscle engaged, enabling the group to be aware of differences between observations, perceptions and projections. Using psychodramatic action methods for this, such as role reversal, doubling and mirroring, promotes empathy and can be utilised at all stages of the groupwork (Blatner, 2004).

The 'warm up' for the group is the launch pad for increased engagement between group members, contributing to stronger group cohesion, and promoting spontaneity and expression. As part of this I must work consciously on my own warm up in connecting to the group participants. This involves being aware of my role, how am I and what am I bringing to the session, attuning to what is going on for participants, reading the group's conscious and unconscious communications as much as I can, promoting deep rapport, trying to be aware of transference and counter transferences. As part of my own warm up I will often initially join in and model playful curiosity. Play helps to establish trustful warmth, deep connection between and within participants, and containment within the group. I find adapting this warm up, making it longer and creating exercises according to the context and culture, helps people thaw more and develops their trust in what can be considered initially for some a strange way of working.

Exploring creative approaches

Initially, each session begins with a different calibration of warm-up exercises and then works with emerging themes though a variety of art forms. Visual art work is most often considered appropriate and accessible for all. In many cultures, activities that promote interaction and physical contact between genders are initially encountered with resistance. In Iraq, Syria and Yemen, the group deemed dance and movement unsuitable for youth or adults but helpful for children. Drama was initially considered sensitive, particularly depending on the story being dramatised. Poetry was valued by both genders and thought appropriate for all ages, although children were not considered able to use this form. So, again, developing trust in different art modalities is not a linear process but requires indirect circling, attunement and intuitive facilitation. Working with stories and single scenes and drawing on Image Theatre, sculpting and embodiment contributes to the development of a language of ensemble. I also draw heavily on Augusto Boal's (1995, 2002) Theatre of the Oppressed approach as it is powerful in promoting trust, imagination, playfulness and physical range expansion. The glue of safety and trust supports the group as it moves between different stages of group formation, and as it moves from warm up into action, and from action to grounding and sharing.

Storytelling through such media, as well as with words, enables members to experience the capacity of stories to promote connection, communication and relationship. The capacity to recognise, value, help and be helped by those perceived as 'other' is the essence of emotional and social capital. Emotional and social capital are central to the restorative process, as the bonds of trust between community members are often deliberately targeted in times of conflict. Conflict can turn us into isolated islands. It is helpful to be mindful of how participants with experience of conflict, adversity and trauma may have had to shut down, disconnect from empathy, learned to hide their spontaneity and survive by not trusting.

> My life goals, my work, is to ensure that I never go back or allow such conditions to ever come near or touch me or my family again. First and foremost is the need for security, land, home and finances. Then I can think of others.
>
> (Male Khmer Rouge survivor, Cambodia, 2009)

So introducing storytelling as a means of connecting people is a good place to start and return to throughout. Stories can be spoken, embodied and enacted. Often, our stories are strangers to us and need time and safety to come 'home'. Aspects of the story may have been exiled to the unconscious or the past, or we may have become stuck and used to seeing and telling only a particular version. Sharing stories also connects us back to our voice, the interface between our internal and external worlds. As all group members are engaged in a similar exploration, this contributes greatly to our courage, motivation and perseverance to stay and bear witness.

I usually introduce a combination of storytelling and action using general, resonant, safe words, such as 'door', 'teacher', 'dinner', or a colour. These words trigger stories and draw from a commonality of cross-cultural experiences. Most will have stories of a teacher that come to mind, or of an encounter with a dog or an animal, that lets us establish our voice in the group. This simple act can provide a sense of achievement that promotes self-worth, a feeling of inclusion and of being heard. Later, the sharing of more personal stories contributes further to reducing the feeling of isolation and of developing trust and empathy between the group members. If stories are too painful, and are not yet ready to be shared, I find working with resonant objects such as clay pots, shoes, scarves, to be a helpful intermediary substitute; anything that promotes safety by working through the object rather than directly can be very helpful for an individual and group.

When participants feel comfortable with a wider range of stories through creative expression, I introduce Image Theatre, working with sculpts, using the body to express without words initially, and later forum theatre. Forum theatre is a form of theatre from Augusto Boal (1995, 2002), wherein a story containing an issue is garnered from the group. A scene is shown once and then repeated to the audience, during which any audience member (Boal called them 'spect-actors') can shout 'stop' and step into the scene, and take the place of one of the characters. The scene then continues in a different way, showing how any audience member can change the situation and gain a different outcome.

The focus may be an individual's story or a weave of combined experiences around a similar theme of oppression. Group members hone this story which contains the moment of oppression, of shut down, where the protagonist is not able to achieve their aim, when they are cut off from personal power or encounter abusive power. Stories of oppression unfortunately are endless and will be there in the group, waiting below the waterline. Once the moment of crisis is reached then the group members/spect-actors are invited to step up and into the role of the protagonist. The scene then is replayed so that other spect-actors can enter the scene and attempt to navigate the block as played by the oppressor, someone using their power to deny the protagonist their aim. This process allows us to also practice new roles unfamiliar to us, or which we cannot envisage and to gain confidence. New roles can be rehearsed, and roles that no longer serve us can be let go. This method helps stretch and flex our imagination and also contributes positively to creating future, preferred visions of ourselves.

I am more confident after being in this group. I did not have the eye contact habit because my ex-husband never allowed me to look into his eyes, he could be angry immediately and he would hit me badly. Now I feel more comfortable to talk to people, and I am living with hope about my future career.

(Syrian woman, 2014)

I have people in my family who always tell me this is what life is like for a woman and so not to expect otherwise. Now I am like bird in a cage that is free. And now I feel so very happy. I'm always very curious and like to ask a lot more questions now.

(South Sudanese woman, 2015)

Using this powerful form of theatre in Cambodia and Vietnam, I discovered that the high values around loss of face and big distance in power differentials made it very difficult for women in particular to inhabit some roles with confidence. To challenge patriarchal power, even in character, felt unnatural for them and so the experience fell flat. The form was not safe enough, more distance was needed, and we found the solution in masks. They provided an extra layer of safety for the women to be someone else, to connect to their own power, and be able to step up into the role and inhabit it with confidence.

Once a level of trust and group cohesion is developed, I usually introduce local myths that contain relevant themes, for example of rejection, alienation, betrayal, migration, endurance, kindness, hope, acceptance. Such symbolic stories offer containment and opportunities to obliquely explore resonant but often banished and buried themes. The indirectness seems to make it easier for participants to get up and act, it is safer than moving from warm up into an enactment of an experienced story. Initially hesitant, most participants delight in the safety, freedom and range of possibilities that playing a character in a myth story affords them.

An Iraqi mother in one session gravitated to a role where the protagonist vents her rage and anger. Being in character, using the safety of distance the role afforded, enabled her to act out her own rage safely, to connect to her own cordoned-off anger and deep reservoir of personal power without fear of reprisal or shaming, to vent with a force that initially surprised her and the other group members, and then delighted her. The ripples of this enactment touched others in the group, and helped others step up and find their own voice.

A similar example from Yemen, not through acting out but through an art image a participant created of herself, wearing her own choice of clothes as she imagined them. Hair flowing, tank top, colourful jeans, and smoking. Just describing the image to the others in the group was energising for her, and a powerful encouragement for them. Another way of affirming and consolidating such an image was to invite the group to then write a poem to the image. This second layer of expression enabled deeper dialogue, and opened the group to further self and shared discoveries, and discussions that went on long after the session itself. Reversing roles with aspects of an art image created can yield further insights for the individual and the group. What one participant shares can connect with the experiences of others. Again, the group's ability to hold each other compassionately through painful memories or associations is integral to this approach.

The last art forms reached usually are the dance and movement sessions, although this can vary according to the context. These were particularly powerfully experienced by a care team group of mostly Syrian and Turkish women. Initially considered a culturally inappropriate art form by the group, they later spoke of the freedom and joy in being able to move and dance according to how their bodies wanted to, rather than following traditional dance moves, and spoke of the feeling of connectedness in witnessing others in the group move and express themselves with no self-censorship or sense of shame.

When I reflect, and saw how we moved and danced, I felt the journey was like the journey of life, we face new lives through the seasons, people come and people go, while we dance accordingly.

(Syrian woman, 2014)

THE INFLUENCE OF CREATIVE APPROACHES ON ADVERSITY-AFFECTED DEVELOPMENT

Adversity-activated developments can emerge following exposure to adversities (Papadopoulos, 2007), and creative reflective practice can play a key role in facilitating awareness of these often-subtle developments. Creative expression enables new perceptions of oneself and others, of relationships, and even the meaning and purpose of our lives, to be made visible and further concretised. Work around these adversity-affected developments, rather than solely through a trauma lens, can be an empowering frame.

I am strong like a tree, deep roots but despite that, just like the tree, I have faced many bad times like the tree faces: snow, rain, wind. I feel I am facing everything and all the challenges of life and I stay strict and strong against all the conditions and bear fruit.

(Syrian woman, 2015)

In this section, I describe some of the resiliencies and adversity-affected developments that I have observed within the groups I have facilitated, using the creative approaches described above.

Spirituality is a cross-cutting theme that infuses so much of strengths-based work, and is integral to identity, power, values and hope. The deliberate intention of a torturer is often to break people's sense of hope and of spiritual redemption. The spiritual shattering for those coming from a strong faith background can be a significant part of the trauma.

Physical expression and range is another theme of focus. A torturer's deliberate attacks on the body, where memory is stored (Van der Kolk, 2014), can further contribute to an internal shattering and loss of hope. The ability to be at home in the body is damaged, which can lead to a profound shattering of the sense of 'self'. Much of the work around hope within the group combines practising self-soothing and mindful body work as well as psychoeducation around neurophysical responses to stimulate an awareness of what is happening within themselves and others. A key aim is for participants to begin to expand their sound and movement expressional range which can become limited after trauma exposure. This supports and helps mirror the expansion of emotional range, and can help with regulation of neurophysical stress responses.

This approach also explicitly engages with concepts of power. Much human suffering emanates from abuse of power, which is often disguised as cultural, state or family norms. In my experience, participants can best explore the nature and impacts of power in its different subtle forms through embodied action, followed by discussion, rather than vice versa. Being mindful of, and explicit with, the group about my own power as a male group facilitator, contributes to the growing group awareness that there are different types of power and that we can have choice in exercising which form we and others use, when we can recognise and discern. Image Theatre and ensuing dramas enable people with little experience of personal power to connect with what are often-dormant and shamed qualities of power within them. A key intention and outcome for members is to become more aware of different types of power, to discover their own personal qualities of 'power' in relation to others, and become aware of and able to practice using their power in accordance with their values.

I feel less guilty and am aware of my power now and how to own and use it. I am able to hold and manage my sadness from [my children and family].

(Iraqi woman, 2017)

A doorway to introduce the theme can be the exploration of local proverbs. These can provide a means to explore culturally specific experiences through common images contained in the culture's mythology. A group of trafficked women survivors in Vietnam enacted a popular local myth in which an ancient queen is thrown out of heaven and has to look after her many children. The members could explore different feelings and states indirectly through the safety and distance of the role. Associations and meanings emerge that can be explored in subsequent group or individual sessions. The focus can then move to exploration of different power types and examination of how societal beliefs and attitudes influence and affect the roles played by women.

> I was surprised at first when I learnt about power-within. I realised that I had had power all along but I never used it. I felt as if I had just woken up.
>
> (Cambodian woman, 2009)

Participants also begin exploring and understanding their emotions and how they relate to them. With a group in Cambodia, members had difficulty discerning and naming different emotions. They were familiar with happiness and anger but few others. We began to explore this playfully by voicing and morphing different emotions identified by the group. Gradually, the focus moved to specifically exploring and naming 'my emotions' and 'where in my body' I experience them. Group members are then invited to dialogue directly with their body images, and to process what emerges with an art form, a letter to self. Understanding emotions and emotional intelligence is often untaught; they are more often avoided and suppressed. Emotive communication therefore can be rife with fear and often interpreted as a precursor for conflict.

A focus on values is another common area of growth. Very often our experiences of 'values' are as culturally accepted moral codes of conduct; that is, rules to be abided by, as opposed to freely chosen roles to be lived up to. In clarifying values, my intention is to co-create an environment that is therapeutic, safe, compassionate, affirming and respectful, and which thus allows members to examine how past experiences can inform today's behaviours.

> I am more sensitive to others after learning about my communication. Independence and being brave are my values. Connecting to my strengths helps my motivation. Before I just talked to the animals on our farm because they never betrayed me.
>
> (Vietnamese woman, 2011)

The therapeutic relationship in any culture is influenced to varying degrees by core values informing relationships, particularly those around patriarchy, gender, stoicism, equality, status and hierarchy. Solidarity, love and forgiveness often emerge as common core values amongst diverse groups, desired but difficult to express and practice. Providing invitation and choice is central to such group practice. Group members will determine the values and guidelines which will support the quality of connection, communication and relationship required to develop and grow.

CONCLUSION

The therapeutic witnessing described above enables members to move at their own pace. It enables connections with what was lost to be organised and re-established. The approach enables self-esteem and adversity-activated developments to be recognised and grow; gives 'permission' for acceptance and mourning; and for the internal compass to begin pointing hope-wards. It is an empowering approach that places the person at the centre of recording, recognising and gauging both their challenges and their own incremental growth in the face of such challenges, contributing to building new resilience.

Imagination is a muscle that enables us to see more of ourselves on paths not yet written – or to rewrite what we believe to be immutable. The ways we re-imagine the past or predict what might happen in the future are acts of deep imaginative power with enormous potential to change our perception and internal experiences and sensations. More than ever, spaces are needed within our health, social and educational systems to offer such opportunities for those living with and through adversity.

REFERENCES

Blatner, A. (1996) *Acting In: Practical Applications of Psychodynamic Methods*. 3rd edition. New York: Springer Publishing Company.

Blatner, A. (2004) *Theoretical Foundations in Psychodrama*. 4th edition. New York: Springer Publishing Company.

Boal, A. (1995) *Theatre of the Oppressed*. New York: Theatre Communications Group.

Boal, A. (2002) *Games for Actors and Non Actors*. London: Routledge.

Jung, C.G. (1983) *The Essential Jung, Selected Writings*. Roermond, Netherlands: Fontana Press.

Okri, B. (1996) *Birds of Heaven*. London: Weidenfeld & Nicolson History.

Papadopoulos, R. (2007) 'Refugees, trauma and adversity-activated development', *European Journal of Psychotherapy and Counselling*, 9(3), pp. 301–312. doi:10.1080/13642530701496930.

Richman, S. (2014) *Mended by the Muse–Creative Transformations of Trauma*. London: Routledge.

Van der Kolk, B. (2014) *The Body Keeps the Score: Brain, Mind, and Body in the Healing of Trauma*. London: Penguin Books.

CHAPTER 12

A MOVE TOWARDS GROUPWORK

Addressing Complex PTSD in survivors of torture through Trauma-Sensitive Yoga and LGBTQ Peer Support Groups

Aisling Hearns

> I was beginning to question who I really am and had lost hope of being happy again but since I joined the group, I am more confident, and I have never been proud of who I am like now.
>
> (Spirasi groupwork client)

This chapter will explore the use of groupwork with survivors of torture in a rehabilitation centre, 'Spirasi', in Ireland. Ireland is a small country on the edge of Europe, which has a regular stream of migrants, many of whom fall under the category of forced migrants seeking international protection. Whilst any form of migration can be considered a stressful experience marked by uncertainty, forced migration brings with it the additional elements of disempowerment and a lack of safety. Most of those who undertake a journey of forced migration do so due to conflict and persecution and it has been observed that the experience of torture is vastly over-represented within refugee populations (Steel et al., 2009). Exposure to compounding instances of traumatic events can lead to complex trauma. This chapter explores how symptoms of Complex post-traumatic stress disorder (PTSD) in a population of forced migrants who have experienced torture are addressed using two different approaches to groupwork. The Trauma-Sensitive Yoga Group demonstrates how Complex PTSD can be addressed by reconnecting with the body; and the LGBTQ Peer Support Group demonstrates the importance of creating safe, boundaried spaces to rebuild trust in interpersonal relationships.

COMPLEX PSYCHOLOGICAL TRAUMA SYMPTOMATOLOGY IN SURVIVORS OF TORTURE

As a psychotherapist and manager working with survivors of torture for many years, I have observed the unique and complex effects of torture on the psyche of those who attend for treatment, and seen the impact of groupwork on presenting symptomology. The experience of torture alone is a deeply distressing event which often leads to trauma disorders. However, when combined with the experience of forced migration, we see both prolonged and compounded instances of traumatic events which can lead to more complex psychopathologies. There are a myriad of potentially traumatic experiences facing forced migrants, which are spread across pre-flight, flight, and post-flight phases of their journey. Termed the 'triple trauma paradigm' (Stevenson et al., 2007), the impact of this has been shown to have a cumulative effect and result in a higher prevalence, and comorbidity, of psychological disorders (Poole et al., 2018). Post-migration trauma contributes to the exacerbation of pre-existing traumatic symptoms (Silove et al., 2017), preventing integration into the host community (Schick et al., 2016).

It has been recorded that up to 50% of migrants in Ireland have suffered torture (Wilson et al., 2013). Given that the psychological impact of torture is often compounded further by distressing events experienced during flight and on arrival in the host country (de C Williams and van der Merwe, 2013), including the international protection process and a loss of autonomy (Crumlish and Bracken, 2011), it is not surprising to find high prevalence rates of PTSD and Complex PTSD within these populations. It has been noted that a diagnosis of PTSD for survivors of torture is too inadequate a description for the complexity and magnitude of the

DOI: 10.4324/9781003192978-15

effects of torture and that Complex PTSD may offer a more accurate diagnosis to describe the psychological impact of torture (Herman, 1992), especially when combined with the refugee journey. Like PTSD, Complex PTSD evokes an overwhelming physiological reaction, marked by intrusions, avoidance, and hyperarousal. However, in addition to these symptoms, it also impacts the sense of self and interpersonal interactions, with chronic difficulties in identity, boundary awareness, interpersonal relatedness and affect regulation. This can often lead to withdrawal from social interactions and can have a profound impact on the identity of the person, causing difficulties with trust and intimacy.

SPIRASI'S APPROACH TO TORTURE REHABILITATION: EMPOWERMENT, CHOICE, TRUST, AND SAFETY IN GROUPWORK

In 1999, Ireland became a signatory to the United Nations Convention Against Torture and Other Cruel, Inhuman or Degrading Treatment (UNCAT) and, therefore, is legally subject to Article 14, which affirms that each state must provide "as full a rehabilitation as possible" for victims of torture within their jurisdiction. Spirasi, Ireland's centre for the rehabilitation of survivors of torture, founded in 1999 as an independent charity, is the primary organisation implementing the obligations of the Irish State under Article 14 of UNCAT. Spirasi provides holistic rehabilitative care to forced migrants who have experienced torture, through the provision of medical assessments and reports, psychotherapeutic treatment, and psychosocial and integration support. Despite efforts to streamline the international protection process in Ireland, the system remains long, arduous, and highly distressing, with applicants spending an average of five years awaiting an outcome.

Abuse of power and removal of control are at the core of torture and are used to dehumanise and disempower the victim. This is often achieved by using techniques which create uncertainty and unpredictability, preventing the victim from building coping mechanisms to tolerate the torture. As a result, we tend to see a shattering of trust in others post-torture and an inability to feel grounded and safe in both the surrounding environment and within the body. The perception of being unable to control or predict an aversive event can lead to low self-esteem, self-blame (Peterson and Seligman, 1983) and guilt (Rees, 1991). Tightly intertwined into the values of Spirasi's approach to rehabilitation are the concepts of empowerment, choice, trust, and safety. During interviews with more than 2,000 concentration camp survivors, Eitinger found that one of the most important coping mechanisms was to maintain some sense of control through retaining the ability to make a few decisions (1974). This understanding plays a key role in Spirasi's approach to rehabilitation. In Spirasi we endeavour to create systems and interventions which are client-informed, predictable, reinforce safety, and allow for growth and healing at a pace which is comfortable for the client.

It has become apparent that Complex PTSD disproportionately impacts survivors of torture seeking international protection (Hearns et al., 2021), as is the case with Spirasi's client group. Herman's 'phase model' approach of (i) safety, (ii) remembering and mourning, and (iii) integration, is widely accepted as the best overarching treatment for working with complex trauma (1992). Although these phases can overlap and be revisited, without establishing the first phase of safety there is no ethical progression to the other phases. In the phase of 'safety', the emphasis is on the importance of restoring control and power to the client. Because survivors feel unsafe in their bodies, as well as in their relations with other people, this initial phase can be supported by interventions which reduce reactivity and hyperarousal, such as body work, and through interventions which encourage peer support. The groups I discuss in this chapter take place in the safety-building phase of treatment but also include elements of the integration phase due to the relational component of groupwork.

GROUPWORK DEVELOPMENT IN SPIRASI

The desire to move towards more therapeutic-based groupwork in Spirasi grew gradually. As the therapy coordinator and a psychotherapist working in Spirasi, I attended the International Rehabilitation Council for Torture Victims (IRCT) Scientific Symposium in December 2016. There, I found several of the workshops centred on the efficacy of using groupwork in the treatment of survivors of torture. From the vast array of international presentations, it became apparent that non-Western countries employ a greater use of groups, showing that healing often takes place in the context of the community and not just the level of the individual. The most notable session was research presented by Dr Boris Drožđek. His use of a phase-based, trauma-informed approach, which used non-verbal (body work and creative) therapies with survivors of torture who sought international protection, ignited my curiosity in how to use groups whilst maintaining a sense of safety with Spirasi's client population.

To initiate the process of group development, the Spirasi therapy team explored what groups would be possible based on our skillsets, confidence, experience, resources, and, most importantly, client needs. From here, therapists put together proposals for the group they felt would be of benefit to the organisation. Giving the individual therapists freedom to develop a group based on their own skills helped to generate motivation and limit resistance. There was some trial and error, with some groups taking off and others evolving into something new. Since then, groupwork in Spirasi has grown from strength to strength and the move to groups has benefited our clients through being culturally appropriate, shortening therapy waiting times, reducing isolation, encouraging integration, helping rebuild trust and providing a more holistic experience. In 2022, there are seven different groups offered in Spirasi. All are mixed-gender groups for adults, which act as stand-alone treatment approaches as well as working well as part of a wider treatment model. A summary of each group is outlined below:

- *Trauma-Sensitive Yoga*: A safe space where we do seated breathing exercises, followed by light movements, to help connect with the body, and reduce stress and tension in the mind and body.
- *Mindful Movement Group:* This group involves gentle physical movements and relaxation activities with a focus on staying in the present, aiding relaxation and sleep.
- *Resourcing Group:* This group offers a safe space to practice stress reduction exercises to help deal with ongoing stress and reduce symptoms related to traumatic experiences.
- *Relaxation Group:* This group is a space to listen to gentle music while doing breathing exercises to relax the body and mind; helping to reduce racing thoughts, sleep difficulty, and anxiety.
- *Psychoeducation Group:* This group combines psychoeducation, cognitive-behavioural techniques, and stress reduction to facilitate a deeper understanding of trauma and its effects and to help identify and develop resiliency.
- *Parenting Group:* This group is a supportive space for parents, where experience can be shared and themes explored.
- *LGBTQ Peer Support Group:* This provides a safe space for people who identify as Lesbian, Gay, Bisexual, Transgender, or Queer (LGBTQ) to meet up and form supportive relationships.

Spirasi's groupwork approach aims to:

- Create a safe space by balancing power dynamics within the group.
- Encourage empowerment and autonomy through choice, control, and knowledge.
- Reduce or manage psychological symptoms through psychoeducation and body work.
- Create an environment which allows for safe relationships, harnessing the rebuilding of trust.
- Create an environment which minimises the mirroring of torture experiences by remaining boundaried and predictable.
- Encourage integration and limit isolation through the group and community engagement.

For the purposes of this chapter, I will limit myself to giving an overview of just two of the groups running at Spirasi: the Trauma-Sensitive Yoga Group and the LGBTQ Peer Support Group. I will outline the functionality of each group and how each aids the rehabilitation process, whilst including client testimony throughout – in keeping with Spirasi's commitment to client-informed practice.

TRAUMA-SENSITIVE YOGA GROUP: SAFETY BUILDING AT THE LEVEL OF THE BODY

As Van der Kolk states, 'the body keeps the score' (1994). Psychological pain is often held at the level of the body in individuals with complex trauma who do not have the resources required to tolerate or alleviate these experiences (Emerson and Hopper, 2011). Clients presenting in Spirasi often have a multitude of somatic complaints and are held hostage by physiological sensations related to PTSD. In addition, clients, on first presentation, do not tend to feel safe enough, or ready, to process their trauma through speech. Most of our clients are actively engaged in seeking international protection and are dealing with stressors related to their protection claim, living situation (i.e. asylum accommodation), and much more. Trauma-sensitive yoga (TSY), an intervention which helps to reduce stress, manage PTSD symptoms, restore sleep and eating rhythms in a safe way, all while aiding the client in feeling empowered and active in their rehabilitation, seemed the perfect fit for groupwork within Spirasi's rehabilitation model.

After receiving some staff training, a Trauma-Sensitive Yoga Group (TSYG) was developed in 2018. The TSYG combined approaches learned through training, which focused on gentle shapes (yoga postures) carried out while seated, and some specific TSY techniques and shapes advised by Emerson and Hopper in their book *Overcoming Trauma through Yoga: Reclaiming Your Body* (2011). The group started out running fortnightly with a small number of clients, facilitated by me, a psychotherapist with minimum yoga experience and my colleague, a non-clinician proficient in yoga. This co-facilitation partnership worked well because it has a foundation of mutual respect for the other's expertise and a recognition of how these different skill sets complement each other. Over the months that followed, more clients were referred to the TSYG. Following the move to online facilitation in 2020, due to the COVID-19 pandemic, the numbers for the group increased to 40 active members. The TSYG took place weekly and was an 'open' group, meaning new clients joined on a continuous basis. For this reason, the sessions began with an overview, communicated in lay terms, of what TSY is and how it can help. Expectations are managed by ensuring clients are aware that there is no 'quick fix' for their symptoms and that the benefits of engaging in TSY are felt over time and vary depending on the individual.

Spirasi's approach to rehabilitation is cognisant of not mirroring practices related to the torture experience. The TSYG functions in line with Spirasi's values and as such is scheduled for the same day and time every week and follows the same format to maximise predictability and a safe environment. If there is a change in our usual process, such as one of the facilitators being unavailable or the introduction of a new shape, this is communicated clearly to the clients in the group. When carrying out in-person sessions, there is no touching involved. The facilitators guide the clients through a demonstration using their own bodies only. No straps are used to enhance postures as this might be distressing and triggering for some survivors.

Managing physiological symptoms: Psychological reactions to torture can become trapped at the level of the body when the instinctual fight/flight responses to danger are activated but fail to be completed, causing the body to continue to respond as if it is under threat long after the danger has passed. This can result in a preoccupation with efforts to minimise and avoid a triggering of symptoms. TSY allows clients to gain control over visceral sensations related to PTSD through curiosity, whilst building resources and coping techniques to manage these sensations (Emerson and Hopper, 2011). When the individual becomes adept at utilising the TSY techniques, it can provide a secure base for the client to return to if they find themselves unravelling at later points in the therapeutic process and therefore can be a useful step in preparation for trauma-processing therapy. The practice of TSY has been shown to reduce physical pain being held in the body, with some clients having noted: "*I felt pain each and every day – trying to take paracetamol – ... not knowing that I need yoga, and* [when] *I did get it ... so relieved*" and

> For now I can say all the yoga sessions were good to me because my body was like it is locked, each yoga has different exercise whereby it will be useful for a certain part in my body, I think it has helped my stuffy body to relax.

All shapes are communicated by the facilitators using invitational language; reminding the clients to always be gentle with their body, never staying in a shape which causes pain, and being mindful of limits within their own body due to injury or physical impairment.

Being present: Time is taken at the beginning and end of the session to focus on grounding and being present. We encourage clients to clear a space in their mind and their day to purely focus on themselves. The use of mindfulness, to gently encourage thoughts and sensations to stay in the present during our sessions, appears to have had a substantial impact. Some clients have reported a renewed connection to their breath, speaking of "*awareness of breath*" and "*better breath*". One client spoke of a reconnection to their body:

> Since I came to Ireland some of my body parts were like dead because I couldn't feel them ... especially my neck and back. I had a severe headache which couldn't stop even if I drink a lot of water, but since with Spirasi I am relieved.

Whilst other clients were focused on increased ability to stay present in all areas of life, with one client reflecting, "[I now] *spend time with my children like before, address my trauma, find pleasure, like bodily awareness and pleasurable activities. Slow down, do less and do it with presence and mindfulness*", and another stating, "*I gain control over my mind by trying to wave out some thought that comes to my mind. It also calms my body and helps in relieving stress*".

Restoring Balance: People subjected to prolonged or repeated distress often experience dys-regulation in their body's arousal systems, resulting in a fluctuation of high arousal or complete disconnection from their bodies. Our clients have reflected on how TSY has helped restore internal biorhythms such as sleep cycles; one stated, "[It] *helps me sleep better and I use less medication now, and I can handle stress and anxiety better"*, and another commented, "*My body is less painful, and I sleep better at night due to this, due to the more relaxed nature of my mind and body it makes sleeping easier"*. Another client reflected on the reduction of intrusive imagery during sleep: "*It has helped me in sleeping longer. I fall asleep faster more especially when I use yoga music. My nightmares have reduced"*.

Making choices: TSY differs from traditional yoga practice in that nothing is forced, and limits are not pushed. Being encouraged to make choices which support personal comfort levels is key to restoring a sense of control. The fear and helplessness experienced from losing control can lead to a submissive response in which individuals fail to become active par-ticipants in their own lives (Emerson and Hopper, 2011). In our TSYG we aim to restore a sense of agency and empowerment in our clients by mobilising choice. This has proven to be an important aspect of how we deliver this group; one client reflected, "*Because some others* [shapes] *are painful or harder, so it gives me the freedom to learn it at my own pace, if a position is painful, I can do it another time"*; and another stated, "*It is important because I can do some of action freely"*. It is paramount that clients do not feel that the shapes we use in the yoga practice mirror any experiences they may have encountered through suspension, bondage or forced stress positions. To ensure a different experience, we overly emphasise the choice to move out of any shape that is not comfortable or safe for the individual at any time.

Healthy relationships: Disconnection from the body can lead not only to an imbalance of internal biorhythms but also external rhythms, preventing connection with others. The TSYG facilitates a safe environment to explore being in sync with others, through breath, shapes, movements, and the shared experience of peers (Emerson and Hopper, 2011). Integrated movement with others can create a sense of connection that goes beyond language. Exploring reconnection can be carried out through groups which have a strong emphasis on safety and boundaries. The TSYG allows for participation in a group setting without feeling pressure to engage verbally with others. Relationships within the group are built slowly at a pace that suits the individual. Clients initially tend to focus on the facilitators until their confidence builds within the group, at which point connection and empathy is observed among clients. One client reflected on the role the facilitators have in providing knowledge and certainty for purposes of stability and empowerment: "*The relationship to the facilitators is very important because it helps in asking ques-tions on some confused issues, they clear communication. And help in advanced preparations. Creating focus and encouraging"*. Another client reflected on the importance of a social connection within the group:

They [facilitators] are very important because for now I see them as my family because … every Thursday I get people to talk to, I feel very special, protected … because if someone thinks of you, even if you in a problem you will be knowing that at least Thursday I will have someone to talk to, this is very helpful to me indeed … I don't have a family here in Ireland, but I have [the group].

The TSYG plays an important role in addressing symptoms related to Complex PTSD. Learn-ing to reconnect with the body in a safe way helps with gaining control over the physical arousal symptoms and affect dysregulation which haunt and immobilise many survivors. In turn, this leads to less avoidance behaviours and a renewed sense of safety at both the level of the body and within the surrounding environment. The boundaried relationships built with the facilitators and the other group members over time serve as a template to rebuild a sense of trust in interpersonal relationships. Being treated with respect and having their attendance in the group valued helps to challenge feelings of low self-worth, prominent in those with Complex PTSD. Self-worth is also improved by the skills developed with regular attendance in the group. Clients comment on how, through practice, they make progress with the shapes, their breathing, and their ability to be mindful.

LESBIAN GAY BISEXUAL TRANSGENDER QUEER (LGBTQ) PEER SUPPORT GROUP: SAFETY BUILDING THROUGH CONNECTION

When torture is committed because the person is part of the LGBTQ community – something which is so ingrained to the person's sense of self – it can have disastrous effects on the ability to trust again. This combined with avoidance mechanisms employed to manage PTSD symptoms and the ongoing stressors associated with seeking international protection in the host country, can result in a withdrawal from the social world and a reliance on isolation to feel safe. Given that rehabilitation from interpersonal trauma requires engaging in interpersonal relationships, it is important that peer support is explored within a group context for this population. Peer support creates a space of equal standing. The role of the facilitator, who is also an LGBTQ peer, is simply to support and put into action the client-led approach.

The majority of Spirasi clients remain in an unstable legal situation for many years. We observe that our LGBTQ clients suffer additional distress living within the asylum accommodation system due to ongoing discrimination. The lack of privacy within the accommodation centres and lack of access to social and integration supports results in our LGBTQ clients feeling fearful, alone, and at times suicidal. For many, joining the LGBTQ Peer Support Group is the first opportunity they have had to connect with peers in Ireland. One client reflected, *"Spirasi LGBT group meetings is my first life experience and I found it very helping"*. Another client stated, *"Spirasi is home to me. They welcomed me. Something which was not considered in my home country"*.

The group began in 2017, as a response to the growing number of clients being referred into the organisation and as a response to the deep shame I observed in some of the LGBTQ clients I was working with through individual therapy. In one session, a lesbian client tearfully pleaded with me to *"fix"* her. It was the catalyst I needed to develop the LGBTQ group. It was slow beginnings with sometimes as few as two clients turning up to sessions. It took a while to figure out what direction the group should take. Initially, I had envisioned a place for clients to meet each other and form connections in a natural way by providing a safe space to do so. However, I found that clients were hesitant to interact socially and distrustful of engaging with anyone other than me, as facilitator. Nonetheless, over the years the group began to grow, and different approaches were tried to encourage engagement, i.e. art therapy projects, games, psychoeducation, cultural diversity discussions, and inviting in external speakers. Some approaches worked better than others. After much discussion within the group, the clients made clear their preferences for the direction of the group. The main theme vocalised was that of support, connection, and belonging, with clients stating that their reasons for joining the group were: *"to meet other members of the LGBT* [community] *and have a sense of belonging which I never had in my country"*, and *"love and support"* and *"to help know that I am important as the person I choose to be"*.

As a result, the LGBTQ Peer Support Group now focuses on empowering individuals through knowledge and information, whilst facilitating a safe space for the exploration of healthy interpersonal relationships. Clients have reflected on their experience of this approach, noting the importance of peer connection and empowerment through knowledge:

> Through the group I have managed to make friends and also to get some information through other people who came in to talk to us about the law and belonging in the LGBT family, i.e. the law about raising kids as gay or lesbian couples.

Another stated, "*I learned about many things, for example about sexually transmitted diseases, tests, test centres, and prevention from HIV; and about our rights.*" In keeping with Spirasi's rehabilitation values it is important that clients feel safe in all Spirasi interventions and interactions. This came through strongly in client feedback, with one client reflecting, "*I feel safe. At least to me it feels like my own community sort of, and I know the people in the group understand me better than any other people who are not from the LGBT family/community*" and another client commenting, "*There is peace of mind, body, and soul*". However, not everyone's experience is the same and some clients are still cautious about how safe the group is. One stated, "*I feel it safe to some extent, but I am afraid someone from the group can tell about us outside of the group to some and which is bad for our privacy.*"

Although there is a steady stream of new clients, there is also a core of long-term clients, who have been active in the group for two or three years. This combination works well as it ensures stability whilst keeping fresh perspectives, which encourages engagement. In 2020, the LGBTQ Peer Support Group moved online, and by 2020 there were 30 clients in the group and more being referred in almost weekly. Rebuilding safe relationships with peers has become central to the client experience in the group. The benefits of the group for our clients have ranged from the individual to the community. Clients speak of belonging: "*I love the sense of belonging*", and restoration of self-worth: "*believing in myself and accepting who I am and what I am*". When speaking about how the group had impacted them another client described, "*a lot [of] self-esteem and being confident about myself*". Clients varied in their views about the role of connection within the group and relationships with the facilitator and with other group members. Some newer clients had yet to trust the relational aspects of the group, with one stating they were not quite there yet but remained hopeful: "*Not really but it's something we still working on.*" Others express a deep sense of belonging and connection to both the facilitator and other group members with comments such as: "*This is home to me*" and "*I feel it as my family, and I feel [the facilitator] as our Guardian*".

What is remarkable is the sense of connection and powerful bonds which are enabled through the group. Some clients remarked on the impact participating in the group has had on forming interpersonal relationships and being confident in who they are with statements such as, "*We are all like a family and found brothers and sisters I couldn't find before*", and "*I was beginning to question who I really am and had lost hope of being happy again but since I joined the group, I am more confident and I have never been proud of who I am like now*", and also, "*In knowing that I am not the only one – acknowledgement by people of the same sexual group [is the] uttermost mental support*". The LGBTQ Peer Support Group helps pave the way for interpersonal connection and integration outside of the group; a client reflected, "*LGBT group of Spirasi helped me to integrate by communicating with different people*". It can help clients to feel a sense of belonging in their new community; one client stated, "*I now fit in the society without being judged by my sexuality*" and another remarked, "*With the help of LGBTQ in Spirasi, I see Ireland as home now*". All of these aspects go towards treating the psychopathology associated with Complex PTSD. Spirasi's values of empowerment, choice, trust and safety, have provided a strong foundation for building a space for group members to explore who they are without the threat of shame or rejection. Being part of the group has helped to normalise being LGBTQ, thus challenging issues relating to low self-worth and ensuring a gay-affirmative approach, as promoted by Spirasi.

MY LEARNINGS AS A FACILITATOR

My learnings focus mainly on the role of a group facilitator. The relationship with the facilitator forms an important template for how to approach building new, healthy and boundaried relationships. As such, power dynamics must be continuously monitored by the facilitator(s) to ensure clients maintain a sense of control, autonomy, and choice. As facilitator it can be easy to slip (or be placed) in the position of expert, or, as one client notes, the position of the parent:

> [The facilitator] is very professional, and she is giving equal importance to all the group participants and if she is not there, we will not be able to have such wonderful meetings. I consider her as our mother who accepts us as gay. I regret that my actual parents never accepted me as a gay or a transgender.

Being seen as a mother, in relation to a caring, supportive and stabilising presence can be beneficial for the group; however, the mother is also traditionally a powerful position in the family group and, therefore, as a facilitator, I need to remain consistently mindful of the possible imbalance of power. To ensure the generation of healthy equal relationships the facilitator needs to be aware of implementing a client-led approach and communicating vulnerability in relation to who they are as a person, as well as curiosity about the clients' experiences and an openness to learning client-informed approaches to healing. Co-facilitation, as in the TSYG, is also helpful as each facilitator can observe and help address any unconscious bias or issues with power and boundaries. I have learned that remaining humble and retaining a sense of humility are key.

ONLINE DELIVERY OF GROUPS

During the COVID-19 pandemic we saw an escalation in need within our client group and an exacerbation of psychopathology. Due to the pandemic, Spirasi's services moved to online platforms in March 2020. This was a learning curve and came with many challenges as well as possibilities. The challenges centred on a myriad of technology difficulties and privacy concerns. However, some positive outcomes emerged. Due to the geographical spread of clients throughout Ireland some clients travel five hours each way to attend appointments, often missing meals, and having to find childcare support for long periods of time. The move to delivering group sessions online has created ease of access for these clients. In addition, because we are not limited in physical space when using an online platform, we have been able to offer more clients a place in the groups. This has helped reduce waiting lists, ensured a speedier engagement for rehabilitation, and helped tackle the heightened isolation experienced during the pandemic. The online format has allowed us to offer additional choices to clients in terms of engagement. Our clients are encouraged to honour their comfort level regarding participation in the group. Some silently observe the group dynamic for as long as they require, whilst others actively participate. Being able to control being seen, by use of their camera, has allowed for clients to be present without feeling exposed. It has also facilitated more control over the client's physical environment, i.e. temperature of the room and level of light. Also, if a client is feeling triggered by something that arises in the group, they can mute the sound for a period until feeling ready to re-join or opt to leave relatively undetected (in which case the facilitator would follow up privately with this client afterwards). Some of these elements to online groupwork have been so successful that Spirasi plans to include a blended approach post-pandemic, where clients can choose to attend in person or online.

CONCLUSION

The shift in focus to non-Western approaches to healing has expanded the way we look at the impact of traumatic events on the psyche and the body. Interpersonal trauma requires healing at an interpersonal level. Human beings have always lived communally, having developed and evolved in the context of relational belonging, due to our prolonged period of helplessness from birth (Yalom and Leszcz, 2005). It makes sense then that treatment for trauma benefits from a relational setting. Rehabilitation centres in Western counties tend to work with clients that are culturally diverse, with the overwhelming majority coming from cultures which are more collective, than individualistic, in nature. Given that collective cultures often engage a group approach to healing, it is helpful for group interventions carried out in Western countries to modify their approaches to allow for a more inclusive, diverse style which is culturally informed (Yalom and Leszcz, 2005). Groupwork in Spirasi, exampled by the two groups discussed above, remains an evolving process. New information, new learnings and new situations continue to reveal fresh challenges and solutions. For these reasons we are conscious of remaining open and flexible whilst still relying on our core values of empowerment, choice, trust and safety to keep us grounded in our approach.

REFERENCES

Crumlish, N. and Bracken, P. (2011) 'Mental health and the asylum process', *Irish Journal of Psychological Medicine*, *28*(2), pp. 57–60. doi:10.1017/S0790966700011447.

de C Williams, A. C. and van der Merwe, J. (2013) 'The psychological impact of torture', *British Journal of Pain*, *7*(2), pp. 101–106. doi:10.1177/2049463713483596.

Eitinger, L. (1974) 'Coping with aggression', *Mental Health & Society*, *1*(5–6), pp. 297–301.

Emerson, D. and Hopper, E. (2011) *Overcoming Trauma Through Yoga: Reclaiming Your Body*. Berkeley, CA: North Atlantic Books.

Hearns, A., Hyland, P., Benninger-Budel, C. and Vallières, F. (2021) 'ICD-11 PTSD and CPTSD: Implications for the rehabilitation of survivors of torture seeking international protection', *Torture Journal*, *31*(3), pp. 96–112. doi:10.7146/torture.v32i3.125780.

Herman, J. (1992) *Trauma and Recovery: The Aftermath of Violence--from Domestic Abuse to Political Terror*. Herman, MD: Hachette.

Peterson, C. and Seligman, M. E. (1983) 'Learned helplessness and victimization', *Journal of Social Issues*, *39*(2), pp. 103–116. doi:10.1111/j.1540-4560.1983.tb00143.x.

Poole, D. N., Hedt-Gauthier, B., Liao, S., Raymond, N. A. and Bärnighausen, T. (2018) 'Major depressive disorder prevalence and risk factors among Syrian asylum seekers in Greece', *BMC Public Health*, *18*(1), p. 908. doi:10.1186/s12889-018-5822-x.

Rees, L. (1991) 'Psychology and torture – Edited by Peter Suedfeld', *Stress Medicine*, *7*(2), 137–138. doi:10.1002/smi.2460070223.

Schick, M., Zumwald, A., Knöpfli, B., Nickerson, A., Bryant, R., Schnyder, U., Müller, J. and Morina, N. (2016) 'Challenging future, challenging past: The relationship of social integration and psychological impairment in traumatized refugees', *European Journal of Psychotraumatology*, 7:1, p. 28057. doi:10.3402/ejpt.v7.28057.

Silove, D., Ventevogel, P. and Rees, S. (2017) 'The contemporary refugee crisis: An overview of mental health challenges', *World Psychiatry*, *16*(2), pp. 130–139. doi:10.1002/wps.20438.

Steel, Z., Chey, T., Silove, D., Marnane, C., Bryant, R. A. and van Ommeren, M. (2009) 'Association of torture and other potentially traumatic events with mental health outcomes among populations exposed to mass conflict and displacement: A systematic review and meta-analysis', *Jama*, *302*(5), pp. 537–549. doi:10.1001/jama.2009.1132.

Stevenson, K., Rall, J., Bussey, M. and Wise, J. (2007) *Transforming the Trauma of Torture, Flight, and Resettlement*. New York: Columbia University Press.

van der Kolk, B. (1994) 'The body keeps the score: Memory and the evolving psychobiology of post-traumatic stress', *Harvard Review of Psychiatry*, 1:5, pp. 253–265. doi:10.3109/10673229409017088.

Wilson, F. E., Hennessy, E., Dooley, B., Kelly, B. D. and Ryan, D. A. (2013) 'Trauma and PTSD rates in an Irish psychiatric population: A comparison of native and immigrant samples', *Disaster Health*, *1*(2), pp. 74–83. doi:10.4161/dish.27366.

Yalom, I. D. and Leszcz, M. C. (2005) *The Theory and Practice of Group Psychotherapy*. New York: Basic Books.

CHAPTER 13

HOMELANDS AND NEW LANDS

Artmaking with refugee survivors of human rights abuses

Amanda Bingley, Emma Rose and Macarena Rioseco

I feel good to do art together with other people. The people inspired me to get out again … I make art about my country, my home, my city. I feel sad because of so many bad memories. But I feel good to do art together with other people. Alizia.

(AoR1)

As Alizia explains, it can feel good to do art together and this may be an inspiration to connect with others beyond the group. In this chapter, we draw on our research on art in recovery designed to contribute to better understand how group "participatory" artmaking can support improved mental health and recovery from human rights abuses. We describe and discuss the process and experiences of participatory artmaking that facilitated the artworks and group interactions.

The participatory art groupwork was based on working with different groups of participants, who were survivors of torture seeking refuge in the UK over several years, from a wide range of countries of origin. They were all in psychological therapy with Freedom from Torture (FfT) as part of a comprehensive rehabilitation approach. We outline our definition of participatory art and the specific context of the groupwork. We explain the thinking and values behind the development and direction of the participatory artmaking and describe the action research "co-design" model we used for the projects, and how this was applied to the groupwork. We note how these approaches and theories can be applied in this and other community and participatory art research. The outcome and impact of the art group is discussed and explored from the perspective of the participants, the interpreters, and therapists. We contribute our reflections as the research team noting the importance of the dynamic of the group, the use of a range of art materials and the facilitation of the artmaking. We describe the ways creative expression appears to work for people as they share their images and thoughts. We stress the need for a supportive and calm space for the artmaking and to have well established links with other therapeutic support.

ART OF RECOVERY PROJECTS

These two small projects explored how participatory art contributes to therapeutic recovery for survivors of torture: "Art of Recovery: Supporting Refugees Traumatised by Torture" (Rose et al., 2018) and in 2019, "Art of Recovery: Migrating Landscapes". Both projects were designed by a research team based at Lancaster University UK in collaboration with the Manchester FfT Centre. The design drew on an earlier pilot study of participatory art with a small refugee group based in Liverpool, UK (Rose and Bingley, 2017). Members of the team brought skills gained from other participatory artwork with a range of groups, including older people in the UK, children and young people exploring resilience in disasters in five European countries, children and young people recovering as a community from flood disasters in the UK, and adults exploring landscape perception through tactile art. The Art of Recovery (AoR) projects were designed in response to the need to explore different approaches of support specifically for a refugee population, many of whom are at risk of severe mental health issues (UNHCR, 2018) and considered to be a global priority (WHO, 2019). There are, as yet, few examples of

DOI: 10.4324/9781003192978-16

research in participatory arts with refugees, but these have shown benefits (Stavropoulou, 2019; Andemicael, 2011). There are more examples of research with community arts, especially in mental health, that have demonstrated the value and support of participatory artmaking (Stickley, 2011).

The research was designed as participatory action research or "co-design", where the research team set up the basic design and then met with therapists, staff, interpreters, and where possible potential participants to discuss the research design, ensuring this addressed the needs of the group. The design allows a continuous reflection over the project, through discussion and debriefing during and after sessions, with the research team, participants, interpreters and therapists. The participants often take their reflections about their artwork into therapy sessions and build on this in subsequent art groupwork. The basic premise is to facilitate and support the process of the artmaking.

The first AoR1 project ran for five weeks. The second more substantive project, AoR2, involved the research team designing ten consecutive weeks of participatory art workshops. Data collection, although including a well-being questionnaire as a quantitative measure, was primarily qualitative (artwork, interviews, and discussions) and it is this aspect we draw on for the chapter. Participants could make paintings, drawings, and collage from acrylic paints and tactile materials, such as clay, sand, felt, wool, stones and feathers. In each workshop participants were invited to explore their imagined or real spaces and places experienced as healing and supportive, either recalled from their country of origin or experienced on their journey towards safety. The places could also be imagined as somewhere they experience now or would like to go in the future. During each workshop session, we ensured that there were interpreters for the languages spoken by participants and a therapist was present if extra support was needed.

Recruitment was undertaken by the charity: therapists invited participants they felt were at a stage in their recovery where they could benefit from participatory arts, especially those who were reluctant to join other group activities. Participants originated from Afghanistan, Cameroon, the Central African Republic, the Democratic Republic of Congo, Iran, Rwanda, Sri Lanka and Togo. Over both projects the team and therapists noted that the group did not work for everyone, particularly if they were still in a highly vulnerable stage of their recovery. In that situation, being in the group as well as taking part in the artmaking could feel overwhelming. This emphasises the importance of ensuring participants have therapeutic support and a chance to discuss taking part in the groupwork, and have some interest in arts and crafts. To this end, before the start of the workshops the team met with the interpreters supporting their clients in the sessions, to explain and discuss the research, the consent process and art activities. We also discussed possible cultural differences in interpretation of artworks. Ethical approval was obtained from the Lancaster University Ethics Committee and from FfT. Informed consent was given by all participants, all names used here are pseudonyms.

THEORIES AND INFLUENCES

Therapeutic landscapes

The idea of a therapeutic landscape suggests people attribute qualities of healing to certain spaces and places. Initiated by Gesler (1993), the concept at first focused on spiritual sites and health settings, and others then explored how different types of landscape, places and spaces, can benefit health and wellbeing (Williams, 2007). By 2021, the concept reflects 30 years of wide-ranging research around material, physical, psychological, social and symbolic spaces associated with healing (see Rose and Bingley, 2017 and Bell et al., 2018). Key texts informing our approach include Perriam (2015), who examines the relationship between place, spirituality and healing, exploring healing as a search for wholeness, implying potential for re-assemblage of a fragmented self. Here healing is not a cure, but an alleviation, a possible reduction in the severity of symptoms and improvement in the quality of life.

Therapeutic landscape literature also indicates the wellbeing potential of *imagining* beneficial places (Kearns and Andrews, 2010; Rose, 2012) in addition or instead of their physical encounter. This concept provided another dimension to our approach, as we encouraged participants to imagine, re-imagine, or remember a past or present place experienced as a safe haven, or journey towards safety, a place they felt had some therapeutic potential. The work of Gestaldo et al. (2004) was relevant in prompting us to consider aligning therapeutic landscapes with experiences of migration and strategies to improve mental wellbeing through artmaking. Gestaldo et al. explore how personalised place-related memories, particularly those associated with "home" and safety evoked through memory, narrative and artistic representation, provide migrants with therapeutic coping strategies beneficial to mental wellbeing. The therapeutic landscape concept provided the underpinning premise that re-imagined representations of landscape, realised in the form of artworks, might provide participants with the experience of a mental and physical place with potential to contribute to healing.

Herman's three-stage model of recovery

We drew on Herman's (1992) three-stage model of recovery from trauma (for more detailed explanation, see Rose et al., 2018) to frame how group artmaking contributes to recovery for survivors of torture. Herman identifies three key stages in the process of recovery, namely: safety; remembrance and mourning; and reconnection. The model emphasises empowerment of the survivor and the creation of new connections, supporting processes of re-integration. We recruited individuals who had established a relative level of security and safety in their new environment and were receiving individual therapy. This facilitated the safety of using imaginary scenes or being able to see real traumatic events at a distance outside of the body, making them less emotionally distressing. Participants' artworks reflected various representations of their past and present lives; sometimes they reflected on past events, and at other times they explored their present circumstances, and the ongoing task of forging relationships within their new land. At different stages, each individual made artworks about their present lives and experiences of reconnection and/or re-integration, conveying the changed person they had become.

Therapeutic holding

Psychoanalytic theory refers to Donald Winnicott's idea of "holding" and the "holding environment" (1953) that describes the optimal environment for "good enough" parenting, a concept that also informed the group workshops. Briefly, an infant provided with an adequate environment for emotional development allows them to become progressively aware of thoughts and feelings as their parent/carer relates to them, in ways that meaningfully mirror feelings as they occur. The child is supported to regulate, manage and tolerate their feelings. The parent handles the child's projection of painful, angry, unbearable feelings, returning them to the child in a modified, contained way (Winnicott, 1967). The therapist provides a similar function helping an adult client work through their emotions.

We identified similarities with Winnicott's concept of holding and the process of working in group artmaking. Through artmaking, experiences and thoughts can be reflected upon and explored, enabling an individual to contemplate them without being overwhelmed. Participants can set their own pace in introducing and re-framing a range of different images of the past and present without being overwhelmed. This may include positive or poignant, joyful or painful experiences and their associated mental states. In this way, through the artwork we suggest individuals in the group could be supported in the "holding environment" to re-think emotional experiences. This was also helpful in individual therapeutic sessions, where they were engaged in learning to contain their feelings, even when facing traumatic memories associated with remembrance and mourning.

PARTICIPATORY ARTMAKING: CREATING AND HOLDING THE SPACE

Successful groupwork requires careful attention to the group environment. Both AoR projects were held in a quiet space, familiar to the participants and large enough for everyone to work in small groups with tables for the artmaking. The room was set up with art materials ready for the start of each session. The research team brought a range of practical art skills and expertise in painting and in tactile 3D artmaking. The first session included basic painting skills, with each small group working on the same large table-sized sheet, trying out different brush strokes in their painting and exploring collage materials. This helped to lay the foundation for everyone to begin to build technical art skills and gain confidence, regardless of any previous experience of artmaking. Anyone joining the workshops later in the project was taught these basic art skills. In these ways, we aimed to offer a space where participants felt supported and "held" as they worked with their art. In other similar artmaking groups, another first exercise found to be relaxing is sandplay and 3D collage; an approach also later used in the AoR sessions.

The prompt for the artmaking maintained the same theme throughout (except the final session), to portray a landscape as space or place, real or imagined, from the past or present that represented healing. As the images were completed the participant could talk with a member of the research team about the images they created. This reflection on their images, the feelings and thoughts evoked was as important to the groupwork as the artmaking. We also found that when participants are sharing thoughts on their artworks, interpreter support is as crucial a role as in therapy situations (Mirdal et al., 2012).

There are three aspects integral to these experiences that emerge. First, participants' thoughts about the artmaking, gaining practical art skills and learning how to work with the materials. Second, the kinds of artwork they produced, prompted by the suggestion to portray a healing space or place, and the significance of their images in the context of their current lives. Third, reflections on joining and becoming part of the group as a social experience with participatory art as an opportunity to share artmaking.

ARTMAKING IN THE GROUP

The painting shows a baobab tree, a single bird flies around its canopy. This is Claudia's memory of the place where the villagers gathered to talk, share food, resolve troubles, and consider community issues (Figure 13.1).

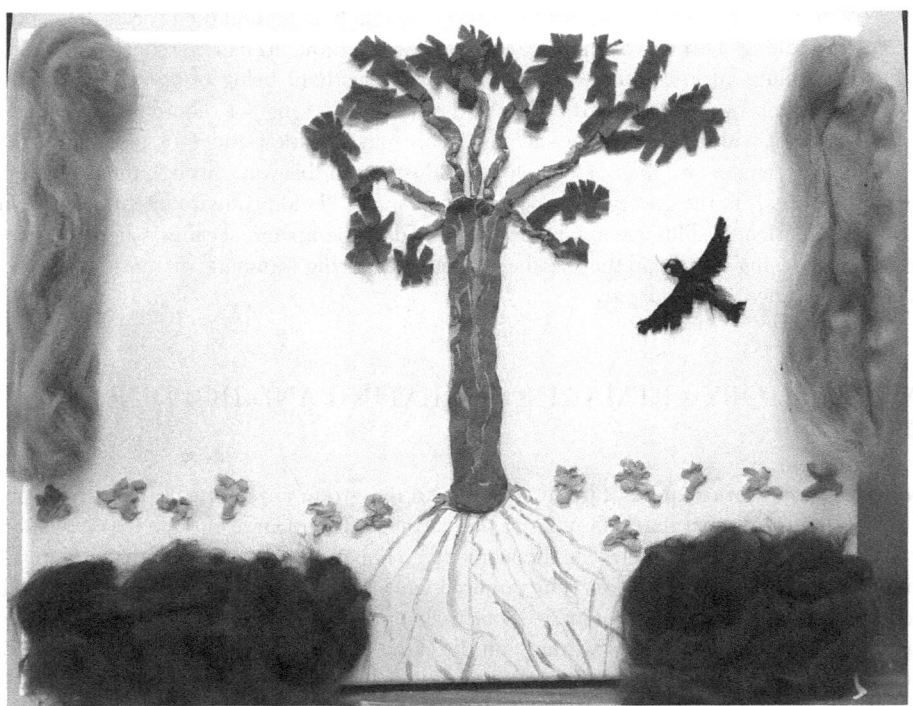

Figure 13.1 Claudia: the baobab

Claudia had participated in the art group for nearly two months. The baobab, as a meeting place, appeared to reflect both the poignancy of her lost home and also the present experience portrayed of the art group, as a shared space to participate in artmaking. The journey of these artworks is both deeply personal and reflected a group endeavour in artmaking as a shared healing. This process inevitably drew out a range of poignant memories of home, the tragedies that led to each person's current situation as a refugee, and the challenges of their present life. Recovery and healing are expressed in myriad ways. The art group evolved over the weeks to arrive at the place of the baobab tree.

In Workshop 6, one of the group participants created a clay and sand model of a cassava grinding and cooking pot, a memory of their community where everyone joined to cook and eat a meal. The scene was one of sharing, and suddenly in the art group, sitting around the table together, the participants started to interact and share imaginary food. They laughed together – this was a first – the interpreters translating their jokes, and for moments the mood lightened. They had been meeting for six weeks before this point of breakthrough into a shared present, emerging unexpectedly in a group where people had gradually gained confidence in their art-making, and through their artwork created many scenes from past and present. Up to this point, the emphasis tended to be on the individual's art, not immediately related to being in a group, though held in the supportive collective space. The clay, sand and collage artmaking represented a shift in the group dynamic, allowing individuals to feel part of a group in a playful space, to take a risk of interacting together through the powerful medium of their art. The evolution deepened further in the last session of the ten-week project when we focused on creating art around food – eliciting a sense of group nourishment in playful modelling and painting of fruit and vegetables grown on allotments, or memories of favourite foods from their home countries.

In interviews, and discussions during sessions, people reflected on these artmaking experiences:

It is good, make[s] me happy and it's good and changed my mind when I've been here. Totally is different. Think about other thing [s] when I come here and enjoy it. It's very good for my mind and … it really relieves me [to] come here and join the group because all [my] mind conjured up art … so I really enjoy it… Wasim.

(AoR2)

Yeah definitely [coming to the art group helped] because I've never done that, where in doing that I feel like it's very something very good to do sometimes … when sometime maybe you are depressive you can try and do that and get away from the bad things, thoughts on your head, so yeah it was nice. Claudia.

(AoR2)

Claudia also reflected on talking about and sharing pictures together in a group: "…*it was a very good experience … it's sometimes nostalgic, and at the same time it's… educative sometimes, somehow and you know nostalgic and educative…*" (AoR2)

Many participants had no experience of artmaking prior to this groupwork. For instance, in AoR2 only four of the twelve participants had studied or even played with art materials, such as painting or drawing, in school or college (three in school and one in college since being in this country). Two participants had experience in wool, hairdressing, or cookery crafts. For most people, this was the first time in their lives they had an opportunity to learn art skills, as explained by Karnou and Pierre when asked if or how the experience of the group artmaking might or not have changed them.

Karnou reflected:

Yeah, I feel different about the picture. I made it because I never made any painting before. This is my first time, so make me feel myself, maybe I can do more than this …

(AoR2)

Pierre explained:

I never do something like that before, to draw something out put on the paper and all, this is my first time just to imagine something to do it so this is my first time so for me it's fine, so I would like to just keep it going you know.

(AoR2)

Having support to gain confidence in trying out art ideas was found invaluable, and enabled people to engage with the group, especially if they arrived feeling particularly sad and without many ideas. For example, one interpreter observing that one person *"had a slow start, didn't feel she had any ideas what to do, unmotivated and low…"*, she then … *"asked for help from M* [research team artist] *and started to engage with the art and with the others on her table, laughing together and she enjoyed the art"* (AoR2).

This emphasised the importance of the convenors of the art group having art skills and/or experience of convening these kinds of creative art groups using 2D or 3D materials. Gaining skills means there is a general sense of the group sessions becoming more aligned as a shared, non-judgemental supportive activity, which also allows a certain playfulness in the artmaking.

Images created in the artmaking

As noted above, people created images of their homeland and these could be nostalgic, evoking sometimes difficult feelings, and also portray the range of challenges and positive experiences of current life as a refugee. The act of sharing these past and present times through the art was an opportunity to tell a piece of their story, to recall past times, to share the challenges in the group. As we discuss below, participatory art has a storytelling function that is shared, supportively witnessed and often expressing spaces and places that have not been shown before. Images can be highly evocative, telling people's stories through the medium of art, the colours and tactile memory, the shapes and different elements of landscape (trees, animals, people, villages or towns, past village customs or events). A number of images were created depicting the organisation's building or representing the support and safety of the charity, as Wasim explained in his picture of a man walking with an umbrella surrounded by birds (Figure 13.2):

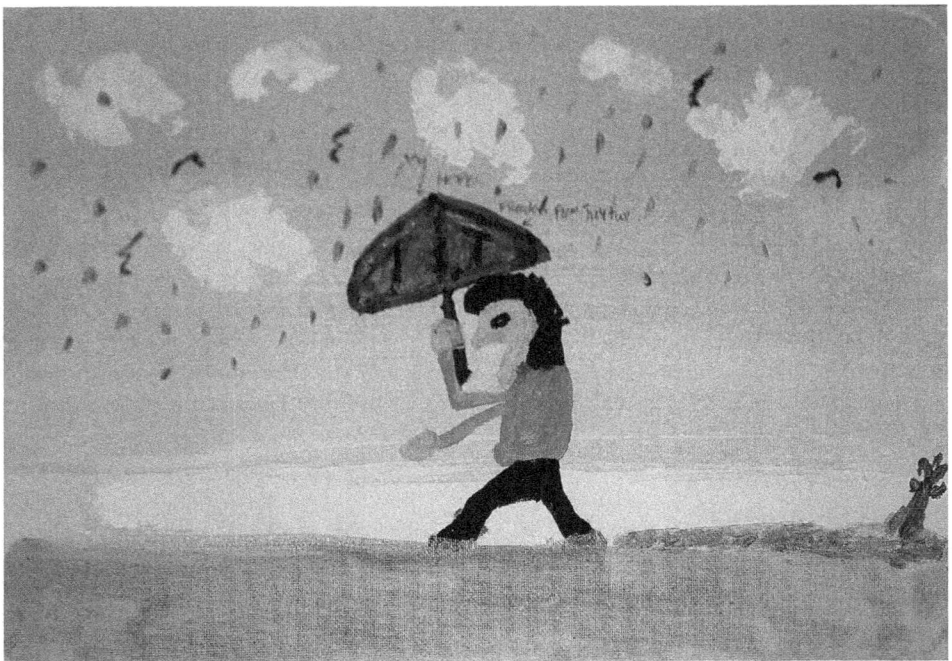

Figure 13.2 Wasim: the umbrella

> The umbrella still is [the charity supporting him]. Without [it] I'm nothing. So, clouds/rain/ sun saved by [it] from anything. The tree is distant, 19 years ago green – but now brown. Still walking and if go out from under the umbrella I'm not safe … keep walking – couldn't reach my own place. Not free now, keep walking, to get anything … so difficult. The umbrella is the safe place – when I have this, I'm safe.
>
> (AoR2)

These images often include tragic memories of conflict, loss and migration. For instance, this is vividly portrayed by Claudia, who created a collage of a boat with people falling off the sides. She commented on the contrast with this picture to her earlier one of village life around the church.

> With the church [picture] is something that I like going, it's happy. Then this one is something that makes me annoyed all the time, this one [points at her boat picture] … You see many people are dying crossing this one, the sea, to come abroad.
>
> (AoR2)

Likewise, Maria painted a series of pictures illustrating with great poignancy the loss of her children, including this painting depicting the distance between her and her children. Over four weeks her story emerged through her artwork, shared in the group (Figure 13.3).

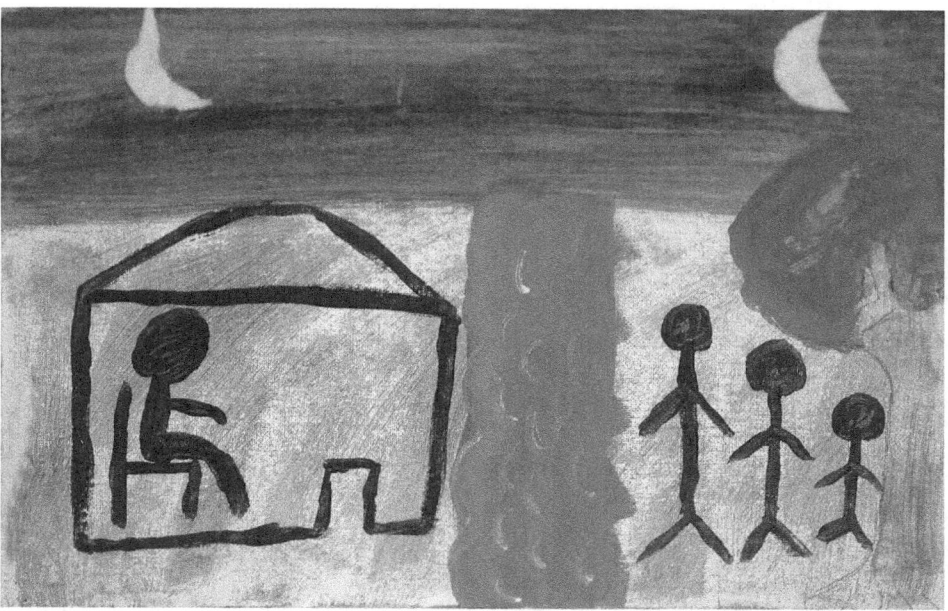

Figure 13.3 Maria: the distance of her children

> The story behind my painting is telling about the distance between me and my children. I am in the UK and the ocean separate me and my children, I do not know when I will be able to be reunited with them. Even though I am in the UK, I am safer here than I was in my country, But I miss my children a lot and the same for them I am lonely, isolated without them.
>
> (AoR2)

In later sessions, she started to touch on some positive aspects of her present life and found ways to imagine and share these memories in the group through her artwork. In the first, she modelled a collage of a Moses basket, where the infant may find safety. In the second, she painted a rainbow flag sharing a celebration of her current life.

These images are often a powerful depiction of people's experience of that space and how it feels to share the story in art. The images of positive and healing spaces are also how individuals can feel supported to hold and share that memory and integrate it into their current lives. As Karnou pointed out as he talked about his picture of a huge sun:

> it help[s] to tell other people about it, they can think about it now. You can find the beautiful sun like that. Maybe if I'm there I'll remember this place, because it can be different, travel anywhere, [and] maybe I can't go this place anymore so…
>
> (AoR2)

As people described some of the images, they emphasised not only the importance of the art-making but also their pride in having created these powerful images. Pierre, for instance, was describing his picture of his past life as a miner in a rural area of his homeland. He was clearly proud of not only his past work in the industry but in his artwork: *"You see that picture I made for our village, when the people work about diamond, so now it feels very, it looked like the real one, exactly a similar one we have so very nice."* He later reiterated the importance of sharing these past memories whether good or bad:

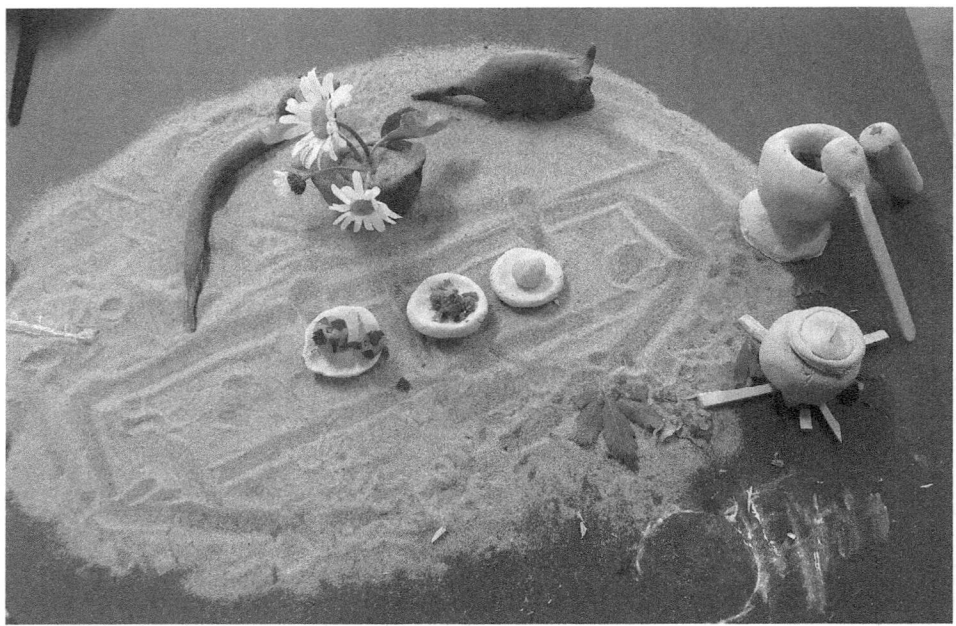

Figure 13.4 Karnou: The whale, cassava grinding and cooking pots

> Yeah, just remind me the good past we had before, before we enter this country, so we had a good past and we had a bad past as well, so all of that is to, used to remember everything, so that's fine.
>
> (AoR2)

In the later sessions, more playful elements occurring in the making of some images are seen. Karnou describes creating his 3D artwork of past times in his village making and sharing food. He explains that first he made a large model of a rat being chased by a snake round a flowerpot – the model is *"out of my head"*. Then he modelled a whale in a blue wool river around the house in the sand with the flowerpot. As he worked on his model there was laughter in the group as he added the blue wool for the river. Using clay, he modelled a pestle and mortar to grind cassava paste with palm oil and fashioned a cooking pot, with an imaginary fire underneath and a dish of food with meat. He went on to share the imaginary food dish with Claudia, who was sat next to him in the small group. This created lots of laughter around the table and the atmosphere became lighter and the group relaxed in a new way together (Team reflections AoR2) (Figure 13.4).

The theme of food was specifically worked with in the last session in AoR2, and Karnou painted a picture of his life now, of a stove and frying pan to cook fish, saying that this was reminiscent of cooking his favourite fish in his homeland.

Evolving social aspects of artmaking in a group

Being part of the art group was considered an important, if not essential, aspect of gaining the art skills and creating these artworks. The group was felt to have a social function that evolved and was helped by the participatory nature of the artmaking; this was emphasised by many participants in both projects. As Karnou reflected in his interview at the end of the project:

The more important for me to meet with the people, I want to be friends with people. I don't want to be alone, 'cos when I be alone too much thinking and then maybe some bad thing can come in my in there, so I can do something wrong to myself. I want to be with the people and in this group, I'd like to be in this group all the time.

(AoR2)

Pierre talked about how bringing a group of people together to do group artmaking supported him to gain art skills, and also encouraged people to enjoy the art and share their laughter:

The point is very good, is very important to people one, two, three, five, more than that, to sit down, to change your idea of, to design. To do something is very good than yourself, when you are yourself you can't do nothing. But when you talk, you're laughing, we do something we enjoy, this is perfect, in that way I want to yeah, I want there to be a community too.

(AoR2)

Samuel commented on the therapeutic and creative aspect of being part of a group, in his case football as well as the art group. He felt that these groups are especially helpful for other refugees. As he says:

It helped me better, it complete[s] my therapy, like all time to do or take your medicine it complete[s] that. Even though I all time I like to play football, to join art group or do something creative thing or learn another thing. … I really appreciate if it you are a new refugee to have a new relationship to other people … yeah very welcome to me.

(AoR2)

The therapists commented on the impact of the group artmaking for some of their clients, opening up new aspects of their past and present lives and helping their therapeutic process. They gave an example of one participant who had created a past scene in their artmaking that they had not shared before, and this opened up new elements in their therapy.

The social aspect of groupwork, in particular, was felt to contribute to people gaining confidence. In AoR1, Fahad reflected that being in the group was: *"Positive, helped me feel confident and comfortable among others … it is a good distraction, it also helped me to socialise and mix with others."* Other people in that art group raised the point that the very effect of working together and sharing ideas and the stories behind their artworks was an important part of the group experience. For example, Mahamadou found the experience: *"… very motivating, because we exchange ideas"*. This was echoed by Errolvie, who explained how motivating it was … *"as we were sharing stories behind our drawings"*. Chathuri pointed out that it was very interesting: *"because we discuss what is very special behind our drawings"*.

See the Project 'toolkit', a series of cards about running participatory art groups for more of the artwork and information about the AoR Projects. In the next section, we discuss what our team and the participants involved learned from these participatory art groups. We note how artmaking as groupwork appears to support people who are in recovery from serious human rights abuses.

DISCUSSION: BENEFITS AND CHALLENGES OF PARTICIPATORY ART IN A REFUGEE CONTEXT

Exchanging stories, sharing what is special behind the art, feeling gradually more skilled and confident, means that over time the art group becomes a place of shared enterprise – a creative recovering as part of a supportive group that facilitates collective healing. This is what our participants have told us and what we also saw evolving over the workshops. Integral to the design of the AoR projects was the importance of the group in participatory artmaking, and the focus on art as the medium for expression of spaces and places associated with safety or healing. There are several important aspects to this phenomenon that revolve around the concept of the potential for healing and recovery through a shared experience of gaining art skills and artmaking as storytelling within a group (Gavron, 2020; Rose et al., 2021). The active witnessing of a shared story in artmaking by the group is key to this process, as well as the making and doing around the same table, sharing art materials and ideas for design, all that is involved in artmaking as a group activity and the group as a social interaction. An essential aspect is the potential for people in the group to re-discover their playfulness and sharing their laughter in the artmaking. Other participatory art and craft projects have noticed these benefits. For example, Smith (2021, p. 151) described a similar potential for recovery in a craft group for people with long-term mental health issues, where the group sharing of craft skills "emphasised wellness through making" and in "curating a space of recovery" supported "social flourishing".

As described above, we drew on different theories in designing the participatory art projects and in helping to make sense of participants' experiences in their artmaking. This included how we set up the room as a supportive space; co-designed the sessions and worked with the theme of healing spaces and places; the way we facilitated the sharing of the art during each session; and explored our interpretations of the group's artwork and participants' individual reflections. We specifically took the approach of the therapeutic landscape, where individuals or groups may ascribe certain qualities of healing to spaces and places. This appeared to support people to re-frame their past and move from a sole focus on places that had become associated primarily with trauma and loss. Instead, the focus was to encourage people to find ways to create artwork that allowed positive memories to be expressed alongside the losses.

Participants followed their own pathway, sometimes a clear progression of past events, other times a patchwork of past and present, as they worked through various experiences. Often their artwork depicted extremely difficult and poignant scenes. However, the act of sharing those spaces using paint or collage appeared to be an important moment of trust, most particularly if received supportively and empathetically by the group. Likewise, when people created an image of a place from their past or present that represented healing or some positive memory that they found sustaining, they emphasised the value of this sharing, despite the nostalgia and losses these places represent. As our participants explained, this process was a mix of nostalgia but also educative for themselves and for others in similar situations. Importantly, participants could share those visual narratives and allow some treasured memories to emerge. In turn, others in the group (whether participants, research team, interpreters or therapist) who witnessed the artmaking and heard the stories, were often profoundly touched by this process.

CONCLUSION

From images of lost landscapes, village communities, and losses of family and work to images portraying the challenges and hope of new places and spaces, participants in the art groups re-imagined and shared their stories. During this process, there were important points of learning for participants, and for the researchers. The artwork expressed in paint and collage demonstrated the capacity for individuals to start to trust and share their memories with others, and participants spoke about the benefits of these opportunities for creative and social interaction offered by group artwork. They also explained how they discovered new-found confidence in gaining art skills, which was a positive experience, not just during sessions, but with potential for new, creative opportunities that could transfer into other parts of their lives. Through their artwork they were able at times to express a range of feelings, from nostalgic and difficult memories to present challenges and healing with hope for the future, that they may not have been able to express in other situations. Some participants were able to take these experiences back into their therapy as a contribution to their continuing recovery. At another level, artmaking gave participants a creative space to experience playfulness and sharing together, and this was a point of learning for them, and an important insight for us as a research team. Playfulness is an essential element of artmaking and within a group has a role in recovery.

The art in recovery projects were designed to contribute to better understanding how group artmaking can support the mental health needs and recovery of people who have experienced torture and human rights abuses. We conclude that taking part in a well-supported participatory art group can be sociable and creative, with potential to contribute to recovery for people with mental health needs. Participatory art can encourage the sharing of a dynamic and evolving reflective relationship to the past, present and potential future.

REFERENCES

Andemicael, A. (2011) *Positive Energy: A review of the Role of Artistic Activities in Refugee Camps*. Geneva: UNHCR. Available at: https://www.unhcr.org/4def858a9.pdf (Accessed: 28 March 2021).

Bell, S., Ronan, F., Houghton, F., Maddrell, A., and Williams, A. (2018) 'From therapeutic landscapes to healthy spaces, places and practices: A scoping review', *Social Science & Medicine*, 196, pp. 123–130. doi:10.1016/j.socscimed.2017.11.035.

Gavron, T. (2020) 'The power of art to cope with trauma: Psychosocial intervention after the tsunami in Japan', *Journal of Humanistic Psychology*. doi:10.1177/0022167820982144

Gesler, W. (1993) 'Therapeutic landscapes: Theory and a case study of Epidauros, Greece', *Society and Space*, 11, pp. 200–223. doi:10.1068/d110171.

Gestaldo, D., Andrews, A. and Khanlou, N. (2004) 'Therapeutic landscapes of the mind: Theorizing some intersections between health geography, health promotion and immigration studies', *Critical Public Health*, 14(2), pp. 157–176. doi:10.1080/09581590410001725409.

Herman, J. L. (1992) *Trauma and Recovery: The Aftermath of Violence from Domestic Abuse to Political Terror*. New York: Basic Books.

Kearns, R. and Andrews, G. J. (2010) 'Geographies of wellbeing', in Smith S.J., Pain R., Marston S.A. and Jones J. P. III (eds) *Handbook of Social Geographies*. London: Sage, pp. 309–328.

Mirdal, G. M., Ryding, E., and Essendrop Sondej, M. (2012) 'Traumatized refugees, their therapists, and their interpreters: Three perspectives on psychological treatment', *Psychology and Psychotherapy*, 85(4), pp. 436–455. doi:10.1111/j.2044-8341.2011.02036.x.

Perriam, G. (2015) 'Sacred spaces, healing places: Therapeutic landscapes of spiritual significance', *Journal of Medical Humanities*, 36(1), pp. 19–33. doi:10.1007/s10912-014-9318-0.

Rose, E. E., (2012) 'Encountering place: A Psychoanalytic approach for understanding how therapeutic landscapes benefit health and wellbeing', *Health and Place*, 18(6), pp. 1381–1387. doi:10.1016/j.healthplace.2012.07.002.

Rose, E. E., and Bingley, A.F. (2017) 'Migrating art: A research design to support refugees' recovery from trauma – A pilot study', *Design for Health*, 1 (2), pp. 152–169. https://doi.org/10.1080/24735132.2017.1386499

Rose, E. E., Bingley, A. F., and Rioseco, M. (2021) 'Art of transition: A Deleuzoguattarian framework', *Action Research*, pp. 1–26. doi:10.1177/1476750320960817.

Rose, E. E., Bingley, A. F., Rioseco, M., and Lamb, K. (2018) 'Art of Recovery: Displacement, mental Health, and wellbeing', *Arts*, 7(4), 94. doi:10.3390/arts7040094.

Smith, T. S. J. (2021) 'Therapeutic taskscapes and craft geography: Cultivating well-being and atmospheres of recovery in the workshop', *Social and Cultural Geography*, 22(2), pp. 151–169. doi:10.1080/14649365.2018.1562088.

Stavropoulou, N. (2019) 'Understanding the 'bigger picture': Lessons learned from participatory visual arts-based research with individuals seeking asylum in the United Kingdom', *Crossings: Journal of Migration & Culture*, 10(1), pp. 95–118. doi:10.1386/cjmc.10.1.95_1.

Stickley, T. (2011) 'A philosophy for community-based, participatory arts practice: A narrative inquiry', *Journal of Applied Arts and Health*, 2(1), pp. 73–83. doi:10.1386/jaah.2.1.73_7.

UNHCR. (2018). *Health*. http://www.unhcr.org/uk/health.html. (Accessed 28th March 2021).

Williams, A. (ed.) (2007). *Therapeutic Landscapes*. Aldershot: Ashgate Publishing.

Winnicott, D. (1953) 'Transitional objects and transitional phenomena', *The International Journal of Psychoanalysis*, 34, pp. 89–97.

Winnicott, D. W. (1967) *Mirror-Role of Mother and Family in Child Development*. New York, NY: Routledge.

World Health Organization (2019) *The WHO Special Initiative for Mental Health (2019-2023): Universal Health Coverage for Mental Health*. World Health Organization. Available at: https://apps.who.int/iris/handle/10665/310981 (Accessed 28th March 2021).

CHAPTER 14

THE ART OF HEALING IN A TRANSITORY CONTEXT
Groupwork with people seeking asylum in asylum centres in Kosovo

Ardiana Bytyçi, Malisa Zymberi, Besnik Rustemi, Ejona Miraka Icka and Feride Rushiti

The war of 1998/1999 led to thousands of Kosovo Albanians fleeing Kosovo or being internally displaced. Many are still living with the consequences of this war. The Kosova Rehabilitation Center for Torture Victims (KRCT) was established in response to the devastating impact of conflict and torture on families and communities.

Dr Feride Rushiti founded KRCT in 1999 following her work with refugees at the Kosovo–Albania border. KRCT provides multidisciplinary rehabilitation, treatment and reintegration for traumatised victims of torture, particularly survivors of sexual violence during the war. In 2006, KRCT expanded its remit to include human rights advocacy, by protecting and promoting the human rights of all people deprived of their liberty in correctional facilities, detention centres, police holding cells and mental health institutions.

In 2008, the Department of Citizenship, Asylum and Migration (DCAM) was established due to the increase in numbers of people passing through Kosovo on route to Europe or choosing to claim asylum in Kosovo. In 2012, the first asylum centre was set up to accommodate the majority of these people. The exceptions are those that can fund their own accommodation or vulnerable cases whose specific circumstances cannot be managed within an asylum centre. The asylum centres are semi-open residential settings.

In 2012, UNHCR approached KRCT to become involved in supporting people seeking asylum initially at the asylum centre in Magure/Lipjan and then at Vranidoll/Podujeva. This was our first experience of working with people seeking asylum.

In December 2019 KRCT introduced a groupwork programme within the asylum centres for two main reasons. Firstly, the team's therapeutic goal was to work with as many people seeking asylum as possible. Secondly, in KRCT's experience of providing therapeutic services to survivors of war and torture, groupwork had been an effective method to identify individuals who had experienced potentially traumatic events as well as provide an opportunity for people to support each other, share their painful experiences and gain a deeper understanding of their symptoms and responses.

This chapter will focus on KRCT's groupwork programme in the asylum centres. We will briefly describe the post-conflict context in which KRCT delivers all its services and the adaptions made to working in the asylum centres. It will share the team's experience of co-designing a groupwork programme alongside people seeking asylum that aims to improve their mental and physical wellbeing. The chapter describes a range of activity-based groupwork and its impact and explores how groupwork and group activities have enabled the clinical team to identify people in need of psychological treatment as well as enhancing opportunities for the team to offer rehabilitation and support to a larger group of people who are often still in the midst of flight.

SHARING OUR HISTORY OF DISCRIMINATION AND CONFLICT

Political repression and economic deprivation of Kosovo Albanians increased Albanian/Serbian tensions in the 1990s, leading to an escalation of the conflict between the majority ethnic Albanian population and the Yugoslav military of primarily Serbian forces by the end of February 1998. In 1999, Serbian forces engaged in a campaign of ethnic cleansing against Kosovo Albanians with thousands killed and hundreds of thousands displaced to neighbouring

DOI: 10.4324/9781003192978-17

countries (Bastick et al., 2007). In 2021, the consequences of this conflict still remain a challenge for Kosovo society.

Though war atrocities in Kosovo are widely documented, their consequences, including the mental health impact, did not receive the deserved institutional response. Up until 2021, these consequences have only been addressed by non-governmental organisations (NGOs) using pharmacologic and/or psychotherapeutic interventions.

Efforts to measure the impact of the Kosovo war from a psychological perspective started immediately after the end of the conflict and there have been a number of studies. Research indicated a high prevalence of potentially traumatic events among Kosovo Albanians, with large numbers experiencing multiple traumas (Cardozo et al., 2000). In one study, 28%–53% of respondents had experienced torture (Morina et al., 2010).

KRCT mental health practitioners have had similar experiences of war and displacement as their clients. Most of the authors of this chapter experienced the 1998/1999 Kosovo war as children and were refugees seeking psychosocial support from international organisations and local NGOs in the neighbouring country camps designated for Kosovo Albanians.

The rehabilitation programme at KRCT was designed based on a simple question that the authors wanted to be asked years ago after leaving their homes: What would make you feel better? They asked this question frequently with people seeking asylum in the centres, who have now become active contributors in developing the rehabilitation programme, especially the groupwork component.

KRCT practitioners recognised that their own processed memories from the conflict often contributed to a greater empathy and vigilance in identifying and working with resident's psychological difficulties, adapting the programme and taking into account their needs at all times. The team now deliver what they needed to be offered in similar circumstances at a different moment in time.

TRAUMA AND VULNERABILITY AMONGST THE ASYLUM-SEEKING POPULATION

People seeking asylum or in transit in Kosovo are a diverse group and have different vulnerabilities. Many children and young people are unaccompanied. There are women at risk, single parents, survivors of violence and/or trafficking, people with physical or mental impairments and others who need special protection. People seeking asylum in Kosovo have fled countries such as Syria, Palestine, Algeria, Afghanistan, Libya, Iraq, Morocco and Turkey (DCAM, 2020).

Traveling to Kosovo via unsafe routes means that, as well as the persecution and/or war that led people to flee, many have been exposed to stressful and potentially traumatic events during the journey. Furthermore, remaining excluded from basic services, being in a new environment and without a social network, adds to the stress of exile (Hameed et al., 2018).

The residents of the asylum centres, whether or not they fulfill the criteria for international protection, are all potentially in need of mental health support. There are high levels of depression, anxiety and post-traumatic stress disorder (PTSD) (Richter et al., 2018).

TIME TO CHANGE OUR APPROACH: COMBINING INDIVIDUAL COUNSELLING WITH GROUPWORK

In the early stages of KRCT's work in the centres, individual counselling was used as the only intervention, but the brief length of stay made it challenging to offer ongoing treatment for psychological difficulty. Most people stayed for a couple of days, with others staying for a few weeks or months. A small number of refugees chose to stay in Kosovo and receive subsidiary protection or refugee status, leaving the centre to live within the community.

It was time to integrate a new approach into our rehabilitation programme, in response to the movement of the population within the centres. We wanted to make the most of the often time-limited opportunity by offering an intervention and a sense of connection that would make an immediate difference, as well as equip people for the challenges that lay ahead. Not only have the numbers of people seeking asylum increased since 2019, but the composition of the asylum-seeking population has also been changing continuously. For example, there has been an increase in the numbers of families and unaccompanied adolescents in 2021.

The team decided to offer groupwork and group activities due to the known social benefits of groupwork as well as increased therapeutic results when combined with individual counselling.

THE GROUPWORK PROGRAMME

The groupwork programme was designed to respond to the needs of those who seek help for a short period of time. It also takes into account those who stay longer because they are reviewing their travelling options as well as those who see Kosovo as their final destination. The programme includes psychosocial activities and groupwork for women and girls, children, families and young men. No one is excluded from our programme; each and every person is entitled to benefit from mental health services based on their situation, preference or mental health difficulties.

The programme is organised on a daily basis within both asylum centres and the regular presence of the team is supported by the institution and the asylum officials working directly with people in the centre. The presence of mental health practitioners has positively changed the institutional perception of mental health, and our contribution has been acknowledged and encouraged.

The groupwork programme is fluid and flexible, changing frequently in response to the composition of those who are living at the centre. Our collaborative approach means residents lead the team to what's best for them. Many use art to express what they feel; others prefer using groupwork to share their stories and some use games to cope with their suffering. The programme does not represent a linear direction for addressing distressing events and vulnerability. KRCT use groupwork to complement individual counselling or individual counselling to complement groupwork.

Activities with children are focused on enhancing social skills and addressing emotional problems using interactive games. They are offered on a regular basis within the weekly programme and are more intensive compared to other groups, given that play has a significant impact on children's development and psychological health. Women's groups and activities are based on promoting self-awareness and empowerment and are often more diverse in terms of the types of activity, because of the range of skills and interests that women bring. Activities offered to adolescent boys and older men are mainly sports based (indoor or outdoor) and often require a more structured programme.

AIMS AND VALUES OF THE GROUPWORK PROGRAMME

Coping with potential trauma in the country of origin and facing a series of survival challenges along the way can be manifested in physical problems and psychosocial difficulties. In addition to individual treatments, we have tried different ways of working in groups to heal emotional damage and increase self-understanding and understanding toward others. We have noticed that groupwork (artistic or sports) has helped people seeking asylum to become more self-reflective, reduce stress symptoms and change behaviours and unhelpful ways of thinking.

The aim of the groupwork in this transit context is not only to encourage social interaction and the sharing of personal stories but also to contribute to the overall wellbeing of people in the centre as well as preventing psychological deterioration. Groupwork also gives the team opportunities to observe and assess areas of strength.

We have often encountered self-injurious behaviour among residents, especially amongst young separated boys. Many people who self-harm describe it as an attempt to cope with overwhelming emotional or physical distress that they feel powerless to manage. In addition to offering individual therapy to recognise and cope with emotional or physical distress, their involvement in group activities has increased their connection to other residents of the centre, created a sense of purpose, and reduced the incidences of self-harm.

Psychosocial groupwork activities help people seeking asylum learn about self-care. This was particularly important for families due to the high level of stress experienced by parents and children on the move. Many of the residents in the centre came from a similar cultural context to Kosovo with a focus on family and community. This shared culture helped the team to co-design groupwork priorities and topics for meetings because of their own histories and cultural understanding (Weine et al., 2021).

There are many occasions when psychological distress and PTSD symptoms are naturally manifested in groupwork, whether it be psychosocial activity or a workshop. Sometimes group-work can be more effective in identifying psychological symptoms than individual assessment and counselling. There are no set rules, guidelines or specific techniques that are applied to every individual. We are flexible at all times and respond as situations develop.

Groupwork participation has helped to reinforce social skills, and removed the feeling of isolation by giving residents the opportunity to engage with others. Also, bringing, sharing and treating group concerns becomes easier when everyone is in a similar situation. Talking with others during a shared struggle, restores and strengthens a sense of belonging somewhere again, which has been lost in the process of fleeing.

The programme of activities is designed to create a healthy routine among residents. The activities have the potential to become life-changing habits that can help to bring calm to both the mind and body in times of stress, anxiety or pain. The more residents engaged in activities, the more we observed their levels of stress and anxiety decrease.

Activities are helpful, but they also stimulate creativity and distract the focus away from distressing events and negative emotions to more positive ones.

EVALUATION TOOLS TO ASSESS PSYCHOLOGICAL DISTRESS

Psychological symptoms are identified mostly through using adapted and validated tools. Iden-tification of needs and mental health difficulties are done through questionnaires included in the Guidelines for Reception Conditions of Applicants with Specific Needs initiated and devel-oped by KRCT in partnership with UNHCR and the asylum centre: (1) A questionnaire for assessing the specific needs of applicants for international protection, which was developed by the KRCT team; and (2) a PROTECT-ABLE questionnaire (2011) (PROTECT-ABLE, 2021).

The questionnaire for assessing the specific needs of applicants for international protection is a simple tool designed for non-professional staff in the asylum context to assess the needs of people seeking asylum. It collects information about the specific circumstances/needs of people to be taken into consideration, as well as recording where and how these should be addressed. The PROTECT-ABLE questionnaire facilitates the early identification of people who have suffered distressing experiences, e.g., victims of torture, psychological, physical or sexual violence.

Psychological assessment is conducted using various tools such as the Harvard Trauma Questionnaire and the Hopkins Symptoms Checklist for anxiety and depression. KRCT use the translated or adapted versions of these tools in Albanian.

GROUPS AND CULTURAL CONTEXT

Most of the people seeking asylum originally came from collectivist societies with their own cultural traditions and customs. Group activities have been developed or directed by residents' own preferences and so they have naturally integrated cultural and traditional elements. Most residents said that they preferred to meet as a group and participate in activities, rather than attending individual counselling. Sharing personal stories during different types of group activities was common, and self-disclosures were often followed by the offering of support from others in the group. As a result, group activities became a tool for establishing a supportive network within the centres.

The culture of returning the favour or reciprocity is very common in most of the residents' cultures. Therefore, specific attention has been paid to ensuring a fully equipped creative activity room where residents can be productive and are able to offer something of worth to others who have helped them.

> The first moment I got needles in my hands, I knew that finally I had the chance to create a GIFT thanking you for your work with us. It's been a long time since I am living in the Asylum Center and your support has become the only hope I live with. After every session or activity finished, I had this disappointing feeling of not having anything to give in return, as a thank you symbol. Fortunately, this activity allowed me to knit these beautiful socks where I can finally give them as a gift and show how thankful I am for the support I receive every single day – now I can feel some peace.
>
> (Yasmin, who knitted a pair of socks as a gift for a KRCT psychologist)

The asylum-seeking population in Kosovo is mainly young men, who usually stay for a shorter period of time at the centres. There are less women and children, but they stay longer and participate more intensively in both individual therapy and/or groupwork. Almost all groupwork offered is single-gender, which is often more culturally familiar and comfortable. Women report that they felt safer and more able to explore their experiences within a women-only setting, including their experiences of gender-based violence. We have observed that men also benefit from being in a group together and are able to participate more freely than they might in mixed-gender groups.

We outline below the key themes embedded in our groupwork programme and share some of the activities on offer at the centres that have been found to be beneficial.

COPING THROUGH PLAYING

Various activities are designed as group games to help residents cope with their psychological difficulties. Playing usually takes various forms while working with children; however, games were also used as a tool to help the team identify psychological difficulty in different age-groups. These games also help the team observe biopsychosocial functions.

Playing a game usually does not require any special skills, and because of this every resident can join in. The difficulties and challenges encountered during the journey impact on people's ability to trust others and build new relationships. This can lead them to isolate themselves within this setting. The games have been effective in helping residents become social beings again as well as building trust in others.

One of the most important circadian rhythms is the sleep-wake cycle, and we found this to be very important when working with boys and young men. The lack of activities and structure in the lives of many of the young men has led many to feel their days are empty. Many struggled with sleep and stopped paying attention to self-care. Therefore, it was important to create a new routine, using the stimuli of various well-known board games such as cards, dominos, chess and tumbling tower (Lam, 2021).

The purpose of introducing these board games was to stimulate concentration, competition and encourage residents to get to know one another, hearing about different values and sharing experiences from the past. One example was two young adolescents from Morocco and Syria who played chess together; through their play, they learnt different chess methods, techniques and tricks. The team saw the mental health of these young boys improve as a result of this new routine and friendship.

Depending on the composition of the group, most activities last one and a half hours and there are no age restrictions. The only requirement the team asks from residents is that they choose to join freely, and they participate. We try to create some cohesion between different age-groups and ethnicities.

The games selected are international and not culturally specific, so that they can be easily played and enjoyed by everyone. Because many of the residents are men, play is effective in getting to know them in a relaxed way, enabling the team to develop trusting relationships with residents.

Playing games is used as a tool for making connections between adolescent boys and older men from different countries. Increasing a sense of belonging among these young men has created a feeling of personal security for many, and, as a result, a feeling of security in the group.

The group then learn to act as a group and accept new members. One example is Ali, who was diagnosed with multiple mental health disorders and had experienced several crises within the asylum centre. Alongside psychiatric treatment, the activities helped Ali learn to socialise and he valued being accepted by the group. His participation in the group helped group members understand the psychological difficulties that people experience following distressing events and challenged the negative stereotypes about mental illness that some group members carried.

Most of the young men have been on the move since their childhood or adolescence and have experienced distressing events and/or torture, not only in their country of origin but also during the journey. All have been separated from their families and have tried to integrate in many countries throughout their journey. Having this supportive network available in the centre has directly influenced their overall wellbeing and reduced their levels of agitation and aggressivity.

Healthy competition is a normal part of growing up for young men in most cultures. However, being in survival mode for a long period of time had diminished this feeling for many. The team found that creating a stimulating environment to safely trigger competitive spirit has been important. Whether it be outdoor or indoor activities, adolescent boys and older men left the small space of their bedrooms and engaged in groupwork that used different skills and achieved a specific goal. Though simple in their nature, these activities required structure, effort and adaptation to the needs of the group.

After establishing the group and building the trust between each member, the asylum centre officials and/or NGO staff based at the centre often joined the games, which helped in building trusting and beneficial relationships with staff.

The existence of the group is secure, and older members take on leadership of the group and welcome new members as people come and go. This tradition has been embedded and is very effective as it ensures group cohesion and continuity.

CREATING TO BE PRESENT

KRCT has facilitated a number of mindful creative activities for women, where they have created hand-made items as a way of expressing their feelings and representing their internal worlds.

Knitting and embroidery frames

The knitting group was introduced to the women at the beginning of 2020, and it immediately changed the atmosphere inside the asylum centre. Knitting first started as an idea to help women socialise together, as well as to create a routine where they can enrich their day and create a warm environment within an institutional setting. It became much more than that, and women started to create long term knitting projects.

> When I started to knit this scarf, I didn't really know to whom I was knitting it for, or even what it would be. I wasn't sure if it would be a scarf, socks or a hat. I was just tired of my disturbing thoughts that reminded me every second of my dreadful past. I needed a break! While knitting, I actually got the break. I started to think about how I've forgotten the existence of Mahmut, my husband. It's been years since we left Afghanistan and are traveling from one country to another. We are all the time worried for our children, their future and their safety. I forgot the love I've got for him. I forgot we used to care about each other. Made some more stitches and decided to knit this scarf for him. Swam into each memory we created together and knitted a super long scarf as a celebration of our love.
>
> (Emine)

Picking up a pair of needles and a ball of yarn was a very calming activity for women, who also enjoyed spending time together, helping and listening to each other. This has positively impacted on their wellbeing and created an opportunity to be resourceful. The women began to gather in groups of four or five and started knitting items for their loved ones, such as hats, scarves and socks.

Knitting and embroidery has many therapeutic benefits and it has helped to relieve anxiety and stress, enhanced social connection and built self-esteem. Women described feeling at ease as they knit together, sharing stories as they work.

Air-dry ceramic clay

Working with clay requires delicacy, concentration, time and dedication. It benefits psychological health and can trigger positive emotions and peaceful moments for women. Creating ceramic items not only brings joy, but at the end of each session, women were more relaxed and less anxious.

Working with clay to make a ceramic piece required a longer period of time as a group, enabling the space for women to get to know each other better, and creating an environment where it became possible to talk about distressing experiences. Women began to support each other by sharing coping strategies they had used in managing their psychological difficulties.

Ceramic making created an environment that led to a natural process of a women's self-help group forming. The group was established mostly based on their own initiative and it was the women's ideas that led to any new activity chosen. Even if the groupwork for women was designed in a specific way by the team, the activities changed as new women arrived and defined their needs within this structure.

Women introduced 'pieces of home' to these ceramic sessions. Uma is from Syria. Most of her jewellery was burned during the conflict and what was left was sold to fund the journey to Europe to flee the war. The handmade clay jewellery she made during the first session was an improvised piece that she wore on her wedding day as a gift from her parents. The newly recreated jewellery served as a memory from her wedding day to keep with her for the rest of her life. This link to painful memories and precious items created some closure for Uma and re-creating this piece in this setting was part of her healing process.

CONNECTING WITH YOURSELF WHILE BEING WITH OTHERS

The therapeutic aim of the activities is to equip refugees and people seeking asylum with helpful techniques to use in the future, despite the conditions in which they may be living. The structure of the programme is designed to also work with attitudes, people's senses of themselves and connection with others. It aims to facilitate a greater self-awareness and build on people's ability to operate in the world whilst in survival mode.

Yoga classes with women and children

Yoga is known to have multiple benefits on psychological and physical wellbeing (Emerson and Hopper, 2011). However, the team was aware of the cultural differences amongst the women and carefully tested each activity before it formed part of the programme. When introducing a yoga group for women, the team took into account the background of each woman, their knowledge of mental and physical health, and reflected on how they might manage some of the movements i.e., some techniques or yoga positions might not be acceptable for all of them.

> I did hear about yoga classes and how people feel about it, but I was never sure I would be up to enjoying it. I also always had these thoughts of not being able to be good at it. But with our yoga class here, a lot of things changed. I feel more at peace with myself and with people around me. The atmosphere during that one hour of the class is the safest hour of my mind and being.
>
> (Sadije)

Women rarely missed the yoga classes and reported that they felt less anxious and stressed, as well as slept better. Women found the group so helpful that they felt it could also benefit their children. As a result, yoga classes with children were introduced and parents reported improvements in concentration, memory and patience.

Sports activities with young men

Living under the same roof in a stressful atmosphere has sometimes led to conflict amongst the young men. Seeking to create a more positive environment, the team were encouraged when an aspiring 17-year-old footballer, Najeh, proposed introducing football into the programme. He was assigned as the coordinator of sports activities, which then became a regular feature of the programme. Najeh was responsible for setting up sports activity groups for residents and these were organised independently without any supervision from the team.

Asylum centre officials joined some of the football matches, which contributed to the development of trust and created an environment where it was easier for residents to raise and have their concerns addressed by asylum centre staff.

Sports activities were organised with the purpose of creating group belonging and integration, as well as creating moments of joy, triumph and accomplishment when a team played well or won. This helped to build self-esteem and create positive memories to draw on in the difficult times ahead. In these activities, there was a wide variety of age groups represented.

EMPOWERING ASYLUM-SEEKING WOMEN

Asylum-seeking women had built a life in their home countries, which had been destroyed or lost during conflict or for other reasons. Women expressed their grief at the loss of their homes and described the attachment they had to their previous life and the feelings of security it had given many. Being on the move led some women to start to dream of working again, using their different skills.

KRCT reflected on this and initiated a project that would bring 'pieces from home' into the groupwork programme to enable women to use their different skills. Women were invited to organise classes based on their previous professions or sharing skills learned from home:

> I used to have my own school of sewing back home. I had around a hundred students over a year and three employees. I used to lead this school for twenty years. Now, this class here, these women and this setting is making me feel the past – as when I was a normal married woman with a regular job and big dreams.
>
> (Aisha)

Using art was the most commonly used creative activity. One resident, Amira, led a painting and drawing class for women, and she encouraged them to express themselves creatively, and taught them drawing/painting techniques.

Women were keen to learn from other women. One of the women had been a make-up artist and she organised make-up and hairdressing classes. KRCT provided the make-up and organised the classes, but the make-up artist led the session by teaching women how to use make-up and encouraging them to take care of themselves, despite their current situation. It was the first time in a long period that women had the chance to cut their hair and take care of their physical appearance.

All of the activities led by women had one main purpose: to empower each other. From this process of supporting each other, the 'Book of empowering and inspiring messages' was created. In the book are written empowering messages for women who come to the asylum centre in the future given by asylum-seeking mothers, sisters and daughters. The book can be accessed by women residents at all times.

To acknowledge their contribution in Kosovo, women's hand-made items were exhibited within the asylum centre. There was also a virtual public exhibition, 'Know me Beyond Words', where their items and the stories behind them were made available to the public. Raising awareness on the capabilities and skills of asylum-seeking women celebrated their potential to contribute to Kosovo.

STORIES OF THE PAST, LESSONS FOR THE FUTURE

Parenting and family relationships

Despite being a transit country, Kosovo also accommodates families in need of stability and integration. The team again faced a new challenge, as the approaches used with individuals were not as effective with families as hoped. Parenting on the move is a challenge and parents have not always been able to meet their children's basic needs, including emotional ones.

Families began to take part in KRCT's rehabilitation programme and the team began to observe different parenting styles, gender-based violence and child neglect. The consequences of the distressing events the families had undergone was evident in its impact on individual members, but also on family functioning as well as parenting and child development.

KRCT introduced parenting groups that were an opportunity to encourage parents to travel into the past. Parents were invited to explore their childhood memories and share stories with the group. The most emotional part of these discussions was when they connected their own childhood experiences of being parented, with their current parenting styles. One example was Muna, who reflected on her mother's model of parenting and her own parenting approach. Muna's mother was an inspirational woman fighting in a patriarchal society to empower other women, including her two daughters. Muna came to an understanding in the group that she was modeling her mother by constantly working to shape a positive future for her children.

Sharing stories of how people were parented raised awareness amongst the group of how important their role was on their children's development and future life, despite the struggles of being a family on the move.

THE ROLE OF FOCUS GROUPS

The rehabilitation programme has been designed based on the feedback from focus groups that were organised regularly. Focus groups were offered when groups with similar characteristics formed at the centre, such as a group of young men all speaking the same language.

The purpose of the focus groups was to listen to and understand the needs and hopes of people seeking asylum, as well as to assess their difficulties at an individual and group level (European Migrant Advisory Board, 2019). The team aimed to find out more about their future goals as well as ask about the new life they hoped to build. They were encouraged to share information about their country, culture, traditions and see if there is something similar in Kosovo that would make them feel at home.

Focus group discussions were a platform for residents to express themselves and not feel judged. Most of the young men were hesitant to express themselves and so to facilitate them opening up, the group discussions were themed e.g., multiculturalism, describing their countries of origin, cultures and traditions.

SUMMARY

The residents of the asylum centres have all had a life that has been interrupted by distressing events causing their forced migration. Leaving home and being on the move for long periods of time and being subject to potentially traumatic events has been the common experience for all who have found help and support from our team. The groupwork programme evolved to respond to this set of circumstances.

As practitioners, whether designing intervention programmes, facilitating groups or offering counselling, we always keep one thing in mind: asylum-seeking people need the team to hear them and use their skills and experience to assist. Being alone and not having a social network and trying to fit somewhere new in the world is an exhausting experience. It can be particularly hard for parents who are trying to keep their families together, without a protection system that guarantees their children will access public services and education wherever their journey takes them.

Sometimes just the presence of mental health practitioners in this environment encourages people to seek help. KRCT believe that the team should always be part of the daily routines in the asylum centre, so that the pathway to support is made easier. This is particularly important in transit countries where the goal is not only to alleviate distress, but to make people aware that seeking psychological support wherever they go is not a weakness. Indeed, it is the most important thing to do in the new world that awaits them.

Introducing groupwork was challenging, but the provision of individual counselling at the beginning of our work at the asylum centre was not possible, even though we wanted to listen to each story. The pilot programme of group activities was not initially structured to take into account the transit context; as it developed, however, we saw that it enabled us to identify those in need of treatment in a helpful way that benefitted all residents.

The writers' own experience in 1998–1999 has shown that war and displacement are undeniably life-changing events, but resilience is also a power to move on and become active citizens wherever life leads us.

All names of people seeking asylum included in this chapter are fictional to protect confidentiality.

REFERENCES

Bastick, M, Grimm, K, Kunz, R (2007). *Sexual Violence in Armed Conflict: Global overview and implications for the Security Sector.* Geneva, Switzerland: Geneva Centre for the Democratic Control of Armed Forces. Available at: https://dcaf.ch/sites/default/files/publications/documents/sexualviolence_conflict_full.pdf (Accessed: 19 June 2022).

Cardozo, BL, Vergara, A, Agani, F, Gotway, CA (2000). Mental health, social functioning and attitudes of Kosovar Albanians following the war in Kosovo. *JAMA*, 284(5):569–577. doi:10.1001/jama.284.5.569.

Department of Citizenship, Asylum and Migration (2020). Annual Statistical Report. Available at: https://mpb.rks-gov.net/Uploads/Documents/Pdf/EN/359/WEB_Raport_2020_Eng.pdf (Accessed: 12 January 2022).

Emerson D, Hopper E. (2011). *Overcoming Trauma through Yoga.* Berkeley, California. USA. North Atlantic Books.

European Migrant Advisory Board (2019). Ask the People: A consultation of migrants and refugees. Available at: https://ec.europa.eu/migrant-integration/library-document/ask-people-consultation-migrants-and-refugees_en (Accessed: 12 January 2022).

Hameed, S, Sadiq, A, Din, AU (2018). The increased vulnerability of refugee population to mental health disorders. *Kansas Journal of Medicine*, Feb; 11(1):20–23.

Lam, M (2021). Playing this board game will challenge your ideas about refugees. *The Conversation.* Available at: https://theconversation.com/playing-this-board-game-will-challenge-your-ideas-about-refugees-97538 (Accessed: 21 December 2021).

Morina NN, Rushiti, F, Salihu, M, Ford, JD (2010). Psychopathology and well-being in civilian survivors of war seeking treatment: a follow-up study. *Clinical Psychology and Psychotherapy*, March-April; 17(2):79–86. doi:10.1002/cpp.673.

Protect Able. Available at: http://protect-able.eu/resources/ (Accessed: 20 December 2021).

Richter, K, Peter, L, Lehfeld, H, Zaske, H, Brar-Reissinger, S, Niklewski, G. (2018). Prevalence of psychiatric diagnoses in asylum seekers with follow-up. *BMC Psychiatry* 18: 1–7. doi:10.1186/s12888-018-1783-y.

Weine, SM, Arënliu, A, Görmez, V, Lagenecker, S, Demirtas, H. (2021). Conducting research on building psychosocial support for Syrian refugee families in a humanitarian emergency. *Conflict and Health* 15:31. doi:10.1186/s13031-021-00365-6 (Accessed: 21 December 2021).

CHAPTER 15

STONE FLOWERS

A music group with refugee survivors of torture

Christine Adcock, Jude Boyles, Lis Murphy and Emmanuela Yogolelo

'Stone Flowers' is the English translation of the traditional song 'Gole Sangam' in Farsi. A Stone Flower symbolises the symbiotic nature of two apparent opposites, resonating with the balance of beauty and strength, resilience and fragility and the brilliance of nature to be both everlasting and renewable.

Stone Flowers is a group of refugee torture survivors who meet weekly to write poems, lyrics and melodies, learn new instruments and perform songs.

The Stone Flowers project was created in 2011 by Freedom from Torture North West (FFTNW), a torture rehabilitation charity and Music Action International (MAI). MAI is an NGO delivering music programmes with refugees in exile, displaced communities, refugee camps and post-conflict settings. Stone Flowers is a collaboration between music facilitators and torture survivors with a shared learning of music, language and culture throughout the creative process.

The initial project team consisted of an FfTNW clinical psychologist/cellist, MAI's music facilitators including musician-interpreters with lived experience of torture and/or seeking asylum, volunteer musicians and a team of five interpreters. Survivors were usually referred to the group by their therapist but any survivor attending FfTNW could choose to join the sessions at any stage in their treatment. The music group was an open group and membership changed from year to year. Stone Flowers is diverse in gender, age, sexuality, faith, wealth and class. What participants have in common is that they have all sought asylum in the UK and experienced torture, and this is what connects them.

In the UK, most music projects with torture survivors and people seeking asylum are choirs which learn composed songs. In this chapter we share the methodology that was developed for running a music group that composes and performs their own melodies and lyrics in the languages of its members, including Arabic, English, Farsi, French, Kikongo, Lingala, Sango, Swahili, Ewe and Tamil. The methodology was initially inspired by music programmes created in post-conflict Bosnia-Hercegovina.

We will demonstrate how this approach gives survivors control over their creativity, and agency and ownership of the group. We will describe the core values that underpin this collaborative approach and examine the psychological and physiological benefits of music.

The authors reflect the range of perspectives and roles within the group. Lis is a musician and the creative director of MAI. Emmanuela is a professional musician with lived experience of seeking asylum. Jude was the manager of FFTNW and supervised the project team throughout their time at the centre. Christine is an amateur cellist and was the clinical presence in Stone Flowers.

The song lyrics in this chapter were developed from the group collective process and therefore are not attributed to any one individual. All quotes are from group members unless otherwise stated.

> We didn't cry in front of them
> We didn't show any weakness
> They didn't listen to us
> They destroyed our whole world
> They took our dreams away

DOI: 10.4324/9781003192978-18

Torture became our memory
Prison became our life too
                    (The Memory)

IMPACT OF MUSIC ON MENTAL HEALTH

I didn't have much confidence before, but when I joined [Stone Flowers], it helped me find my confidence and express myself.

It helped me gain my feeling of trust in others, to be with others and helped me be myself and trust myself. It helps me express my feelings and not hold it all inside.

There is a large body of evidence on the positive effect of music on quality of life. Anyone who has attended a live music performance or learnt an instrument describes an experience which involves physicality, emotional intensity and a concentration that is hard to define. Experientially, we are "taken out of ourselves", "flooded with memories", having heightened emotions. The nearer to live music we get, the more intense the experience.

Historically and culturally, the importance of music has long been known and it performs many tasks in the transmission of culture. Music has been used as a rhythm to accompany and drive physical work, to tell stories, to express emotions, to relax, to connect with cultural heritage. It has numerous functions that incorporate so many parts of the body and reflect a person's sense of self. As one group member from the Democratic Republic of Congo said, "*we have a song for everything*".

Research has shown how music is experienced by individuals. It demonstrates the responses from neurotransmitters in the brain (Hodges, 2010, Fancourt et al., 2016) to the affect on behaviour and emotions (Clift, 2013) and shows how music can increase mental wellbeing. In this way, anxiety, depression and confidence are improved by experiencing music.

In this chapter, we are particularly interested in research that helps us see how music can ameliorate some of the mental health challenges that torture survivors' experience. For instance, many of the group members were very distrustful of others and were fearful of any group activity. Research has shown that singing in groups can increase our feelings of connection, bonding and positive wellbeing. Interestingly, singing also stimulates the release of endorphins that can affect pain threshold.

Beyond all pain
Beyond all fear
Live in the moment
Live in the moment
                    (Aram Bash)

Almost all of the survivors were anxious. Therapists at FFTNW worked hard to communicate the value of breath control or relaxation to ameliorate some of the distressing symptoms of anxiety. Teaching this skill and ensuring it is practiced is difficult with people who are hypervigilant, frightened and feel under threat. Conceptualising the role of physiology in anxiety and panic attacks is not always easy across cultures and languages. Encouraging people to practice these skills in the context of their stressful day-to-day lives can be challenging. Singing offers the possibility of using helpful skills but within a context of creativity and positivity. People can practice for a reason not linked with their 'problems'. The improving quality of singing acts as a natural biofeedback loop and can eventually be generalised (Hodges, 2010).

Many survivors manage a chronic pain condition (Weinstein et al., 2016). Some research shows that music can help with pain management and symptom relief (Hanser, 2006). Research has also shown that depression (Hanser and Thompson, 1994), PTSD (Beck et al., 2018), and sleep problems (Jespersen and Vuust, 2012) can all be mitigated through participation in music.

Music performance alone can be an important vehicle for healing trauma and impacting on negative feelings, through helping people forget distress and allowing them to communicate hope, as well as reducing isolation and loneliness through integration (Muriithi, 2020).

> Through our songs we try and spread the word and send out our messages and use the power and beauty of music to emphasise our message and express our feelings. When they get our message, I feel proud. It is so rewarding.

HOW AND WHY WE STARTED

In our early planning sessions, we made an active decision that Stone Flowers would develop a new and different approach to traditional music therapy. Music therapy was formalised in the mid-20th century to harness the long-recognised power of music as a vehicle for delivering specific therapeutic models. There is a large body of research on the impact of music therapy, which has its own theory and methodology.

Stone Flowers focuses on the inherent properties of creativity and music-making, therapeutic in itself, but extends this to offer group members control and the empowerment of performing and recording. The aim was to create a collaborative process where each member could influence the process, could take ownership of the group and their place in it, as well as learning new skills from each other and from the music facilitators.

The project team offered a session structure of relaxation and energisers, song-sharing and singing, non-verbal body percussion and collaborative songwriting leading to rehearsals and public performances of original music.

Although MAI music facilitators had experience of working in mental health and refugee settings, they were offered trauma awareness training to support them to reflect on the potential negative impact that certain activities might have on group members. The training explored the potential emotional and psychological impact the sessions might have on the project team and promoted self-care. This was supported by a monthly supervision group facilitated by a therapist at FFTNW.

This training and support enabled musician-interpreters with lived experience to prepare and protect themselves. The supervision group and the clinical presence of the musician-therapist throughout the life of the group at FFTNW provided containment for the project team and helped the music facilitators manage the impact of the stories they listened to. The clinical overview was also needed to safeguard group members. Furthermore, individual and group dynamics were an important element of the process and so the music facilitation team sometimes needed guidance and support from the musician therapist.

Group planning and de-briefing sessions that were self-facilitated by the project team were built into the process and took place before and after every session. Planning sessions focused on each group member's engagement. There were discussions about where extra encouragement was needed to develop a group member's creativity and participation; noticing moments where people seemed more relaxed or engaged, or any positive interactions that facilitators could encourage.

Debriefing sessions ensured music facilitators were working coherently and were able to observe and adapt week by week to the emerging music-making. They allowed reflection on covert or overt ways in which group members, including music facilitators, were impacted by the session. They created a space to reflect on whether the project team had been personally affected by a session or if music facilitators were being influenced by unconscious verbal or nonverbal communications from group members.

CREATING A SAFE SPACE

FFTNW worked with survivors whose mental health needs were complex. Many were withdrawn and traumatised and had been refused asylum. Some were facing destitution and/or detention and several had been detained in the UK. Most had lived for several years with uncertainty and the sense of threat that the asylum process engenders. Many group members had not felt able to join other group activities at the centre.

Being part of any group, even being in a room with others, was challenging for some survivors who had high levels of anxiety and fearfulness. The music facilitators needed to co-create a space that was safe for people who were oppressed by the psychological and physical damage from their past and harmed by their experiences of the asylum process in the UK. Access to the positive experiences of music and connecting with parts of themselves beyond damage and pain was paramount.

Music facilitators considered how potential group members could be met and introduced physically into a room of strangers and how to enable them to feel comfortable enough to choose to stay silent or not actively participate.

At the beginning it was important there were separate groups for men and women. Most of the women had experienced sexual violence perpetrated by men so creating a women-only space was vital. It was also important to frame the beginning of the group as 'taster' sessions to demonstrate to survivors that they had some control over participation and commitment to the group.

To create an inclusive and equal space, sessions began in a circle (as do many ancient traditions of music-making). People could leave the room at any time and the door was always slightly open. Members could get involved when they felt able; and could do as little or as much as they liked; they could stand or sit. If anyone was in pain, they were encouraged to be mindful of the movements and not to do anything that hurt. Everyone was welcomed to join in or just to listen. Music facilitators explained what would happen in each session to reduce anxiety and prepare everyone for what lay ahead.

The music facilitators co-created a group agreement at the beginning of the project, which included statements such as: "we listen to each other, we respect each other's opinions even if they are different to ours, we support each other", as well as practical things such as "mobiles on silent, try to be on time". This culture of supporting each other developed over the years as lasting connections between group members were formed.

The music facilitators aimed to create an environment of music-making that was inclusive and emotionally safe, sharing and writing new music in different languages, and working towards a professional album and public performances. This was unchartered at the time, but the project team felt confident survivors would want to perform in the future.

My best memory was the last performance. It was special and it was in a church. In that performance, we also gave our stories to the people that came. They didn't know about asylum people and so it was good because we educated them.

Most group members had not played an instrument before, some had experience of singing, but most had no formal experience of playing, performing or creating music. It was important that the team used a human rights, participant-led approach with an initial focus on wellbeing, before the process of making music.

THE ROLE OF INTERPRETERS

Interpreters played a key role in the creative process. They ensured that each member communicated their ideas and enabled the group to understand and support each other's contributions. Not all groups have the luxury of multiple interpreters and many of MAI's programmes work without this support. In these groups, music facilitators use more non-verbal techniques, translate lyrics outside sessions and encourage survivors to support each other with interpretation in the session. However, interpreters add an extra level of inclusivity and immediacy.

Qualified interpreters were trained in working with torture survivors in a group setting and were offered an initial briefing session and then short debriefs after each session by a member of the project team. Group members were encouraged to talk freely, to say what they thought and felt. With support, interpreters learnt to interpret everything, and grew to trust the process of the group and the skills of the music facilitators to manage any difficult dynamics that emerged.

The role of musician-interpreters

Having musician-interpreters who had lived experience of the asylum process and who were from the same communities as survivors was important. Musician-interpreters had the dual role of being musicians but also acted as interpreters throughout the process. They were often caught between their professional role and their community membership, sometimes having to manage a complicated range of expectations from survivors in the group. At times, they described feeling concerned when a group member from their community was struggling to participate and feeling some pressure to support that person to engage. Trusting group members to find their own place in the group in their own time could be challenging.

> I remember when we started Stone Flowers, we were saying "if you don't want to be in the circle, of course you can grab your chair and be in any place as long as you are here together with us in the room. If you feel like you want to leave to go outside, you can do that, if you want to come back you can". There was one participant who would always sit out of the circle in a corner. After three sessions I noticed now they are between the corner and the circle, they are moving towards us bit by bit, slowly, slowly, until the day they joined the circle. That was powerful to me, really powerful.

(Musician-interpreter)

STONE FLOWERS METHODOLOGY

Relaxation and energisers

Sessions started with easy physical movements that participants could copy. This relaxed the body, created a sense of group movement and shared focus. As the group developed, these activities were led by members, so they emerged as individuals, and gained confidence and could share creative ideas non-verbally. People began to connect, relax and laugh together.

Physical relaxation was also important to prepare for playing or singing music without tension, improving the sound created.

The movements then developed into body percussion where music facilitators clapped, stamped, clicked or made percussive vocal noises in rhythm. This began as call and response and then they repeated a rhythm as a group and played with layering different rhythms; stopping and starting different people together and using body gestures to make louder or quieter sounds. Later in the process, survivors led this part and created their own rhythms that people joined in with, even in performances. The sense of play experienced by survivors being in the role of conductor, gesturing people to start and stop or play loud or quiet created a sense of communication, control and connection, all without anyone needing to say anything.

> The good memory is, during a session, they were all clapping, I was playing the drum, so it was making me feel … it was making me feel free.

Next, there were simple breathing exercises, again to calm people's nervous systems, but also in preparation for singing. This needed to be done gently as singing can make people feel exposed or embarrassed. They may have been told they can't sing or feel uncomfortable with the physical feeling of their body resonating. Call and response using gentle humming was a way to ease into this process. Vowel sounds (Ahh, Eee, Ooo etc.) were then added to the hum on different pitches. If the response was good, the facilitators used short phrases, scales and modalities from different music styles and built to singing a warm-up song with uplifting lyrics in English or in a language of a group member or music facilitator.

INSTRUMENTS AND IMPROVISATION

The project team used accessible instruments that could be played well with a little practice such as hand percussion from Brazil and Africa, mbira (West African thumb piano), shruti box (similar to Indian harmonium), bazouki (played in the Balkans and the Middle East). The music facilitators and interpreters also played instruments familiar in participants' home countries such as saz (Middle Eastern), tabla, keyboard, guitar, violin and bass.

Instruments were laid out in the centre of the room for members to choose from, followed by a series of exercises where people could explore the sounds of the instruments and create sounds together or copy call and response, eventually leading to an improvisation with someone conducting non-verbally, indicating when members should start and stop playing. This is reminiscent of music-making in many different cultures. In African music traditions, improvisation is common:

> When we sit in a circle we can sing together, we play percussion together, you can feel something wants to burst out of you. That is allowed and nurtured; and we have a lot of that in Stone Flowers, which is also about supporting people's feelings.

Reading the energy of the room was important. If the energy seemed low, the music facilitators might start more calmly with their movements, tone of voice and choose slower, quieter music, perhaps moving to more energetic styles later in the session, and vice versa. Bringing the group dynamic to a similar level was sometimes challenging if some members were energetic or anxious and others exhausted. The music facilitators learnt to communicate effectively and sometimes non-verbally with each other to change the flow or plan of the session in response to the members of the group.

Attention was paid to body language and gestures. Often facilitators sat on the floor and were physically below the group members. No pointing or strong gestures were used, but gentle encouragement and enthusiasm through considered movement and facial expressions.

The project team later encouraged survivors to teach the group songs in their own language or show the group music that they loved on YouTube. Each song was then broken down by speaking the words line by line, led by members and repeated together as a group. The group then slowly learnt the melody through call and response in sections. Teaching and sharing with others encouraged a sense of worth as well as improving confidence. All of these steps led to the next phase of the process which was creating their own songs collaboratively.

THE CREATIVE PROCESS

> I started to enjoy myself and enjoyed expressing myself and my feelings. Then we got to that creativity part and then every bit of the group, its full of joy and happiness. I love every second of it.

It was important not to expect survivors to create music to 'tell their story' or for music facilitators to choose the topics, but to provide an open forum where survivors could choose to sing about whatever was meaningful to them. This was also important in supporting people to connect with their pre-torture selves.

Group members were split into language groups with an interpreter and a music facilitator to discuss possible topics together. A common starting question was '*What message do you want to give to your audience?*'. In the beginning, themes were around peace, hope and, later on, lyrics became more political and about peoples' individual stories.

> We lost our right
> We lost our loved ones
> Should we lose our feelings too?
> Should we lose them too?
> (Motherland)

> Will my children eat today?
> WIII they go to school?
> Will my children be well?
> Will they be washed?
> How will they manage without me?
> (I Cry Without Tears)

Awareness raising through music became important and the lyrics began to reflect the activism and experiences of multiple oppression of the members. The general public in the UK has been exposed to negative rhetoric about 'asylum seekers' since the 1980s, and the opportunity to listen to refugee voices in a creative setting was powerful. A commitment to awareness raising by the group informed the project team's performance planning, reaching audiences who may not have met refugees before.

> Children turned out to be weapons in Rwanda
> Democracy turned out to be dictators in Congo
> The continent is rich but the people are poor
> (Oh Africa)

> People sleep on buses
> There are beggars in the streets
> No food or even shelter
> People call you 'terrorist'
> (Fantasy Island)

A refugee is a lawyer
A refugee is a doctor
A refugee is a musician
A refugee is a human being

Refugees ask for freedom
Refugees ask for protection
Refugees ask for respect
(A Refugee is a Human Being)

The role of the music facilitators was to take creative ideas from the groups and piece them together by asking questions and offering suggestions of ways to sing or play the song. The expertise of the music facilitators was a means of supporting, not leading, the creativity of the group. They aimed to give equal space to survivors to co-create songs that could be performed together. Often, one group would share their lyrics with another group, which inspired them to write about the same theme in their own language. Survivors then taught everyone how to pronounce the lyrics in their language and the songs were split into solos, chorus, spoken word and instrumental.

> This group has given me so much of opportunities which I had inside me, so many frustrations, stress. Whatever I had, I was able to say my idea and share my idea with this group. There are so many people that are talented here and they are given a chance.

> When we started to encourage survivors to participate in song writing, they would say "No no no, you do it, I'm just watching", "Use your ideas, I don't have any ideas", but the same person in the next session, they have an idea. Now they feel that they can also control their thoughts, they can express themselves.

> (Musician-interpreter)

GROUP OWNERSHIP

It was important to ensure that each group member had a unique role and contribution in the creative process and in performance. This could be a section in their language, either as spoken word or sung, an instrumental solo or a role in introducing the song and explaining the song's meaning to the audience. It was important for members to feel that if they were not present in the group, there was something missing, and this encouraged people to feel an essential part of the group and to attend regularly. Members found it important to speak out on behalf of others who did not have a voice, as well as to be visible as torture survivors and as people seeking asylum.

Stone Flowers chose the name of their group, created their own logo and made batik material with beautiful patterns designed by group members. This was made into costumes which are still worn at every performance.

REHEARSALS AND PERFORMANCES

When a group of songs had been composed, Stone Flowers began to work towards performances. At this stage the project team brought in other professional musicians from diverse backgrounds and worked together to tighten up the song arrangements and add more instrumental parts, making the final product as professional as possible. Sessions turned into rehearsals. In the early years, music facilitators would sometimes sing during performances. However, as the group progressed, music facilitators would play instruments and support vocal harmonies, while survivors were the lead vocalists and instrumentalists.

The professionalism of the performance was important for survivors, they wanted to create good-quality music that stood alone and that they felt proud to perform. MAI always documented performances through films and photographs which were shared with group members. This contributed to members using these positive memories of performing as a coping strategy for reducing stress and intrusive memories about torture when they were away from the group.

Live performances gave some survivors' roles and identities that were beyond their traumatised selves. For others, they re-connected with aspects of themselves that had seemed distant or lost. They again enjoyed the position of being centre stage when introducing a song or provoking an audience response. The act of performing educated the audience about the politics and reality of their experience.

CHALLENGES

Attention to creating balance between language groups was important to ensure fairness. Some members experienced perceived slights from others and attention had to be given to laughter if seen as mockery. On one occasion a member felt another was laughing at their creative sharing. The laughter was actually about something unrelated, but the person felt humiliated. In response, the facilitation team were more proactive about ensuring that everyone listened when members were sharing, and they encouraged everyone to applaud after contributions.

Some survivors wanted to write religious songs, which required careful facilitation as there were often strong views on religion in the groups and religion could also be the focus of persecution and torture. Such issues were discussed, and agreement was sought so individuals could choose to sing or not.

There were a number of gay survivors in Stone Flowers, and some of the songs featured powerful lyrics about homophobia. At the time FFTNW were a diverse team and there were lesbian, gay and bisexual staff and volunteers who worked within a team atmosphere that was gay-affirming. There were posters in the centre about LGBT+ events and staff and survivors attended Gay Pride annually. This commitment was shared by the Stone Flowers project team and care was taken to support gay survivors attending the group. Gay survivors found it difficult to be completely open about their sexuality in the group, but for some the process of writing songs about their experiences of oppression enabled a 'coming out' process to the group through music.

> Pain must stop!
> Hate must stop!
> Homophobia must stop!
> Only love shall remain
>   (Pain Must Stop)

IMPACT OF STONE FLOWERS

After each project phase, group and individual testimonials were collected from survivors to determine the impact of the music sessions. Survivors were asked if they wanted to make any changes to the project and what they would like to do in the future. Audience members were asked for feedback at performances via a questionnaire that was put on every seat at the venue. Audiences were asked to feedback on what they had learnt from listening to Stone Flowers songs, as well as their opinion on the music and performance.

What survivors said about impact

The consistent feedback from members has established that the group impacted on many levels, not just on improving general mental wellbeing but on self-confidence and self-awareness, as well as the ability to manage distressing memories and trauma symptomology. Members were less isolated, felt more able to connect to others and described a new curiosity about finding out and valuing other cultures and traditions. The group enjoyed performing with professional musicians and this inspired many to learn an instrument or to make music in other settings.

Survivors described how they used music to distract themselves from their physical and emotional pain outside of the sessions. For some it helped with their sleep problems and nightmares by giving some emotional and physical material to use as 'grounding' techniques. The facilitators also noticed that their concentration and memory improved as the sessions proceeded.

Survivors talked about feeling proud of their creativity and how the process of music-making, recording and performing improved self-confidence:

> Well, the first time I sang a song that I created. I created the poem and the music with the other members. I knew it was mine and I had created it. It was mine. I just felt so proud. I always in my whole life wanted to do this and I did it. I don't know how it was, but I did it. It was so amazing.

> Recording, well I just feel so proud. When people bought the CD and tell us they enjoy our songs and play them with their children. That people sing along and play them over. It's amazing.

Survivors talked about how they supported and protected each other and that for many, Stone Flowers felt "like family":

> I had to push myself to come out of my shell. I created a shell to protect myself, but we are like a family together. We protect and support each other. That's so supportive. I love to sing, play instruments and know about making music.

> It has been 8 years and it has helped me find myself and helped me overcome my difficult experiences. It helped me write and stand on my feet again. It's been a big support in my journey. We are a big family. It is probably what I would have received if I had my family here. Mental and moral support, it helped me live my life and rise again. It's been huge.

Many survivors talked about how the group had impacted on their mental wellbeing, not only supporting them to relax during the music-making process but to lift mood, distract from distress and create new and positive memories:

> Music has helped me feel better. I can't wait for the sessions; it has made me more relaxed and comfortable than I was before. It has helped me relax with others. I can be myself and feel comfortable. I can't imagine not having this group in my life. I feel like the good things started happening in my life when the group started, after all the bad things.

> Music helps me so much. It lifts my spirit all the times I go. If my mood is low, it helps. It helps me forget all my stress. It is so helpful. I have not got [asylum] status, but the group has value for me. For me the best part is learning new songs and performing. Music has helped me too much. To be honest it was our best therapy. We sing another countries language, we love each other. We share everything.

It is uplifting for our mental health, some sort of happiness and forget things. It cannot be explainable, happiness that we have, it's really memorable.

It was very helpful because although I was getting a refusal letter [Home Office] ... I've started composing a song which we're going to sing in a few months, I can't just give up on that. I have to go to the group, and it will make you feel release for all the bad news you were getting, and it was like ... calming down my mental health and just pushing me to go, to keep singing to keep singing.

Many group members had been tortured because of their activism in their country of origin and others were politicised by their experience of seeking asylum. All were committed to educating the public about their experience of being tortured and of living in exile, with all its challenges:

It is so nice that people come to see us. Outside, nobody listens to us, we feel that nobody cares. But here to have people come and respect us, and hear what we have to say, it gives us hope. Music is the way to make them give us attention, learn about us, and respect us.

Audience feedback

Performances enabled audience members to understand and emotionally connect with the experiences of refugees in a direct way that "made it real". This was very important for survivors.

The performance was really moving and powerful. The music was fantastic. Showing the experiences of asylum seekers was really affecting.

It is the first time I've put myself in their shoes. I felt very emotional.

Moving and poignant. A story and a truth for our times that needs to be seen by many. Thank you to all the performers for sharing this.

SUMMARY

Stone Flowers now work independently with MAI and existing members help to invite and welcome new people to the group. Stone Flowers have produced two studio albums and inspired live audiences across the UK. They regularly give presentations at universities and NGO forums across the country and internationally. They have featured in music magazines, local and national newspapers, on the radio and TV.

Their songs and stories have become part of creative music programmes delivered in Ireland, the UK, Georgia, Sierra Leone, Bosnia-Hercegovina and Palestine. Activism and raising awareness of human rights abuses remains at the heart of the Stone Flowers ethos. www. musicaction.org/stone-flowers

REFERENCES

Beck, B. D., Lund, S. T., Sogaard, U., Simonsen, E., Tellier, T. C., Cordtz, T. O., Laier, G. H. and Moe, T. (2018) 'Music therapy versus treatment as usual for refugees diagnosed with posttraumatic stress disorder (PTSD): Study protocol for a randomized controlled trial', *Trials*, 19(1), p. 301. doi:10.1186/s13063-018-2662-z.

Clift, S. (2013) 'Optimism in the field of arts and health', *Perspectives in Public Health*, 133(1), pp. 1–18. doi:10.1177/1757913912469306.

Fancourt, D., Williamon, A., Carvalho, L. A., Steptoe, A., Dow, R. and Lewis, I. (2016) 'Singing modulates mood, stress, cortisol, cytokine and neuropeptide activity in cancer patients and carers', *ecancermedicalscience*, 10, 631. doi:10.3332/ecancer.2016.631.

Hanser, S. B. (2006) 'Music therapy research in adult oncology', *Journal of the Society for Integrative Oncology*, 4, pp. 62–66. doi:10.2310/7200.2006.003.

Hanser, S. B. and Thompson, L. W. (1994) 'Effects of a music therapy strategy on depressed older adults', *Journal of Gerontology*, 49, pp. 265–269. doi:10.1093/gronj/49.6.P265.

Hodges, D.A. (2010) 'Psycho-physiological measures', in Juslin, P. N. and Sloboda, J.A. (eds.) *Handbook of Music and Emotion: Theory, Research, Applications*. Oxford: Oxford University Press, pp. 279–311.

Jespersen, K. V. and Vuust, P. (2012) 'The effect of relaxation music listening on sleep quality in traumatized refugees: A pilot study', *Journal of Music Therapy*, 49(2), pp. 205–229. doi:10.1093/jmt/49.2.205.

Muriithi, B. (2020) 'Music as the medicine of trauma among refugees in Arizona', *Voices: A World Forum for Music Therapy*, 20(2). doi:10.15845/voices.v20i2.2891.

Weinstein, D., Launay, J., Pearce, E., Dunbar, R.I.M. and Stewart, L. (2016) 'Singing and social bonding: Changes in connectivity and pain threshold as a function of group size', *Evolution and Human Behavior*, 37(2), pp. 152–158. doi:10.1016/j.evolhumbehav.2015.10.002.

CHAPTER 16

SEEDS OF HOPE

Mary Raphaely and Martha Orbach

"*My life is like a leaf blowing in the wind.*" May was enslaved in her own country, trafficked to Britain, and held captive in a rural town before escaping. How could she begin to recover? In a group, working in a garden, she began to put down roots.

"The garden could be said to stand at the crossroads of nature and culture, of matter and consciousness" (Nitschke, 1999, p. 238); this intersectionality is key to its therapeutic potential. In this chapter we share a way of working therapeutically in the garden, looking at the fundamental principles of our practice, describing methods we use and highlighting examples from our work.

We work both physically and metaphorically in nature. Being in nature is inherently mindful, engaging all our senses, reminding us that things change, today is different from yesterday, helping us to stay in the present. In nature the soul can breathe. The garden provides a place to connect with the miraculous in the everyday, and to reconnect with ourselves. Here we can see the beauty that is possible right where we are; and that, as in the Zen tradition, what we find in the garden depends on what we bring. In this space healing can take place.

Here we have developed our model of therapy for those who have suffered torture, political violence, trafficking, rape and other gross human rights abuses.

A group therapist and an artist and community gardener, we have both worked with a number of refugee and migrant-led charities in community gardens and allotments. These organisations act as supportive networks and provide vital practical assistance, with colleagues carrying out assessments and casework, and ensuring that group members' basic needs are met.

The descriptions of our work in this chapter reflect the experiences of many people we have worked with. In order to protect confidentiality, we have changed all names and identifying details, and in some cases created composites involving different people working through similar challenges.

Typically, our groups have functioned organically with people joining and leaving as they wished. There is usually a core of around five group members changing over time, sessions varying from 3 to 12 people. Thus, there are always more experienced members welcoming and guiding newcomers.

Survivors frequently find it initially difficult to articulate their distress and explore its origins, exacerbated by a lack of a common language and limited English. Combining our skills in group analytic psychotherapy, art, horticulture and community work, we bring together ways of working which rely less on words and more on our universal connection with nature and each other.

Outdoors in a small group, we plant, weed, prune and tackle the tasks needed to tend the garden. As the garden grows so do the participants' confidence, connections and wellbeing. The weekly rituals of work build trust, the group providing containment which can evolve into a sense of family, the physical activity and sensory experiences providing temporary respite from inner anguish and developing resilience.

With individuals from Afghanistan, the Democratic Republic of Congo, Burma, Mauritius, Iran, Cameroon and Albania amongst others, we work without interpreters. Communication challenges are many with this mixture of language, culture and history. But collective memories of plants and landscape help connect people who otherwise have little in common.

We are part of nature and have a visceral connection with our environment. "There is increasingly compelling evidence showing that access to greenspaces really matters for our

DOI: 10.4324/9781003192978-19

health" (Public Health England, 2020, p. 10), particularly for deprived communities. The COVID-19 pandemic highlighted this alongside the inequality of access to green spaces. There is an "inverse association between surrounding greenness and all-cause mortality" (Rojas-Rueda et al., 2019, p. 469) and anxiety and depression "go up as we go away from the green and into the grey" of our increasingly concrete environment (Cameron, 2016). This increased understanding has led to an expansion of the use of therapeutic gardens from hospitals to prisons.

SOIL – GROUNDWORK

As with other creative and non-verbal approaches, ours is a hybrid of several systems, combining garden work with group analytic principles, therapeutic input and a community context (Raphaely, 2010). How someone engages with physical tasks in nature reveals much about their inner landscape, allowing for interpretation and growth. We avoid the strict application of a Western psychoanalytic model and delivering lessons in horticulture. Focusing on nature and concentrating our interaction in the present, we remain vigilant for clues of deeper resonances as we dig and sow together, finding parallels between nature and the internal world.

Nature is universal; although we are based in the UK, our methods can be adapted and scaled to entirely different contexts. During COVID-19, we worked remotely and packs containing pots, seeds and compost were sent to housebound individuals. The seedlings grown during difficult times and in spaces with little access to nature provided signs of new life and hope, as did the online communities which formed around them.

A vulnerable man living in poor housing with his family became increasingly disturbed. We suggested he place a head of garlic on the surface of a pot of soil in his room, that he water it lightly and observe it for some weeks. This served as an interesting transitional object, and he sent frequent photographs of its changes. After some weeks, he was advised to gently lift it; to his amazement he found that each clove within the garlic head had formed its own roots.

He was then encouraged to carefully separate the cloves and plant them apart, where they continued to thrive and develop into independent plants. He linked this to his own family and their need to develop independently; now he could begin the process of changing their accommodation. Nature had spoken louder than words.

In the garden, we always work as a group, enabling a broader, deeper engagement with the land and the material. When lives are fragile and uncertain the sole responsibility for care of even one plant could be a burden, particularly when it might not lead to fruition. Here the caring responsibilities are shared, as is the joy of harvest.

Sprouting broccoli leaves created unexpected joy in the group, as they or similar species are widely grown across East Africa. "*We eat that back home!*" came a shout from one woman. Usually reserved, she called over the other African women, "*Look, look! Sukuma wiki!*" Gathered around this plant, they shared recipes, and that its name means "*stretch the week*". They had forgotten themselves, no longer shy, but excitedly talking over each other. For displaced people in a strange city, there is something revelatory about discovering a familiar plant growing – a small part of home, thought lost, now recovered.

Our purpose is not to create a beautiful garden, but to find links in nature with group members' experiences and feelings. Plants are evocative and can provide an instant link to the past, something which could take years in a conventional therapeutic setting. Growing vegetables together activates non-threatening connections to the past, providing new sustenance.

In nature we all stand equal, having an essential entitlement to this earth. People often bring more knowledge of the land than we possess, helping to flatten the hierarchy. We are facilitators rather than teachers or experts, this requires careful listening for where members' interests and enthusiasms lie, enabling them to achieve their ideas. If material brought by participants indicates it is important to prune something in a particular way, we do this regardless of whether it is good horticultural practice. Thus our approach differs from traditional horticulture, becoming a clear psychotherapeutic pursuit.

We aim to facilitate healing and create sustainable connections with the environment, helping people to increase agency and ownership. In the words of one member:

> I have witnessed a big change here, so I am very pleased. This garden has been part of my life, I have really enjoyed the way we were planting and harvesting … and I am really proud to have been part of the group which made it possible.

We listen carefully to ascertain the most helpful task for each individual each day. This is an important flexibility the garden offers, allowing people to feel met and held by the work. We tailor tasks to nurture participants' interests, and to respond to emerging themes quickly, adapting pre-made plans when necessary.

We do not work with single-sex groups. A very high proportion of both women and men we work with have been raped. This might make it difficult to tolerate being with others in close proximity indoors, particularly with mixed-gender groups. Working alongside each other in nature, however, it is possible to moderate both physical and psychological distance while approaching a shared task. This greatly helps to rebuild trust.

We aim to build and facilitate community in the garden and to create the conditions for this. People have different reasons for coming: some enjoy how *"we laugh all the time in the garden"*, others need quiet sanctuary and mindfulness. As part of creating a shared space, we begin a session sitting and talking in a circle and end with tea, reflecting on our work and discussing next steps. This allows for collaborative planning and supports engagement. It is important to respect decisions taken, ensuring that for the next session the promised seeds or materials are provided.

We often have deep connections to our childhood landscape, and associated sensations can house many memories. Group visits to botanic gardens provide access to specific ecosystems; plants like coffee, tea and palms define landscapes but do not grow in England. They give opportunities for sharing stories: building with latanier palms, drinking from coconut pith, growing yam.

Reconnection provided by a familiar plant or climate, even in miniature, can help repair the break caused by trauma between members' pre-traumatic lives and the present. Cut off in exile from the sights, smells and sensations of childhood, the opportunity to walk amongst banana trees and feel the humidity can be joyful. Standing in a huge conservatory at Kew Gardens in London, one man observed: *"This is the closest I've been to home for years!"*

The garden must be relevant and grow plants with meaning for the group. This can be as simple as buying spinach instead of radish seeds. Seeds travel with diasporas, carrying a wealth of knowledge and resource.

In one group, there was a clamour to grow okra, although it was unknown to several members. Exploring the urgency of the request, we understood why the seedlings were so carefully nurtured in the greenhouse: *"In my country, if someone comes to your house and you do not offer them okra, they won't feel welcome. When my grandmother visited and my Mum didn't cook okra, she would leave, angry."*

Often, proposing a new idea is a fragile but powerful expression of hope and belonging, and must be treated with care. People who have lost everything cannot always trust easily or allow themselves to hope. A group member explains how a core healing the garden offers is the slow joy of relearning that if you plant a seed, fruit will come and the harvest will follow:

Being in the garden makes you switch your attention from the bad things that have happened that you want to put aside, to the things that you want to keep alive. Then there is also some hope. You know a plant will flower, you will get the fruits.

In a group the fruits of our work are celebrated together, and the wider ecosystem enriches our efforts, with plants such as callaloo, rocket, and poppies, self-seeding and popping up all around.

ROOTS – DISPLACEMENT, SEEKING SAFETY AND BUILDING TRUST

Survivors' needs are many and complex. Most experience precarious housing and enforced moves to remote and substandard accommodation, undermining any grounding they might achieve and exacerbating already high levels of stress and trauma. Contact with nature is usually very limited, along with any sense of place where one could begin to put down roots.

We addressed this directly in one of our gardens. Group members identified privacy as an issue as we could only use a section of land belonging to a community centre. We discussed creating a barrier, what it should keep out and what could be allowed in, in this very different context from many peoples' past experiences.

As a group, we planned a screen of living willow to shield us. Planting the cut willow stalks we considered: how close must things be to each other to offer support? Is it possible for a plant to grow when it is severed and distanced from its original root? Will it grow strong? In shaping and tying the willow, would it break if forced to bend too much? The metaphorical aspect of these issues was quickly accessible to all.

This screen featured in the group for months: on their own initiative, members carefully interwove new shoots, delighting in the privacy it quickly offered. One member spoke about how he had nothing of himself where he lived; pointing to the willow cuttings he said, "*I need a place to put down roots*". Over tea after the session, we reflected on how much safer this place felt, despite new dangers in peoples' lives. A feeling of satisfaction and tentative hope spread between the members. Together, we could contemplate the future.

We draw on the elements to find points of connection. We have all known open skies, high winds, sunshine and pouring rain, birdsong, growth and decay. In one community garden, our weekly sessions always involved a fire when the weather justified it. Fire is central in many cultures and carries strong associations for many of our members. At Nowruz, the Iranian New Year, the custom of jumping over the fire created much happiness and laughter in the group.

But we must remain always alert as nature can trigger memories of terrible times. In the midst of this jocularity, one of the women recoiled, gazing terrified at the flames, dragged back to the moment her village was torched. Immediate intervention was necessary; she was supported, comforted and accompanied home. At last we understood her reluctance to participate in this session, and why in her therapy group she had mostly sat silently weeping and resisting any attempts to engage further. This experience allowed her finally to speak about what had happened to her whole community.

Working in the garden, she was transformed. A more experienced farmer than any of us, she planted, harvested, and quietly directed others with authority drawn from happier times. For a short while she could reconnect with her former strength and feel safe. Too hurt to engage in much talking, her sense of stability grew slowly as she worked in her group and enjoyed some respite from her isolation.

Torture attacks connections, wholeness itself, often severing and destroying links with all that is positive and sustaining. It fractures the capacity for trust, damaging the roots of the psyche. Violence to the body through persecution causes lasting and often incapacitating damage. Digging and planting, people reconnect with their physical selves, repairing some of this disconnection.

Therapy with survivors of torture and organised violence stands firmly between an individual's external and internal worlds, incorporating and integrating references to both. While working together in nature we carefully reweave the ruptured threads, bearing witness, helping to build trust again, and slowly restoring hope.

SEEDS – HOPE AND NEW BEGINNINGS

In nature we experience the regular turning of the seasons. Cycles of life, death and rebirth are evident in the sowing, growth, harvesting and dying back which nature provides. Engaging with this process can be transformative for someone who has lost touch with a sense of natural order:

> Plants give me courage when I feel very down … when they die, another one comes. Life is there all the time, so I try to stay in the present, and don't let myself go back where the pain is. I feel proud when I see all the shoots turning green, because we planted and harvested them – life is that cycle.

To plant a seed is to have hope for the future, and people have hesitated about doing this. In the greenhouse as everyone chose a packet of seeds, Juliet was happy, pointing to the picture on her pansy packet: "*This is the first time that I can see the future, maybe my life will change and become beautiful.*"

But as she began to make indentations in the soil, her mood shifted, and she took a long time planting the seeds, first placing them deep in the soil, then bringing them back closer to the surface. Asked why, she said, "*these seeds are my children, I need them to come quickly, quickly*".

She started to shake, weeping without tears, and frozen with grief. Forced to flee her country some years before, she had to leave her small children, and she had no idea what had happened to them.

Now Beata put her arms around her, and she led Juliet down the garden to a small group of crocuses, holding a tiny double iris that was found in the compost. She said, "*come, let us plant it together, it is the grandmother and the mother, and we should put it here next to the children to be a family*". Arms wrapped around each other, they shared the terrible pain of not knowing where their children were, and in this moment the group could only bear silent witness. Together they somehow contained their desperation.

It is vital to re-engage with people's pre-traumatic capacities. We encourage recourse anyone makes to their previous knowledge and experience; these memories provide nourishment and increase resilience.

Frank initially hesitated when given a daffodil bulb to plant in the autumn, perhaps doubting that it would grow. He said,

> In my country when I plant a tree, I make a prayer – and I then have to say what I want to see, and that it should grow quickly. If it is a big tree, I will make a bigger prayer. … Like that, people will gather underneath. You don't just put a new plant in the soil, we need to think about it; we need to care for it, to have a relationship with this new thing.

Gardening is care made manifest. Planting and caring for a seedling may be the first step towards rebuilding a self which has been shattered by torture. Gardening also moves participants from being cared for to being carers; this is vital for recovery.

PRUNING – GARDEN WORK

The metaphorical nature of our work can be surprising. We were repairing a garden shed, salvaging what we could from old material. One of the group sat watching, too depressed to participate. Noting this, the men in the group drew her in, and helped her to join in the task.

When we had finished there was much jubilation, and the entire mood had shifted. Later she told the group how strong the experience had been. By discarding the old bits and repairing the shed with the others, it was now protected from the bad weather coming.

She had found a link with her own life; while struggling with all the bad things in her life, this experience had enabled her to think about the healthy parts, and this had given her renewed strength.

We all need to feel useful and to have a sense of purpose; for many this is denied by the asylum system. In enforced stasis there is huge satisfaction to be gained from clearing weeds from a piece of land and preparing it for new growth. These collective endeavours greatly assist forging a new community. As personalities emerge while tackling physical tasks, people rediscover an old sense of themselves, and clearer identities re-establish in the group.

For people seeking asylum, trapped in a dehumanising system, there is special joy in growing and sourcing food to take home. At harvest time, a group insisted we two also take home some produce, delighting in the equalising of this shared bounty.

Core to our practice is to help participants see their lives as connected in some kind of continuum and not as fractured irrevocably by their terrifying experiences. The past can feel like an unscalable wall, cut off, and only something delicate can succeed in opening a door, and letting some light enter the darkness to nurture new shoots.

Tortured in his home country, terrified by his journey to England, and traumatised by his experiences after arriving, Frank had struggled to give a coherent account; words were inadequate. We needed another language, which nature provided. His confidence returned as he began to re-access his considerable knowledge of working the land: planting corn, pruning fruit trees, cutting out dead wood to facilitate new growth. Slowly recovering a fuller sense of himself was vital in strengthening his resilience. Some repair had taken place, and Frank was now able to participate increasingly in the group, emerging as a wise and philosophical elder: "*I've learned that many things from my past are useful – I wasn't looking behind the wall of my past before.*"

A PLACE TO BREATHE – SANCTUARY

Sanctuary, oasis, refuge – these words are often used to describe urban gardens; their meaning is common to many, creating a shared experience with the wider community. This is particularly powerful for those caught in the asylum system. Britain's 'hostile environment' ensures the perpetuation of a sense of extreme unsafety, keeping people trapped for years. The garden represents a radically different place, an escape into a new environment, a parallel world in the heart of the city.

Out in the open, on a fundamental level, there is a feeling of being at home. People subject to state surveillance or forced to live beneath the radar often feel safer as part of a group in a green space.

Herve was initially difficult to understand, repeating, "*I was running all the time … they were trying to silence me*". He came weekly for five years, grateful even in the rain for the space the garden provided. Talking incessantly, but often as if he had been joined in mid-sentence, he would end, shrug apologetically, expecting nothing. Working in the garden, hands in the soil, feet on the ground, helped unscramble his thinking, calm him and provide some relief from his incessant panic.

He slowly connected with others in the group. With jumbled words, he participated, and was accepted. People accepted his way of speaking and he earned respect for his quiet competence and commitment. Enjoying the jokes and participating in the collective sense of satisfaction over tea at the end of the session were a vital part of his emerging sociability and it was in the generous, non-confrontational, non-verbal space of the garden that he slowly re-emerged.

Tea is hugely important in our garden work, providing a gentle way for people unused to being with others socially, to be together, accepted and linked by shared work.

Initially, Herve would always say he didn't know, or couldn't remember how to do anything; but a year or so in he started to realise he did. He began fixing things, taking on small projects, repairing dilapidated furniture, sharpening tools. Before finally being granted asylum and securing a full-time job, Herve made a bench. He researched and chose the design himself; we bought the timber and he constructed it. He would sit on it in the circle of his group contentedly contemplating the garden; it remains in place, a legacy of a beloved soul.

The frequent demand, with each new agency, to retell the same story of trauma and loss binds the person seeking asylum tightly to their dreadful experiences. Working outdoors changes the dynamic; talking becomes secondary. We do not ask when someone arrived in England, how or why. They choose whether to share their story, allowing them to live in the present. Explaining why he took three buses to come and help cut back brambles on cold autumn days, one man explained simply, *"they don't ask me questions here"*. Another, having planted something while thinking about his young son, said, *"I am very happy to have a little place here, it feels like my garden, nobody asks me what I am doing there"*.

ECOSYSTEM – INTERCONNECTIONS

Key to our approach is the idea that establishing a relationship with the land is the first step towards connecting with the group and with the wider community. This will be critical for migrants to begin to feel settled in their host country and find a way to contribute to it. Interactions with local people are important. They may provide cultural connections and routes into communities but might also reveal suspicion or hostility.

Nature can quickly form communities of interest, uniting diverse people. A cherry tree in the garden was laden with fruit, drawing attention. In minutes, David had scaled the tree and was passing armfuls of cherries down through an international relay system to a growing audience. *"We make cherry pilaf"*, one of the Iranians explained; *"I will make cherry pie"*, a local Polish woman cried. A chorus of recipes and memories emerged from the assembled group of locals and refugees.

The shared investment in the garden can build bridges with the local community, particularly where locals may have a shared plant heritage with those seeking refuge. Bonds can form caring for plants they both know.

An elderly neighbour, after discussion with a vulnerable member of our community, brought her a cho cho, rare to see growing in England, but native to many warmer countries. Sarah explained how this made her feel recognised and seen within the garden and the community. She described the connection they had formed, saying she *"respected her as an elder"*, and this gesture helped to reaffirm to her that she existed despite having no passport and being endlessly held in stasis by the asylum process.

When a woman from the neighbouring estate learned that many members did not know what rhubarb was, she baked several pies for everyone to try, providing an unexpected point of connection. She had probably never met a refugee before; nor had they had a kind exchange with a local person. Moments like these create a sense of community and understanding which transcends barriers, and affirms everyone's right to be here, celebrating all contributions.

LAND – SETTLEMENT, SECURITY

How we work is determined by the space available. A protected space is useful, although occasional breaches can provide fruitful learning material. Each context provides different challenges: how secure is the site? Do other people work here?

Often the land we use is rented, shared, and without any guarantee for the future. There are vital lessons in accepting that rights to such land are tenuous, but that much can be gained from engaging with it anyway. Losses in the lives of our members are so great that, for them, there is a risk in engaging with the temporary nature of our projects. Working through the anxieties this induces can prove cathartic.

Inability to control our shared workspace once had potentially devastating consequences. We arrived one morning to find that all the large shrubs that shielded the back wall of our part of a communal garden had been hacked to the ground by a volunteer team. The group were shocked and dismayed. To some, the scene instantly triggered memories of devastation wrought in their villages by rebel groups such as Boko Haram, recalling feelings of panic and fear.

We struggled to persuade them to keep going; they felt exposed and unprotected. The following week only half the group attended. The episode underlined that we staff are not omnipotent, that all that we can know is the present moment that we inhabit. We worked to establish the parallel: setbacks occur and resilience is needed to deal with the asylum experience. Slowly, we set about replanting a shelter for the garden.

Digging and weeding, planting and seeding, people ground themselves, finding roots in this new space. Gardens provide space to engage in different ways, sometimes beginning by observing quietly, and then slowly becoming empowered to bring strengths and ideas to the work. The group aspect is vital in supporting these moments, as people find their feet again, re-connecting with their knowledge and sharing skills, they model what it might feel like to be appreciated by this new family.

Glamorous Laila, an unlikely gardener, always stylishly dressed, was drawn to the garden by her friend Lisbet, a self-confessed farmer. She enjoyed the group banter but remained guarded, a gentle but passive member. She would only forget herself and come alive on occasions like the potato harvest, when she joined in gleefully emptying sacks onto the ground as we all scrabbled for the new potatoes.

It took three years before Laila emerged from her shell, talking about the need to bring beauty to peoples' lives and her love of flowers. She spoke about how the scent transports one to paradise, and that the garden should be made beautiful to lift peoples' spirits. Poring over bulb catalogues, she chose a planting scheme for the terrace, taking initiative and ownership in a new way. When the bulbs arrived, she led the planting, choosing combinations and bringing her sense of style to the garden. The new planting was widely applauded, growing her confidence and drawing her further into the work.

MEMORIALS – A PLACE FOR GRIEF AND REMEMBERING

A vital, but little discussed aspect of our work relates to memorials. Many from our groups have either fled a situation in which they lost loved ones or have heard of the death of a beloved person once in England. There was no time to say goodbye, to reflect quietly on their loss, and no known burial place. Realising the importance of this, we have occasionally planted a shrub as a memorial, creating a ritual around it involving the whole group.

A woman whose baby was murdered in front of her chose to plant a soft pink, sweet-smelling rose. Haltingly, she shared this story with the group, who surrounded her with care and support of the kind practiced in her culture. She continued to visit this plant, watering and sitting beside it as her new toddler played around it; she was clear that she could only risk having another child once her first baby had been properly put to rest.

A man whose wife and young children were killed in reprisal for his having fled his country, was insistent in his choice of plant. "*Its flowers must be white, beautiful and tiny, like their little faces – the leaves must be here always, no dying in the winter.*" Helped by his chosen symbolism, he was for the first time able to speak in the group; with difficulty, he described his desperation each time he thought of their fate. This was met by a profound silence; then tentatively one of the women approached and hugged him. Others slowly followed wordlessly; thereafter the group paid close attention to the wellbeing of his shrub, the most acceptable way they could demonstrate their support.

The group agreed on the need for a communal point of reflection, choosing a rosebush called *Blessing*. On specific occasions we gave large white beach pebbles to group members, inviting them to write a prayer, a wish, or simply a name with an indelible pen. These were placed around the rosebush, sometimes with the writing uppermost, sometimes hidden. Members shared whatever they wished to in the group. This plant remained a focus where people returned in quiet contemplation whenever they wanted; we ensured that the supply of stones continued.

CONCLUSION – A DIFFERENT COUNTRY

There is something radical about community gardens in urban environments. They disrupt the norms: property prices make their existence unusual, and the values of shared space and accessibility contrast with the surrounding private and commercial ethos. They introduce a wild element into an otherwise regulated environment, creating a space that allows other versions of oneself to emerge. Here one can talk to strangers; everyone is a friend when watching tadpoles or sheltering from the rain.

We try to bring some of the spirit of farming into the urban environment, where everyone has a job and works together. Even in urban gardens, one can re-create some of the joy of clattering down a ladder to a shared lunch during haymaking.

Jemal was incredulous when we produced a packet with ten tomato seeds. Slicing a large tomato, he squeezed its seeds into a dip in the soil, covered it with dry leaves, and made a tripod of bamboo to contain it. Others, having sown seeds in the greenhouse, amiably teased him that owing to the weather, here in England we start growing tomatoes inside, but he ignored them and visited his creation weekly. Eventually, he conceded defeat and an important discussion ensued: conditions are different here, this is a new country. Drawing on this during his frequent night-time panic attacks served to ground him in the here and now. Recognising this new land was an important part of making new roots.

The garden allows skills to revive after long dormancy. This can be particularly important for men who have lost their traditional role as makers and fixers. A sense of purpose comes flooding back in chopping wood or mending a wheelbarrow. When we needed to build a cold frame, a man who had come to the garden every week quietly took over. Following the instructions and carefully organising and laying out the pieces, he brushed aside any help from us, directing members of the group, with only the occasional "*Do you have a ...? What is that thing ... for bolts ... to unscrew? Ah a spanner, I never knew that word in English, I have been here 17 years and never had the chance to use one.*" A qualified engineer, he was forbidden to work during a protracted asylum process. Now at retirement age, he was using his skills again.

Some words from Markus encapsulate our collective work. One day he arrived breathless, showing a lovely photo on his phone. He said,

> I never knew this before; it is called a daffodil, and it tells us that the hard time is nearly finished, winter is now over. In my country I had never heard of spring, we do not have this in Africa, but this is the flower that tells us that it is coming. At home, we only ever put flowers down when someone dies.

He had finally arrived in England; and now he added, "*My country has beautiful sun but rubbish human rights; yours has rubbish sun but here we have human rights.*"

Working in the garden is not the solution to a specific problem – it is more a place of metaphors, sensory experiences, work and discovery.

And May, her life no longer a leaf floating in the wind, worked with the garden group, joined a library, went to college, qualified and now works as a nurse.

REFERENCES

Cameron, R. (2016) Urban Horticulture – repairing the rift, John MacLeod Lecture 2016, Royal Horticultural Society. Available at: https://www.youtube.com/watch?v=C2FPUll2xbM (Accessed: 22 January 2022).

Nitschke, G. (1999) *Japanese Gardens: Right Angle and Natural Form*. Köln, Germany: Taschen.

Public Health England (2020) *Improving access to greenspace: A new review for 2020*. Available at: https://assets.publishing.service.gov.uk/government/uploads/system/uploads/attachment_data/file/904439/Improving_access_to_greenspace_2020_review.pdf (Accessed: 22 January 2022).

Raphaely, M. (2010) 'Routes to the unspeakable: working with victims of torture', in Gautier, A. and Sabatini Scalmati, A. (eds.) *Bearing Witness: Psychoanalytic Work with People Traumatized by Torture and State Violence* (1st ed.). London: Routledge, pp. 13–26. doi:10.4324/9780429472213.

Rojas-Rueda, D., Nieuwenhuijsen, M., Gascon, M., Perez-Leon, D. and Pierpaolo, M. (2019) 'Green spaces and mortality: A systematic review and meta-analysis of cohort studies', *The Lancet, Planetary Health*, 3 (11), pp. 469–477. doi:10.1016/S2542-5196(19)30215-3.

CHAPTER 17

FOOTBALL THERAPY GROUPS FOR SURVIVORS OF TORTURE

Terry Hanley

This chapter introduces the practice of working therapeutically through football with individuals who have survived torture. It begins by providing a background to this approach, making specific reference to the way that sports have the potential to offer therapeutic interventions that are biopsychosocial in nature. This is then considered in relation to how therapists might make sense of integrating such activities into their work and how this relates to common theoretical understandings of the way that those who have survived torture may reconstruct and rebuild their lives. It is proposed that activities such as football can play an important part in helping individuals who have experienced significant trauma develop trust with services and therapeutic alliances with those offering support. To end, the concepts that have been introduced throughout the chapter are illustrated through the description of an existing football therapy project. Here the collaborative work between a specialist service that provides psychological support to refugees who have survived torture (Freedom from Torture) and a small community focused football club within the Manchester area of the United Kingdom (FC United of Manchester) is presented. The challenges and opportunities associated with running this project are described and discussed.

FOOTBALL AS A FORM OF THERAPY

Football, or soccer, has an important place within the culture of many countries. It can unify individuals towards a common cause and polarise differences. People hug strangers as if they were their extended family if they support the same team. In contrast, they may also threaten or want to fight with others if they do not. Whether you, the reader, love, hate or are ambivalent towards it, it is difficult to ignore the passion that football can rise up within people. The 'Beautiful Game', in the words of the Brazilian footballer Pele, can be both a destructive force and a creative one. Within this chapter, we acknowledge the divisive nature of the sport, but focus primarily upon the constructive growth that can occur by using football as a therapeutic tool.

The French existential philosopher Albert Camus is famous for writing some of the most thought-provoking work of the twentieth century. He was also known to be quite a good goalkeeper. Within an alumni magazine for his youth football club, Racing Universitaire Algerios, he even proclaimed that all he knew about morality and obligations he owed to football. The sentiments of his words highlight the way that, for Camus, as with many fans and players, football can act as a way of learning about the world. It provides a world within the world for individuals to learn about themselves, and to learn about the way that they engage with others. Whether a person watches football, or plays football, the activity does not occur in a vacuum. It is constantly in dialogue with others around them and the broader community.

So, how can playing football be therapeutic? When we consider mental health and wellbeing, the biopsychosocial perspective first proposed by Engel (1978) is a helpful starting point for considering the way that sports might integrate into health care. This perspective highlights the way that biological factors (e.g. our physical health and genetics), psychological factors (e.g. our personality and coping skills) and social factors (e.g. our peer and family circumstances and relationships) all play a role in keeping us healthy and impact upon our overall wellbeing. Fundamentally, inherent within this view is the notion that humans are embedded within a series of complex systems that interact with each other. This systemic perspective can be aligned to ecological theories, which argue that the individual cannot be taken out of their

DOI: 10.4324/9781003192978-20

socio-political context (Bronfenbrenner, 1979), and combined with humanistic theories, such as the person-centred approach that places great emphasis on the quality of the relationship between the therapist and clients (Rogers, 1951). Notably, such theories propose that when an individual is provided with a warm, safe, and accepting environment, constructive growth can occur. This ecologically informed humanistic psychology (Hanley et al., 2019) can provide a helpful base for understanding the ethos of many group or community interventions and can arguably provide a means of understanding therapeutic work facilitated through football.

With the above framework in mind, this chapter makes the case that football can be therapeutic where the group in question is fundamentally safe and supportive to its members. Football groups are unable to change the broader society, but they can provide microcosms of support in which people can connect with others, learn about themselves, grow constructively and, in some cases, flourish (Joseph, 2015). As referred to earlier, however, football is far from a safe space for many who play it. Team sports, as with other group activities, can be fraught with difficult dynamics. Within the footballing context, players might compete with others to be the best at a position, argue about decisions they viewed as unfair, or feel annoyed towards other members of the team who make a mistake. Football is typically a competitive game, and the opportunities and challenges associated with it can lead to strong emotions. In many contexts, issues such as these might be left to sort themselves out or be managed by a coach. Increasingly, however, there are instances where football groups are being proactively supported by mental health and wellbeing professionals.

WHY USE FOOTBALL THERAPEUTICALLY?

Given the evocative nature of football, the question 'Why try to utilise football therapeutically?' might be asked. The answer, in short, is that football appears to be a successful means for offering support. It has already been used effectively as a therapeutic vehicle to work in a number of ways and with a wide variety of groups. For instance, the language of football can be used to support therapeutic conversations in more traditional therapies (Jones, 2009) and many football clubs provide information about mental health and wellbeing initiatives (Pringle, 2009; Curran et al., 2017). The potential for football to harness therapeutic discussions can particularly be seen in how national football associations, such as the Football Association in the UK, provide guidance for coaches about how they can support individuals struggling with their mental health and wellbeing (The Football Association, 2019). Such guidance provides practical information to coaches about how to identify those who may be struggling and how best to support them in obtaining the help they need.

In addition to providing information and signposting individuals to services, numerous football groups have started to emerge that have an explicit therapeutic element – activities that are being increasingly referred to as 'Football Therapy'. Within the current literature, groups and tournaments have been set up and evaluated for those who have a mental health diagnosis (Darongkamas et al., 2011), refugee groups (Tribe, 2002) and those who are currently homeless or vulnerably housed (Sherry, 2010). These projects provide a significant shift from many of the more community-focused projects as, instead of the development of football skills, mental health and wellbeing are placed well and truly in the foreground. As such, although developing footballing skills remains important, they are by no means the major goal of the activity itself. Instead, ensuring that the participants have a positive experience in an environment in which they feel safe proves pivotal to the work. Given this change of emphasis, it is notable that projects that do prioritise the therapeutic element of the work are commonly overseen by a therapeutic practitioner, as well as a football coach or sports psychologist (Twizell and Hanley, 2021).

INTEGRATING FOOTBALL INTO THERAPY

The idea of integrating an activity such as football into therapeutic work will not come naturally to many therapists. It is a messy activity that is difficult to control and can lead to physical injuries. Further, although it involves huge amounts of communication during football sessions, arguably it does not involve much talking. It is, therefore, a long way from much of the therapeutic theory that encourages practitioners to proactively work to provide a contained physical space for individuals to explore the life situations that they find themselves in.

Given the above, many therapists will baulk at the use of sporting activities in the therapy that they offer. However, many will integrate a variety of different therapeutic methods into the way that they work with clients. Such integrative, or pluralistic, perspectives commonly prize the idea that one size of therapy can never fit all, with the acknowledgement that those who seek support come in all shapes and sizes and want to work through all manner of difficulties in therapy. Therapists are therefore encouraged to work responsively and consider what their clients' preferences and goals are when considering a way forward (Hanley et al., 2017). Typically, a therapist might consider whether they offer a psychological approach such as cognitive-behavioural therapy or person-centred therapy, but why should this stop there? Alternative ways of offering therapy have become commonplace in the therapeutic landscape. Many therapists utilise expressive techniques, online therapies have proliferated, particularly since the pandemic, and telephone counselling has been a staple service for decades. With this in mind, it is therefore argued here that, just as art can act as a medium for expressing emotions and the Internet can increase access to therapeutic support, so can alternative media such as football (or indeed other sporting activities such as horse riding or surfing – approaches that are also used therapeutically).

One of the arguments for working therapeutically through football is that it is a context that is familiar and comfortable for many people. Indeed, for some, accessing traditional, in-person talking therapies can prove incredibly difficult. In its simplest form, it is notable that many football therapy groups highlight the potential of attracting male clients who might not typically be drawn to talking therapies. Similarly, many groups that have been written about, and referred to above, focus upon work with male groups. Such assumptions reflect trends within broader society, but as football becomes increasingly popular for all genders, the scope of such provision will potentially increase too. What is important to note is that football is a context that some people feel is more accessible than other formats. We return to this issue below when considering the role of football in supporting survivors of torture.

FOOTBALL THERAPY FOR SURVIVORS OF TORTURE

This section reflects briefly upon some key elements that relate specifically to working therapeutically with survivors of torture through sporting activities. These are: (i) the physical nature of both torture and sporting activities; (ii) football therapy as a part of a broader ecosystem of support; and (iii) the role of the football therapy group in the process of moving beyond the impact of torture. To end, a brief overview of a recent evaluation of a football therapy project with survivors of torture is provided.

The first element is the physical nature of both torture and sporting activities. The impacts of torture on survivors are known to be multifaceted, with the psychological and physical impacts being difficult to separate (van der Kolk, 2014). On a surface level, this wisdom is evident in the titles of books that examine the subject matter, for instance 'The Breaking of Bodies and Minds' (Stover and Nightingale, 1985) and 'The Body Keeps Score' (van der Kolk, 2014). Alongside this understanding runs the assumption that the support that is provided to survivors also needs to be multifaceted. Football therapy offers group members the opportunity to reconnect with their physical selves in a safe and supportive environment. This may be through the personal physical challenges associated with exercise, or indeed the robustness of the competitive element of sports.

The second element to highlight is that football therapy groups with survivors of torture are only part of a broader support package. Where services catering for this specific group have been set up, they are commonly supported by additional one-to-one evidence-based interventions. For instance, individuals may also receive support by a therapist providing trauma-focused CBT or EMDR at the same time as attending the football group. Such a way of working might be viewed as prizing the broader support ecosystem that people find themselves in. For example, contracted psychological support might sit alongside support from community groups (e.g. that offered by religious groups or obtained through volunteering opportunities) and other essential resources (e.g. general legal casework and medical support). The world of therapy, which so often views therapy in isolation, can therefore potentially learn from the world of football. Pele said, "I'm constantly being asked about individuals. The only way to win is as a team. Football is not about one or two or three star players." Looking after the mental health and wellbeing of ourselves and others might therefore be similarly best viewed as a team sport.

When considered alongside the three stages (1. establishing safety, 2. remembrance and mourning, and 3. reconnection) of moving beyond traumatic events articulated by Herman (1992), two of these stages appear particularly relevant. These are discussed in turn below:

Establishing safety: One way of making sense of the use of football therapy groups with survivors of torture is that the group can act as an anchor point for its members when accessing multiple sources of support. As individuals may find themselves moving between the various stages described by Herman, football therapy groups can play an important role in the development of a constructive alliance throughout any therapeutic work. For instance, as many individuals who have survived torture are also commonly seeking refuge in other countries, the culture of therapy can be unknown and potentially unsettling to those being offered support. The trust required to feel safe within therapy should therefore not be taken for granted. Running groups that survivors are comfortable in can enhance relationships between the services and those using them. Specifically in this case, the focus of engaging in football-related activities has the potential to help build trust and aid survivors to feel safer with those in supportive roles.

Reconnection: The 'reconnection' stage, in which individuals begin to look beyond their earlier experiences, also seems very relevant to the role of football therapy groups. Here these groups can provide an important supportive scaffolding for their members whilst they reconfigure their understanding of themselves in the world. They provide experiential encounters with others that can contain conflict, compassion and coaching. The football pitch, rife with all the emotions that it evokes, can therefore provide much opportunity for transformative learning. Finally, the groups can also play an important role in aiding their members to disconnect from any intensive relationships with therapists and organisations that they may have. For some, the organisations they have worked with may be viewed as having provided another opportunity in life. As such, providing constructive safe spaces to disconnect, and potentially supporting individuals to engage in other activities (e.g. other football projects/teams), can therefore be helpful.

Football groups have the potential to offer a safe and familiar place for those involved to engage with others. A recent evaluation of a football therapy group with survivors of torture was conducted with a similar project run by the Freedom from Torture centre based in London (Horn et al., 2019). This project runs in collaboration with a premier league club, Arsenal Football Club. The evaluation aimed to explore the ways that the group contributed to the wellbeing of the individuals taking part and to chronicle some of the key characteristics of the group. In summary the group reported that those involved:

- Developed positive relationships with others

People come from different communities, we speak different languages but when we play we have one language, the language of football.

(Player, p. 103)

- Had a sense of belonging to the group

When I arrived in the UK it wasn't easy to socialise, I didn't know anyone, even I didn't want to talk. But I feel like I belong to the UK because I belong to Arsenal. Arsenal is part of the history of the country, if I belong to Arsenal I belong to the country.

(Player, p. 104)

- Helped to foster hope for the future

When I came to the UK my brain was full of old memories, thinking only of the place I came from. It takes time to start collecting new memories—now I dream about my time here, instead of at home. Coming to the football group gave me a starting point, a way to start collecting new memories.

(Player, p. 104)

- Helped individuals to manage their emotions

The staff are great, I've never seen them angry. Even if you're an angry person, being around them teaches me to be calm. I love the way they control the atmosphere—they know we have problems. They are patient.

(Player, p. 104)

- Enjoyed the sessions

The time you're playing football you don't think about the difficulties in your life. The only thing is, your main concern at that time is to enjoy your game, is to score goals or something like that, that's the only thing you're focused on that day. Probably you might want to think, 'oh my God, my papers', but you see the ball is coming, and you forget about that for at least one or two hours, which is enough for the whole day.

(Player, p. 105)

- Saw improvements in their physical health

I love playing football, exercise is good for my body. I sleep better.

(Player, p. 105)

Please note that the themes and quotes from players presented here come from Horn et al.'s (2019) paper. They are included at length here as many of the sentiments of this research echo the feedback provided by the Manchester group described below.

THE FREEDOM FROM TORTURE FOOTBALL PROJECT IN MANCHESTER, UK

Freedom from Torture are a UK-based organisation that provides specialist psychological support to help refugees who have survived torture move beyond their experiences and rebuild their lives. They have a clinical model that offers evidence-based support for individuals who have experienced trauma. They have a number of centres across the UK and, in addition to one-to-one therapeutic work, run a variety of group-based activities that are open to those using the service (e.g. yoga, poetry, music). As noted within earlier sections, these groups are intended to complement the therapeutic process and are not intended to be offered on their own. The Manchester-based football project is one such service.

Kicking the project off

The football project evolved from a suggestion that was made by the organisation's Experts by Experience group, a service user-led group developed to feed opinions of survivors into the running of the service. This group had become aware of other football projects that had supported refugees and believed this approach had the potential to offer survivors in Manchester another means of keeping healthy. There were a number of people who were particularly interested in football and the suggestion proved popular with the group. In seeking a partner for the project, a local football club, FC United of Manchester (FC United), came forward to offer resources. FC United are a small football club (when considered alongside other Manchester-based football clubs) who have a strong ethos of supporting community projects. They have a compact stadium, which houses a number of changing rooms, and a separate training facility. The training facility includes pitches and equipment such as goals, balls, mannequins (for practising free kicks) and clean kit. Fundraising has allowed Freedom from Torture to provide players with football boots and shin pads (essential safety equipment).

The GOALS of the project

The project is multifaceted and purposefully aims to support people on a number of levels. The overarching goal of the project might be viewed as:

- To provide a safe space in which individuals feel accepted and valued for who they are

Sub-goals to this might be seen as:

- To provide players with a space to exercise and develop their fitness and football skills
- To provide a safe space to experience the psychological ups and downs associated with engaging in sporting activities
- To provide group members with a space to socialise with others who have shared interests

These goals specifically reflect the biopsychosocial perspective mentioned earlier in the chapter.

The players

The group is typically made up of between 5 and 12 survivors who make use of Freedom from Torture's services – this can change from week to week as group members may have other commitments that they need to attend. Those in the group range greatly in age, with some members being in their teens and others in their fifties. It is also notable that, at the time of writing, the Manchester group is solely a male group. This is not a specific rule of the group but reflects those who have been interested in joining to date. If female members were to join, extra changing facilities would need to be arranged and a female supporter for the group recruited.

The group is staffed by one psychological practitioner and a further volunteer supporter, both of whom join the group in the activities. They are also regularly joined by a member of the coaching staff from FC United.

The Manchester group is relatively fluid in its membership. While the groups consist of a core of regular players, it is not an explicitly closed space. As such, the group might see new members join and leave at various times in the year due to the changes in support needs of the individuals. When this occurs, the process needs to be carefully managed so as to ensure that newer members feel included into the existing group.

It is important to acknowledge that each group member also accesses other services offered by Freedom from Torture. The football therapy project is a single cog in a broader support machine, or, for want of a more relevant analogy, a single player on the team.

The day of the match

The weekly football therapy sessions follow a set format. Table 17.1 provides an overview of a typical session.

Whilst the session includes a substantial football focus, it is by no means the only activity that is engaged in by the group. Most of the session is taken up by other group activities.

The group forms: All groups have to start somewhere. Whereas many football groups meet at the pitch where they will play, the Manchester group meets at the Freedom from Torture office. As the training facilities are a little way outside of the city centre, it was viewed as helpful to meet on familiar territory. Taking this approach meant that the group travels together to the training facilities. The journey is made by public transport and is funded by Freedom from Torture. Whilst this poses some challenges, it also allows the group to form and discuss the past week (both life events and the week's football). Further, it provides the opportunity to support people in learning about the public transport system around Manchester.

On arrival at the training facilities, the group goes to the changing room and gets ready for the session. Whilst changing rooms are a standard part of football training sessions, it is also a point where people may feel more vulnerable. Thus, it is vital to ensure that the space remains private whilst individuals get undressed and that any private possessions that are left in the room are safe.

On-pitch activities: Whilst the football element of the work may be viewed as the most novel element, it is almost the most straightforward bit. The sessions vary in content, but typically take the form of a brief warm up and some skills practice, followed by short games. The supporter and psychological therapist take part in all the activities.

The warm up involves asking the group to engage in some jogging and running exercises and then some stretching. As the fitness of the group varies, and some of the members may

Table 17.1 The schedule for the session

Phase	Time	Activity
The group forms	9.30	The group starts to arrive
	10.30	The bus ride
	10.50	The changing room
On pitch activities	11.10	The warm up
	11.20	The skills practise
	11.30	The match
	11.55	Penalty shootout
The group processes	12.00	The changing room
	12.20	Eating together
	12.40	The bus ride
The group ends	13.00	Members leave the group

have physical challenges as a consequence of the torture they have endured, individuals are encouraged to take part with the activities they feel comfortable doing.

The skills practice typically includes passing, set plays (free kicks and corners) and taking part in attack versus defence activities. This is then followed by a brief game. As the groups usually consist of fewer than 15 people, this generally involves dividing into two small teams and playing on half of a typical football pitch. Finally, the session ends with a brief penalty shootout. During these activities, the group laugh, hug, shout, push, pant and celebrate.

Whilst most of this process is football-focused, the staff linked to the project remain attentive to the dynamics in the group. For instance, on occasion members engage less fully in the sessions or withdraw from activities. When this is the case, the staff will proactively discuss with the individual what is going on for them and whether they need additional support at that point in time.

The group processes: At the end of the training session the group returns to the changing room. Whilst changing and showering, the group discuss the session and how it went. As noted above, ensuring the changing room is private proves very important at this stage – having other members of the club enter the room may be disconcerting for some group members.

Following this, the group move from the changing room to a function room in the stadium to eat together, with the food and drink being provided by Freedom from Torture. Once again this provides the men with the opportunity to talk about the session and life beyond the session. In some instances, it may be necessary to discuss and unpack elements of the session that people may have strong emotions about (e.g. being involved in strong tackles or harsh words being said on the pitch). Such conversations are generally facilitated by one of the supporters of the group and reiterate the goals of the group.

After eating the group then return to the Freedom from Torture office via public transport.

The group ends: Once the group returns to the office space everyone goes their separate way. At this stage, there are two major tasks: (1) ensuring the kit gets cleaned (which is organised by FC United or staff at Freedom from Torture); (2) for the psychological therapist linked to the group to share any information related to the group that may be beneficial to colleagues involved in supporting group members. This takes the form of weekly check-ins after the session and monthly clinical supervision.

FOOTBALL HELPS ME BECAUSE...

During a recent consultation exercise, those in the Manchester group were asked to complete the statements 'I play football because...' and 'Football helps me because...'. Below are a number of the comments provided by the group members.

I play football because...

    It keeps me fit and healthy (active as well).

    It keeps me physically active.

    It makes me happy to defend my team.

    I play football because it helps my mentality.

Football helps me because...

    When I come to play I forget everything while I am on the pitch and the most important [thing] is to have fun because it always lifts my mood up.

    It reduces my stress, keeps me fit, makes me so happy and joyful. And also he helps me to practise more my English with other people in the team.

Football helps me to stay strong mentally.

Football = no stress

Football is for a group of people, so I won't be isolated anymore.

These are just a snapshot of the types of experiences reported by the men in the group. As is evident, the comments echo some of the same sentiments expressed in the larger study conducted by Horn et al. (2019) referred to above. The comments also once again reflect the biopsychosocial nature of the football therapy project. For instance, they mention keeping fit, staying strong mentally and not feeling isolated.

REFLEXIVE LEARNING

Working as a therapist on the Freedom from Torture football project has challenged my understanding of where therapeutic work begins and ends. I trained as a counselling psychologist who had worked primarily with individuals and offered therapy in a relatively conventional way – typically working with one other person, sitting in comfortable chairs in a private room that I was confident would have no interruptions. Such spaces are vastly different from a bus or a football pitch. Despite these major emphases in my therapy training, I found myself drawn to the football therapy project. In reflecting on why this was, I highlight two major threads in my thinking: making therapy more accessible and my own personal history of football.

Firstly, for a number of years now, I have been interested in how therapy might be made more accessible to those individuals who could benefit from such support, but don't typically access it. In this case the group setting proves pivotal. As the work of the football group accompanies one-to-one therapeutic work, it provides a helpful space for developing a working alliance with, not just the other group members, but also the organisation. For some, it provides a comfortable home base and enables survivors to meet others with similar experiences and discuss the care they are accessing. For others it provides a space to ask questions that they do not see as naturally falling in the therapy space (for instance, lots of questions were raised about the implications of Brexit following the referendum within the UK). The group setting, combined with the football activity, can therefore be attractive to some people who are less comfortable with the format of traditional therapeutic work and can potentially help to soften its hard edges.

Secondly, during this work I have found that I have drawn upon my personal interest in football. I still enjoy playing football and I have had first-hand experience of the community derived from being part of a football team. Undeniably, the men in the group have vastly different backgrounds to my own, and yet, on the pitch, we have a lot in common. The 'universal language' of football brings the group together through a common activity which is familiar and, in many cases, remains a passion. As a therapist, it is strange to say that I have pushed the people I work with out of the way (on the pitch), celebrated excellent goals/saves with them, spent time in the changing rooms discovering unwashed kit with them, eaten egg sandwiches with them, and even missed or run for buses with them. I have also had numerous conversations about the past experiences of suffering horribly at the hands of others, the sadness and anger of facing racism on a daily basis, and the challenge of getting out of bed every morning when someone has been disconnected from their family who is on another continent. Importantly, the activity is not just about the individuals; I have also been part of the team. I have shared the ups of winning and the downs of losing. Whilst it is not the therapy I was taught in my classes, the relationships I have been involved in have certainly reached depths akin to those developed in previous work. To return to the words of those involved in football therapy projects, "*People come from different communities, we speak different languages but when we play we have one language, the language of football"* (Player) (Horn et al., 2019, p. 103).

REFERENCES

Bronfenbrenner, U. (1979) *The Ecology of Human Development: Experiments by Nature and Design*. Cambridge, MA: Harvard University Press.

Curran, K., Rosenbaum, S., Parnell, D., Stubbs, B., Pringle, A. and Hargreaves, J. (2017) 'Tackling mental health: The role of professional football clubs', *Sport in Society*, 20(2), pp. 281–291. doi:10.1080/17430437.2016.1173910.

Darongkamas, J., Scott, H. and Taylor, E. (2011) 'Kick-starting men's mental health: An evaluation of the effect of playing football on mental health service users well-being', *International Journal of Mental Health Promotion*, 13(3), pp. 14–21. doi:10.1080/14623730.2011.9715658.

Engel, G.L. (1978) 'The biopsychosocial model and the education of health professionals', *Annals of the New York Academy of Sciences*, 310(1), pp. 169–181. doi:10.1111/j.1749-6632.1978.tb22070.x.

Hanley, T., Cooper, M., McLeod, J. and Winter, L. (2017) 'Pluralistic counselling psychology', in Murphy, D. (ed.) *Counselling Psychology: A Textbook for Study and Practice*. London: Wiley, pp. 134–149.

Hanley, T., Winter, L.A. and Burrell, K. (2019) 'Supporting emotional well-being in schools in the context of austerity: An ecologically informed humanistic perspective', *British Journal of Educational Psychology*, 90(1), pp. 1–18. March. doi:10.1111/bjep.12275.

Herman, J. (1992) *Trauma and Recovery*. New York: Basic Books.

Horn, R., Ewart-Biggs, R., Hudson, F., Berilgen, S., Ironside, J. and Prodromou, A. (2019) 'The role of a Trauma-Sensitive football group in the recovery of survivors of torture', *Torture Journal* 29(1), pp. 97–109. doi:10.7146/torture.v29i1.106613.

Jones, A. (2009) 'Football as a metaphor: Learning to cope with life, manage emotional illness and maintain health through to recovery: Commentary', *Journal of Psychiatric and Mental Health Nursing* 16(5), pp. 488–492. doi:10.1111/j.1365-2850.2009.01403.x.

Joseph, S. (2015) Positive psychology in practice, in Joseph, S. (ed.) *Positive Psychology in Practice: Promoting Human Flourishing in Work, Health, Education, and Everyday Life: Second Edition*. Hoboken, NJ: John Wiley & Sons, Inc. doi:10.1002/9781118996874.

Pringle, A. (2009) 'The growing role of football as a vehicle for interventions in mental health care', *Journal of Psychiatric and Mental Health Nursing*, 16(6), pp. 553–557. doi:10.1111/j.1365-2850.2009.01417.x.

Rogers, C.R. (1951) *Client-Centered Therapy: Its Current Practice, Implications and Theory*. London: Robinson.

Sherry, E. (2010) '(Re)Engaging marginalized groups through sport: The homeless world cup', *International Review for the Sociology of Sport*, 45(1), pp. 59–71. doi:10.1177/1012690209356988.

Stover, E. and Nightingale, E. (eds.) (1985) *The Breaking of Bodies and Minds: Torture, Psychiatric Abuse, and the Health Professions*. New York: W. H. Freeman.

The Football Association (2019) *Heads Up: The FA for All*. London: The Football Association and Mind.

Tribe, R. (2002) 'Football for facilitating therapeutic intervention among a group of refugees', in Cockerill, I. (ed.) *Solutions in Sport Psychology*. London: Cengage Learning, pp. 173–183.

Twizell, O. and Hanley, T. (2021) 'Counselling, psychotherapy and training the football elite', *Counselling and Psychotherapy Research*, 21(4), pp. 855–858. doi:10.1002/capr.12463.

van der Kolk, B. (2014) *The Body Keeps Score: Mind, Brain and Body in the Transformation of Trauma*. London: Penguin Books.

CHAPTER 18

AUTHOR DISCUSSION
Body and Soul

Six of the authors who contributed to the 'Body and Soul' section of the book took part in this discussion, representing five of the chapters: Emma Rose and Amanda Bingley; Ardiana Bytyçi; Christine Adcock; Mary Raphaely; and Aisling Hearns. The discussion was facilitated by Rebecca Horn.

REBECCA: Welcome, it's great to have so many of you with us today! You've all seen the three questions we will use to structure our discussion, so let's begin with the first one. What is the core message you would want readers to take from your chapter?

MARY: The message that my co-author, Martha, and I would like to communicate is that nature itself holds people, and this can be enormously valuable. We need to look for ways to engage people physically so that their bodies can speak, as well as what's going on in their minds. Working together in nature stimulates memory, physical activity, camaraderie. Plants can trigger memories. A lot of what we try to do is get behind the trauma to the pre-traumatic capacities; herein lies an important route to healing. For example, the smell of a mint leaf crushed in the hand and held out to someone may remind them of a time with a beloved grandmother 20 years ago. Now they are mentally back in a place before all the trauma, so very difficult to remember, and their latent resilience can grow.

AISLING: Yes, my core message would be similar, that the body-based treatments shouldn't be overlooked. Some people see one-to-one talking therapy as the standard, and then will try other therapies as substitutes, but a lot of the evidence around group therapy is very strong. For the client group that I work with, who are mostly asylum seekers from very different countries and cultures, a group approach which integrates bodywork works incredibly well. It focuses on that connection piece, similar to what Mary was saying, and the camaraderie. It helps to process the trauma without having to go into it. That can be very powerful.

EMMA: Many of the people we worked with were survivors of torture, and working in a non-verbal way in the visual arts was critical for the group dynamics and for their working towards recovery. We enabled them to work with images, and they were empowered to decide what they wanted to depict. So we weren't guiding them, but we were suggesting that they either imagine or remember places associated with safety. Again, this enabled them to think about their homeland and places associated with safety but also their present lives in the UK, and it created a very interesting bridge between traumatic memories in the past and lives in the present. That was really important to many of them, not just expressing what had happened to them or their lives in the present, but also becoming more playful with that and playful with the materials.

AMANDA: Yes, I think it was really powerful to see people be able to access some of the good memories. I was interested in what you were saying, Mary, about going back before the trauma, because we certainly seemed to facilitate the space to do that. And also, as Emma says, as time went on the groups worked in a more playful way, and it seemed to be a very healing place to share things like food and laughter, as well as allowing expression of some of the more traumatic incidents that had happened to them and to see what they were actually managing to develop in their lives. So I think the core message of our chapter is very much about re-emphasising the value of using this expressive mode, and that words come later.

DOI: 10.4324/9781003192978-21

CHRISTINE: I feel that the therapeutic space can sometimes hold people in, and the music that we used allowed them to access parts of themselves that were different to those parts that were locked in trauma. Tonality and tunes are non-verbal and, as other people have said, link back to their homelands and their own cultures and their own memories of being the people that they really thought they were going to be, but haven't been allowed to be.

ARDIANA: It's a great summary and it also resonates with our work. Working with asylum seekers in transit contexts requires us to be very creative, because people are in the transit centres for just days or weeks. In general, you have to just design the programme as the current population group is there, you have to be there in ways that they want to be.

REBECCA: Thank you. Maybe we can go to the second question which we sent you, which is 'Has writing the chapter changed your approach to groupwork in any way?' Sometimes as we write we reflect and we think of things that maybe didn't occur to us previously, and we wondered whether that had happened for any of you?

AMANDA: Writing this chapter was really useful for me because it supported the way we worked in the group. We found that people who benefited most from this were people who were already further along in their healing journey, and the art group came at a certain point in their recovery. If you push people into this kind of group too soon, it's too much for them. I think suddenly expecting people to go into a group, they struggle to cope with the fear that they might be asked to talk about the traumatic experience. So it was valuable to see how groupwork has a part to play, but at different stages in people's recovery. The people that it seemed to work best with were people who had been very isolated, and had not necessarily taken part in some of the other groups they had access to. It was a slow process, but as they got more confident it became a space that they felt comfortable in and enjoyed actually.

MARY: My co-author Martha grew up in and around communities so groupwork was very natural to her, but she's an artist and community gardener rather than group therapist, so she found thinking about our work within this context helped her to refine her ideas. Myself, I trained as a group psychotherapist, so writing this chapter absolutely entrenched for me the idea that people can learn much more from each other, who have been through similar experiences, than they can from us. Also, because we work outside, it is a much less threatening space because people can keep their distance from each other.

ARDIANA: I would also like to add that it was an interesting reflection exercise. We are a team of people who facilitate daily activities with asylum seekers as well as advocacy activities and capacity building, so we are overloaded with work and the space that we had to reflect with each other about the chapter was very beneficial for us. We ourselves were children during the 1998/99 war in Kosovo, and now it's our turn to do what was done in other countries for us. Something that we didn't recognise before writing this chapter was that we were taking into account our own experience of how we wanted things to go back then. We realised that what we wanted when we were refugees was to be understood and to be asked by professionals what would most help us. Therefore, our programme of activities is designed together with asylum seekers; we want people to take part in defining their daily routines that help them to recover.

EMMA: Working on the chapter and remembering just how much some of the people we worked with benefitted, what I take away from this project is the feeling that I really want it to be more sustainable. Once the project ended, we had a group of people who were immensely sad, and with the pandemic a lot of them were going back to being very isolated, having had a glimpse of what it was to be in a group. And that leaves me feeling somewhat sad or guilty as well. I really would hope that organisations can offer more groupwork opportunities like some of those we're discussing today.

CHRISTINE: One of the strengths of the Stone Flowers music group was that it was led by another NGO which is carrying it on. Because that ending is a real tragedy for people when they've committed so much of their emotional life to whatever group it is.

AISLING: My experience of writing the chapter was similar to Ardiana, in that you don't normally get the time to reflect on the work when you are so busy with the day-to-day stuff. When you're running the groups sometimes, and I'm sure you've all experienced this, it just feels too little at times. It doesn't feel like it's enough, until you're able to step back and look at the bigger picture, and at the impact it's had on the clients. So being able to reflect for the purposes of writing this chapter has been really helpful. It's really helped us just to look at what we are doing within the organisation, it's been a nice space for that.

REBECCA: The point that Emma made and then some of you built on leads us nicely to our third question, which is 'what statements or messages can we as a group together come up with to encourage more groupwork opportunities?' It seems that the sadness that you describe, Emma, at the end of the group, and seeing the sadness of the participants as well, emphasises the need for more resources to be put into providing opportunities for the kind of initiatives that you've talked about.

AISLING: I think it's really important for people working with survivors of torture to reflect on their own Western bias in their approach to therapeutic work, which can be quite individualised. I think that's coming more to the forefront, people are adopting an approach with more cultural humility, so I think that would be an important thing to get across, that people should stop, reflect, and move out of their comfort zone to try these different therapeutic approaches. If practitioners are hesitant about trying a new approach, there's lots of research and evidence about these different approaches and creative treatments. They just need to be open to it. However, it always comes back to connection. In my experience, and I'm sure the experience of others, it doesn't really matter what we do. The most important thing is that connection, whether it be a one-to-one connection or the group connection.

MARY: You used a very interesting phrase there: 'cultural humility'. If we think about the sort of cultures that the people we are working with come from, much more group-based, a much more social situation, it is at our peril that we cling fast to a Western psychoanalytic model where 'the doctor knows'. Of course, where it begins to be problematic is if you have very polycultural groups, which we do all the time, but it is amazing how much somebody from Azerbaijan has in connection with somebody from Kinshasa, with somebody from Russia.

CHRISTINE: Within Stone Flowers, one of the major things that everyone came together on is that they wanted to educate the public about what it was actually like to be an asylum seeker, and what it was like to be a refugee. Many of them were political activists, which was why they were tortured initially, but it was really important to them that people understood that they didn't come for a better life, they'd go home in a heartbeat. They couldn't communicate this on their own, they had to say it in a group. They had to say it together and had to say it through music because that was something that the audience could hear. So I think that that the creative arts give that medium for expressing really central experiences.

SECTION 3

TOGETHER THROUGH TALK

CHAPTER 19

HEALING THROUGH CONNECTING

The life of a Tamil–English therapy group for male survivors of torture

Kirsten Lamb

In 1-to-1 therapy, it's only your emotions; in group therapy, it's everyone's feelings; you feel people like you exist, you share together, laugh together. I never wanted to miss the group, to know about how they are all feeling.

(Piriyan)

This chapter uses my work as a therapist with a Tamil–English therapy (TET) group to describe how multi-level healing takes place in a slow, open psychotherapy group. I offer this as an example of an alternative format to time-limited groupwork.

Other authors (Tucker and Price, 2007) have described the therapeutic value of group-analytically informed psychotherapy groups for traumatised refugees and people seeking asylum but mainly with reference to groups with a time limit. I will suggest the benefits of a slow, open group, drawing on group theory, a theoretical model of psychological trauma, and a values-based approach. I will describe events and stories from the group to exemplify how multiple therapeutic connections took place. To give voice to the group members' own experiences, this chapter will provide direct (but anonymised) quotes.

The TET group ran weekly for three and a half years in the North West centre of a UK-based charity. Although the group was the main vehicle for recovery, it sat within a holistic torture rehabilitation programme that included legal and welfare casework, and therapeutic activity groups. The group therapists acted as key workers coordinating these aspects of the rehabilitation programme.

The TET group was started to provide access to psychological therapy to a greater number of survivors of torture. In 2015/2016, Tamils from the Sri Lankan civil conflict formed the largest proportion of our referrals. Consequently, we reserved five places in the group for Tamils and five for non-Tamils who were sufficiently fluent in English not to require interpreters. The group ran with two female therapists and one female Tamil interpreter. My co-therapist was a humanistic and integrative individual/group psychotherapist and psychodramatist; she was of an Indian Tamil background and raised in the UK. The gender make-up of the group and therapists/interpreter was based on staff availability and the fact that the majority of referrals to the centre were men.

THEORETICAL UNDERPINNINGS

The TET group provided an integrative psychological treatment based on Herman's (1997) three-stage model of recovery from trauma; they are described as safety, remembrance and mourning, and reconnection. We adapted the model by reconceptualising the stages as stabilisation, trauma processing, and reconnection and integration. The first stage involves creating a safe space, developing trust, working on stabilising post-traumatic stress disorder (PTSD) symptoms, and developing emotional regulation and other coping strategies. In the second stage, trauma memories are faced and processed. The third stage involves working on reconnecting with positive past memories, developing a stronger sense of identity and self-efficacy, thus enabling a re-integration process both within the person and in relation to the outside social world. The stages are not chronologically distinct or strictly sequential; some processes

DOI: 10.4324/9781003192978-23

will be common across the stages. The final goal of the group is for members to leave therapy and move on to live an ordinary life.

Groupwork facilitates achieving this goal because, as Herman states, "Sharing the traumatic experience with others is a precondition for the restitution of a sense of a meaningful world" (1997, p. 70). Groups, by definition, help members to create new meanings; for example, one member in his feedback said that just by coming to the group, he understood that *"everyone has problems"*; before this, he felt that *"he was the only one"*.

The TET group used the slow, open format of the group-analytic approach. 'Open' refers to the changing composition of the group, i.e. members joining and leaving at different times. 'Slow' refers to the pace at which these 'beginnings' and 'endings' occur (Barwick, 2018a, p. 18). Building on earlier theories of group development (Tuckman and Jensen, 1977), Schlapobersky (2016) developed an integrated framework that gives weight to both individual and group development by outlining a set of five developmental tasks: engagement, authority, intimacy, change, and termination. I will define these tasks as I refer to them in the chapter. With groups that have a changing membership, these tasks are not linear and can be viewed as "oscillating and/or cyclical" (Barwick, 2018a, p. 21). Similar to the three-stage trauma recovery model, the tasks can be revisited with increasing depth as if operating within a spiral framework.

Although a group is a collection of individuals, it is experienced as more than that; in the group-analytic approach, this is conceptualised as the matrix of the group, originally described by Foulkes as "the hypothetical web of communication and relationship" (1964, p. 292). Barwick describes "how each personal story, each interaction comes to have a group meaning as well as a personal one"; thus, the matrix of the group shifts with the addition of interweaving personal stories (2018b, p. 31). Furthermore, Barwick states that "the meaning of an individualised event ('figure') is understood as only becoming fully meaningful in the context of the background ('ground')", i.e. the whole group: this is referred to as the figure-ground configuration (2018c, p. 59). The group therapist needs to attend to the continuous interplay between the individual needs of group members and the needs of the group as a whole. Bhurruth developed the concept of the "social matrix", which recognises that the group boundaries are permeable to past and present societal, political, and cultural events (2008, cited in Barwick, 2018b, p. 32).

For the TET group, we modified the group-analytic approach by using drama-based techniques, non-verbal/physical activities, and a psycho-educational component (e.g. imparting knowledge about trauma and developing skills such as mindfulness). Other additions included developing a peer support component and therapists taking on the key worker role. Refreshments were available in the therapy room and, following the formal group which ran for an hour and a half, the room remained open for an extra half-hour of social time. The therapists left the room unless a member requested casework or psychosocial help, which the therapist (as key worker) provided.

In all therapies boundaries are necessary to create a safe space, but we found that our group sometimes needed more flexible boundaries. Culturally competent practice requires a broader view of therapeutic boundaries, including understanding them from the perspective of solidarity (Speight, 2012). The unstructured half-hour gave the group the opportunity to build peer support and social connections independent of the group.

After the Easter bombings in Sri Lanka in 2019, one Hindu Tamil member could not bring himself to attend the following group session. Subsequently, he explained that he felt so angry that he was worried his words would offend Ritsa, the interpreter who was a Muslim Tamil. Ritsa responded outside of the interpreter role to express her own emotions, as she also knew people who had been killed. They were able to come together as two people struggling to make sense of such a shocking event, no longer separated by their religions. This was a compelling example of how utilising flexible boundaries benefitted the group.

Cowles and Griggs (2019, p. 51) offer the term "boundary crossing" originally defined by Gutheil and Brodsky (2011) as behaviours that are not generally expected in therapy which may be beneficial; in their individual therapy with a woman seeking asylum, these included liaising with other organisations, addressing other needs, managing expectations, giving and receiving gifts, self-disclosure and emotional expression, and endings. In different ways, similar boundary crossings also occurred in the TET group, often bringing more equality into the room. As an example, we had sessions when group members brought in samples of food from their home countries; this positioned them in the role of giver as well as receiver. Whether seen as boundary crossings or having different boundary definitions, these adaptations have to be sensitive to the group's needs. We created a boundary of confidentiality around information shared at assessments or during key worker sessions; for example, sometimes members would delay telling the group about successful outcomes of court hearings or the rejections of asylum applications. As therapists, we had this knowledge but recognised that it was not ours to share.

CORE VALUES

As a clinical psychologist, I draw on the work of Patel, who describes how psychologists can incorporate a human rights-based approach as practitioner-activists:

> The practitioner-activist seeks to uphold and promote the rights of all people to be treated as human beings with dignity. It is a stance which is value-laden, against human rights violations and a role antithetical to being bystanders; a stance which seeks and values the views, experiences and participation of survivors of human rights violations.
>
> (2019, p. 17)

As therapists, we were explicit about our aspiration for all group members to gain refugee status. All but one of the members were seeking asylum. Of those members, the majority had experienced rejections of their initial asylum applications and four had previously been detained in immigration removal centres (IRC). As key workers, we were vigilant in documenting our observations regarding material arising in the group that could provide medico-legal evidence for a further asylum application.

The group members came from Afghanistan, Ethiopia, Guinea, Nigeria, Pakistan, Rwanda, Sudan, Syria and Zimbabwe as well as Sri Lanka; the majority of Tamils were Hindu, and the remaining members were either Christian or Muslim. Given this diversity, we recognised the need to prioritise cultural competence and humility in our practice. Ritsa expressed this well by saying, "*It was my responsibility as an interpreter to convey the message to respect each other's cultures, to translate using words that would not offend anyone in the group*". She witnessed members "*respect and empathise with each other's experiences and current emotional states*"; they offered "*motivation*" to each other. Group therapy gives a unique opportunity to create a safe place for cross-cultural exploration and dialogue.

Using the concept of intersectionality, originally developed by Crenshaw (2005), we can understand how people seeking asylum are multiply marginalised, leading to their experiences of trauma being qualitatively different from those of trauma survivors from dominant cultural groups. It is important to acknowledge this, particularly in relation to their experiences of the asylum process.

We recognised that although being a male survivor of torture was the only referral criterion for the group, we wanted to know and value the numerous other identities group members had – father, son, political activist, farmer, student. It was important not to see group members as only people seeking asylum or survivors of torture. Thus, effective therapy requires an understanding of multiple identities and their intersectionality, recognising that even using the term 'survivor of torture' can be problematic in that it privileges one identity. We valued a strengths-based approach enabling the group members to connect with their positive identities and develop expanded narratives of their life journeys.

Consequently, we gave more space for the exploration of cultural and political histories than would be the case in a standardised trauma recovery group. Furthermore, looking to the future, we hoped to make explicit the benefits of multiracial communities in the UK. We aimed to foster curiosity about difference while at the same time discovering and sharing similarities. This informed the decision not to set up a Tamil-only group. Group members gave their support to this decision, particularly in relation to maintaining the balance of Tamils to non-Tamils when considering new members.

By providing the peer support space at the end of the group, we wanted to de-emphasise our position as 'experts' and to encourage members to build separate, supportive relationships. One Tamil member said he valued his social time with his "*community*" more than the formal group; this confirmed the value of the social space alongside the formal group.

STARTING THE TET GROUP

After accepting the offer of group therapy, potential members were seen for four to six assessment appointments, which enabled them to engage with other parts of the rehabilitation programme and form a therapeutic relationship with the group therapist assessing them. Following this phase, two preparatory group meetings were held a month ahead of the formal group start. This had two functions: to mark the ending of the assessment sessions and to allow for extending the recruitment time.

The beginning of any new group focuses on the 'engagement' task, described by Schlapobersky (2016) as the process of the group member deciding whether to be "in/out" of the group. Members of the TET group were helped by the assessment sessions and their shared knowledge that they were all survivors of torture. The first sessions focused on creating safety, security and containment by addressing boundary and confidentiality issues, and encouraging connections between group members. Whilst the Tamil members immediately identified as a clear subgroup, the whole group was excited to learn about all their countries which were located using a world map. Interestingly, they recognised a similarity in that all the countries, except Ethiopia, had been colonised. The non-Tamils knew little or nothing about the Sri Lankan civil war. The Tamil members shared which part of the island they came from.

We started with simple activities to remember names; these were repeated with members adding details about their current or past life. They would then be asked to introduce each other to the group by recalling the information that had already been shared. Sometimes this caused laughter as members recognised that they were more focussed on what they were saying, not on listening. Members appeared to enjoy the playfulness of these activities and these 'getting to know each other' group activities were often repeated as warm-up exercises.

Early on, group 'rules' and individual goals were discussed, agreed and drawn up into a group contract, which served as a vehicle for orienting new members to the group and for completing annual progress reviews. The 'rules' mainly outlined expectations regarding confidentiality and respect. In relation to non-attendance, it was agreed that a member risked losing their place if they missed three group sessions without any contact. Members were encouraged to phone in and give an explanation that could be shared in the group if they were not attending. It was also agreed that the group would not run with less than three members present so members were encouraged to feel their attendance counted. We noticed that members developed a sense of responsibility to the group as a whole over time. When there were unexplained absences, the therapist would call the group member after the session, as circumstances such as lack of phone credit or, more seriously, being detained could prevent contact.

The nature of a slow, open group means that there will be beginnings and endings throughout the life of the group; over the duration of our TET group, nine members left, allowing for new members to join. When new members joined, the initial 'engagement' phase was shorter; new members tended to quickly adjust to the group culture.

FORMAT OF THE GROUP SESSIONS

Prior to each session, the therapy room was set up with 13 chairs in a circle and refreshments available on a table. Group therapists vary in their preference for keeping empty chairs in the circle to represent absent members; we left chairs empty to enable the presence of members to be felt even in their absence.

Each session would begin with an open invitation to members to check-in and say how they were feeling or how their week had been. This check-in period varied in time depending on the contributions and whether members arrived late. We invited members to repeat their check-ins for late members until we realised that we were prolonging the check-in and avoiding the opportunity for group members to challenge lateness. Referring back to group development theory, we had privileged information sharing, inclusivity and engagement, and inadvertently minimised potential conflict over lateness, reducing the group's ability to manage the 'authority' task described by Schlapobersky. The 'authority' task refers to how group tensions arising from competition, conflict and anxieties about disclosures are managed.

During check-ins, members sometimes just said, "*It was a normal week*", reflecting the tedium of life as a person seeking asylum with almost no money and no right to work. The phrase was readily adopted as a shorthand, a form of avoidance that we struggled to challenge because we accepted it as real.

As the group became more established, late members realised that they were missing the shared news, which led to greater efforts to arrive on time. We also noticed that more explanations were given for lateness and absence, demonstrating the strengthening of relational dynamics. The group moved into managing the 'intimacy' task which addresses trust, attachment and affiliation; members began to describe the group as their "*family*".

We prepared an activity that, if needed, we could use following check-in to encourage communication and sharing, as we did not find it helpful for the group to stay in a period of silence. These activities could be based on getting to know each other more; promoting mindfulness; moving the body; instilling hope, strength and resilience; facing positive and negative memories; or exchanging cultural information and rituals. Apart from the chairs and the space in the room, we had two specific props: a box full of everyday objects, toy animals and small musical instruments that were used to prompt feelings or stories either directly or symbolically, and a bag containing scarves of different colours and textures. The scarves worked as powerful visual triggers to past memories and cultural occasions.

We observed times when members wanted to use these activities as a distraction; they wanted to be able to smile and laugh together. They valued this, but was it a form of collective avoidance of trauma? As the group developed, we shifted the focus of these activities to enable more connection to trauma memories; we found that members often struggled to offer a direct story of their experiences of harm. Sometimes the activities themselves would trigger a past difficult memory that the member was encouraged to re-tell in the group, to engage with the processing of the distress. The activities were also used to connect back to safety after disclosures.

To mark the formal ending of the group session, a ritual was chosen by the group; everyone would stand, form a circle and attempt to clap once in unison. There was no count down to the clap, just a focus on being together and sensing the right time to clap. Sometimes, it took one go to clap together; sometimes, it could be four. However long, there were smiles and a shared sense of achievement that everyone managed to clap as one without words. I only fully appreciated the power of this ritual when Ntwali described how it worked for him:

> Even if you don't take time in the group, you still have time to be connected with others, to focus, to watch others, to look at others to match with others. … Your mind has to be there to clap and match others.

Ntwali was naming the central importance of connecting with others in the room and holding the group in mind. He also referred to remembering the ritual: *"I think about it when I'm alone, always talk about it when I see an ex-member, something I'll never forget."*

VIGNETTE OF AN EARLY GROUP SESSION

This session took place five days after the Westminster Bridge 'car and knife' attack in London in March 2017. At this time, the group had eight members. Of the six present, Layan, Jayish, Piriyan and Parithi were Sri Lankan, Samuel was Nigerian, and Rashad Sudanese. Rashad was the only Muslim group member present.

As usual, every member had the opportunity to check-in, share news and say how they were feeling. Layan had missed a few group sessions and was welcomed back before the check-ins moved on to refer to the terror attack:

> I feel really down about the terrorist attack in London. It's reminding me of home and I'm fearful that tighter restrictions will be placed on us. Brexit is happening now too; this also makes me think I will be deported.
>
> (Samuel)

> I do not believe people place us in the same group as terrorists, we will be treated as individuals with our own unique circumstances by the Home Office. Brexit is mainly about economic migrants not us.
>
> (Rashad)

> We suffer because of the actions of others. Other people use us, as pawns. … Because of this attack, 50 people were returned in Australia. There is no hope for us.
>
> (Jayish)

> Worrying about the bigger world makes things worse. Why should we talk about things we can't change?
>
> (Layan)

Jayish was vocal in expressing his feelings of anger and resentment, as he felt the attack would have personal consequences for him; others presented as worried or low. Piriyan was tired and seemed disengaged; this was often how he appeared at the start of the sessions. Rashad took on a strong, confident position.

The presence of mixed feelings in the group was acknowledged and worked on with a group activity called the seesaw exercise, which involved members standing along the line of an imaginary seesaw. The exercise was used to encourage movement and enable observation of emotions from a more distant position. Members were asked to judge their thoughts in relation to the attack and position themselves on the seesaw, with one side named "heavier thoughts", the other side "lighter thoughts", and the pivot point defined as "the solid place" made up of grounding thoughts. Samuel, Piriyan and Jayish positioned themselves on the "heavier thoughts" side, Parithi and Layan were in the middle, and Rashad was on the "lighter thoughts" side. Then the group members were asked to help make the seesaw more stable by members who were less affected by the London attack helping those more troubled.

Samuel was encouraged to move to the middle position by Layan and Parithi. In this place, he reminded himself of what helps him manage his fear: "*I know the way I think changes from week to week and I change based on what is happening and who I am with. Next week I will think differently.*"

Parithi positioned himself in the middle saying, "*I know many Muslims, we are all individual people some good, some bad. There are good people here. Bad people are stuck in their ways, nothing will shift them; it is better to be open in thinking.*"

Piriyan expressed feeling more fearful since the attack, without understanding why he felt so personally affected. Other members asked questions that helped him understand that his fear was connected to his past experiences. With this new understanding, he moved himself to the middle position having connected himself to his core values: "*I am for humanity and human rights, it is inside me and outside. I want to treat others good, and they will be kind to me too.*"

Jayish was also invited to move towards the middle position, which he refused. When asked what it was like staying where he was, Jayish said, "*I am alone here.*"

The group was brought to a close with members returning to their seats and being invited to reflect on the exercise. This usually involves the sharing of positive sentiments about learning new things and getting energy from being together. Jayish said, "*The group is like a pill, it offers some relief and comfort, but it doesn't last long enough.*"

However, Layan expressed his frustration:

I don't want to waste my time talking about these political things. Things we can't change. I thought the group was to talk about personal things. Like I wanted to talk about why I haven't been here for a month, but there is no space.

Layan looked disappointed and dejected, even though the group responded saying they wanted to know and encouraged him to take time at the beginning of next week's session to share his feelings. Layan did not return to any further sessions and finally responded to the no contact letter, explaining that he did not feel comfortable in the group.

From a theoretical stance, it may be that focusing on the impact of this external event was too problematic for the group, as they had not yet experienced negotiating the 'authority' task; it was too early for members to deal with conflict and competing needs. As such, they had not been able to challenge Layan by saying that there had been space for discussing his personal concerns in his check-in. Additionally, when he had spoken emotionally about his helplessness and loss of control, as therapists we probably missed the depth of his individual despair by focusing on a group activity. On this occasion at this stage of the group, maybe we did not address the figure-ground configuration sufficiently, resulting in the loss of a group member.

WORKING WITH CONNECTIONS

The vignette above illustrates the complexity that a single group session can involve – members navigate not only their relationships with each other but also their relationships with their own physical states, individual memories, cultures and religions. Work needs to be done to heal bodies, heal memories, rebuild relationships with self and others, and find different ways of belonging.

Some members struggled with the physical impact of their torture; they held the pain in their bodies. Physical activities were used to encourage a change in their relationship with their bodies as well as to change the energy levels in the room. We tended to use physical activities to aid engagement, and revisited activities when a new member joined. Sometimes, we combined a physical activity with a problem-solving task. For example, we asked the group to hold hands and tangle themselves into a knot, each member took turns to be outside of the group and give instructions to untangle the group. This light-hearted activity gave members the opportunity to connect safely in a physical way. Physical activity can be used to shift the atmosphere in the room, as it often lightens the general mood, taking members away from their thoughts.

Early in the group, members found it easier to share positive past memories, and they especially enjoyed describing the natural environment of their countries. They moved on to share stories about family experiences and cultural rituals, and these gradually involved the members facing more distressing memories that involved the loss of loved ones or the disclosure of relatives who had gone missing. Members explained their grieving and mourning rituals. One member spoke of his sister's husband's death in a bomb attack and the pressure to remarry quickly. Another member responded by saying that in his culture a widow had to wait five years until she was allowed to remarry.

As the group became established, members began to refer to the group as their "*family in this country*". Members were in relationship with each other as part of the group. This enabled them to stay in the group even when things seemed stuck or difficult. In contrast to the earlier vignette, at a later stage, when Syed absented himself from the group following a difficult session, he did not drop out. Abdii had narrated in detail a terrifying event during his time in an IRC. Briefly, he described being taken from the IRC and put on a removal flight, during which he was handcuffed and escorted by two security guards onto an empty plane. He described the physical pain and mental terror he experienced; as the co-pilot said he would not fly the plane with him on board, he was returned to the removal centre. Syed had also been detained, but he had not shared this with the group. Listening to Abdii took him back to his own experiences; he left the group with his trauma responses re-activated and was too frightened to return to the next session. The phone call to him afterwards provided the opportunity to revisit the stabilisation techniques that he had previously found helpful. He was also reminded of the positive outcome for Abdii, who was subsequently released from the IRC. Syed returned to the group learning that it was safe to speak about an experience that he had previously held within himself.

MOVING ON AND LEAVING THE GROUP

Apart from two members who left the group prematurely, there were seven members who were able to decide their individual leaving dates after obtaining refugee status. Over time, leaving the group became associated with obtaining refugee status.

Droždek et al. (2013) reported that obtaining refugee status during trauma-focused group therapy for PTSD appears to improve treatment outcomes; refugee status was hugely significant for everyone in our group. When a member obtained their status, it was a time of celebration for them and a time for hope for others – hope that it would be their turn next. We used a creative drama activity to mark the occasion – each member stood up from their seats to give the member granted refugee status an imaginary gift. The member then gave thanks for the gift and described what they imagined they had been given. Even in imagination, the act of giving and receiving is extremely powerful. Members sometimes shared actual sweets/dishes associated with celebrating from their own cultures.

Members largely self-determined their notice period; for some, they were ready to leave the group as soon as the practicalities associated with being granted protection were dealt with. For others, the transition to establishing their life as a refugee was challenging and stressful. This meant that they still relied on the support of the group as they faced experiences that were often re-triggering, for example, the threat of homelessness, delays in state welfare benefits, or rejection after a job application. They continued to experience racism and racial discrimination in their efforts to establish their lives as ordinary citizens. Two members felt that they needed more recovery time to build up their self-confidence and trust in their abilities to manage their new life. So, for different reasons, practical and emotional, the moving on and ending period could take up to one year. Giving members the right to choose their own way of ending offers benefits not available in fixed-term groups.

We emphasised the importance of a planned ending for anyone who was leaving and for the members who would leave in the future. This is a unique feature of a slow, open therapy group: that members can prepare for their own departure from a group by observing others that have gone before them.

In group therapy, the ending phase involves facing the loss of attachments and relationships within the group that may have been a considerable struggle to build, especially for survivors who have experienced interpersonal violence. So many people seeking asylum have experienced multiple losses, usually sudden and without the support of cultural rituals of mourning. This was the case for several of the TET group members, especially for Sadi, who fled Afghanistan in 2002 alone as a young teenager, and Ntwali, who was brought up in a UN refugee camp before seeking asylum in the UK. Ntwali said, *"In our group we are a family, though we came from different culture, religion and country."*

Leaving the group involved losing a place where they had felt part of a family. As current losses like this "resonate with every other loss experienced" the therapeutic work of the ending period in the group was both challenging and rewarding (Barwick, 2018d, p. 165). Members were encouraged to take time to name and process past losses; they were also encouraged to see the planned ending as a time to take back some control and find new ways of giving meaning to their experiences. Adbii and Rashad both spoke of the comfort they felt in recognising that by losing their place in the group they were giving another person who needed help the space to join.

REFLECTIONS ON THE GROUP

The group stopped meeting in March 2020 due to COVID-19 and formally ended in May 2021 with a goodbye meeting on Zoom. During this interval, the group members were supported individually by a group therapist through weekly telephone calls offering psychological support and psychosocial assistance in line with the key worker role. Two more members were granted refugee status; their asylum applications included a medico-legal psychological report using evidence from the group sessions. Over time, all members were given smartphones to facilitate sessions over Zoom. Despite the long gap, members still identified as being members of the group and waited for the last meeting.

At this meeting, attended by six members, when asked about what they found helpful during the group, it was striking that, rather than mentioning anything that they had learnt from the therapists, they instead spoke of what they had learnt from each other and how they had benefitted from the experience of being together like a family.

This feedback was significant as, during the life of the group, idealisation of the therapists and the charity had often been a theme; we felt put on a pedestal. Although this was uncomfortable at the time, it was perhaps helpful as a transitional stage that allowed the members to maintain hope and belief in a positive future. By the end of the group, the members identified themselves as their own vehicles for change and healing.

Habib said, *"the weekly sharing"* of the check-ins was most helpful for him: *"I could hear about what others were going through, and I was getting advice from others in a similar situation to me"* and *"I keep some conversations as memories for me"*. For example, Habib recalled Parithi saying how he benefitted from *"putting the rubbish [of life] out into the group"*.

Abdii explained that *"being with others in the same situation made [him] stronger"*, illustrating the power of collective healing. Parithi also recalled the strength he got from hearing Adbii's account of the removal flight described earlier, which helped him learn how to keep himself during his asylum rejections; he was able to internalise Adbii's qualities of strength and resilience so that they became part of his way of being.

Our role as therapists was to enable the group to work safely so that the members could be together, form meaningful relationships with each other, and learn to move on from their distressing past experiences. Exploring the concept of family further, Parithi explained that, in his culture, if difficulties arise within the family, *"there is a boundary around the family, things are not spoken of outside the family"*. Confidentiality within the group helped members to disclose distressing memories and rebuild trusting relationships across gender, religious and cultural differences. As happens in some family groups, we were aware of certain dynamics remaining under the surface and unexplored, such as possible envy when refugee status was granted. Likewise, although running a male-only group with female therapists (and one being white) was not examined, we recognise this would have had an important influence in the group dynamic.

Learning to live an ordinary life after experiencing human right abuses is a process of self-discovery and reconnection. A slow, open psychotherapy group gives time for the journey to take place at a pace that fosters personal growth within a safe environment using the knowledge, strength, resilience, and diversity of its members.

REFERENCES

Barwick, N. (2018a) 'Core concepts: What goes on in groups? (Part one)', in Barwick, N. and Weegmann, M. (eds), *Group Therapy: A Group-Analytic Approach*. London and New York: Routledge (pp. 18–30).

Barwick, N. (2018b) 'Core concepts: What goes on in groups? (Part two)', in Barwick, N. and Weegmann, M. (eds), *Group Therapy: A Group-Analytic Approach*. London and New York: Routledge (pp. 31–50).

Barwick, N. (2018c) 'Core concepts: What does the conductor do? (Part one)', in Barwick, N. and Weegmann, M. (eds), *Group Therapy: A Group-Analytic Approach*. London and New York: Routledge (pp. 51–69).

Barwick, N. (2018d) 'Endings', in Barwick, N. and Weegmann, M. (eds), *Group Therapy: A Group-Analytic Approach*. London and New York: Routledge (pp. 164–180).

Barwick, N. and Weegmann, M. (2018) *Group Therapy: A Group-Analytic Approach*. London and New York: Routledge.

Bhurruth, M. (2019) 'On the Matrix, neuroscience and dialogue', *Group Analysis*, 52(4), pp. 458–474. doi:10.1177/0533316419839030.

Cowles, M. and Griggs, M. (2019) 'Considering boundaries when doing therapeutic work with people who are seeking asylum: A reflective case study', *British Journal of Guidance & Counselling*, 47(1), pp. 50–64. doi:10.1080/03069885.2018.1507535.

Crenshaw, K. (2005) 'Mapping the margins: Intersectionality, identity politics, and violence against women of color', in Bergen, R. K., Edleson, J. L. and Renzetti, C. M., *Violence Against Women: Classic papers*. New Zealand: Pearson Education, pp. 282–313.

Droždek, B., Kamperman, A. M., Tol, W. A., Knipscheer, J. W. and Kleber, R. J. (2013) 'Is legal status impacting outcomes of group therapy for posttraumatic stress disorder with male asylum seekers and refugees from Iran and Afghanistan?', *BMC Psychiatry*, 13(148). doi:10.1186/1471-244X-13-148.

Foulkes, S. H. (1964) *Therapeutic Group Analysis*. London: George Allen and Unwin.

Gutheil, T.G. and Brodsky, A., 2011. *Preventing Boundary Violations in Clinical Practice*. Guilford Press.

Herman, J. (1997) *Trauma and Recovery: The Aftermath of Violence - from Domestic Abuse to Political Terror*. New York: Basic Books.

Patel, N. (2019) 'Human rights-based approach to applied psychology', *European Psychologist*, 24, pp. 113–124. doi:10.1027/1016-9040/a000371.

Schlapobersky, J. R. (2016) *From the Couch to the Circle: Group-Analytic Psychotherapy in Practice*. London: Routledge.

Speight, S. L. (2012) 'An exploration of boundaries and solidarity in counseling relationships', *The Counseling Psychologist*, 40(1), pp. 133–157. doi:10.1177/0011000011399783.

Tucker, S., and Price, D. (2007) 'Finding a home: Group psychotherapy for traumatized refugees and asylum seekers', *European Journal of Psychotherapy & Counselling*, 9(3), pp. 277–287. doi:10.1080/13642530701496880.

Tuckman, B.W. and Jensen, M.A.C. (1977) 'Stages of small-group development revisited', *Group & Organization Studies*, 2(4), pp. 419–427.

CHAPTER 20

CONNECTING HEARTS AND MINDS
A faith-sensitive psychosocial group model
Weihui Wang

Aida and her family of six were living a relatively normal life in Yemen when the civil war broke out. Her husband was the sole breadwinner and they had financial stability. The family as Aida described was filled with happiness. Like many others, Aida's husband first lost his job and eventually lost his life to a rocket-propelled grenade. Aida was left to care for her family. Grieving her loss and without a stable income, the stressors eventually took a toll on her mental wellbeing.

Over the next couple of months she started to become more withdrawn, was unable to concentrate and lost her appetite. Aida was unable to take care either of herself or her children, and became physically violent towards her children. Despite consulting with numerous doctors, her mental health did not improve. Aida's extended family, including her parents, lost all hope of her recovering, concluding that Aida is "crazy". Eventually they stopped visiting. Her children started begging to support the family financially. Aida was the gossip of her community; her neighbours avoided her, and she became even more isolated.

When Aida first started attending the Connecting Hearts and Minds groupwork programme she had a hard time controlling her emotions, especially her anger. She recalled that the first three sessions were the most challenging. Then something changed; she started to feel happy and optimistic about life and began looking forward to the sessions: *"Since I started attending the sessions, I learned to set aside my problems and was less worried about what others were saying about me. I also became more willing to care for myself and my children again."*

Aida developed more affectionate feelings towards her children and started to feel responsible for them again. Her children also saw a difference in her. Aida's son explains:

> Our mother used to hit us and we preferred to stay away from the house because of her harsh treatment. But she has changed a lot. She would play with us and we would even take walks together When she returns from sessions, she would share what she has learned, and the activities and exercises and we would practice them together. We are a much happier family now and we no longer want to leave our mother.

Connecting Hearts and Minds is a community-based, faith-sensitive group psychosocial support programme, which began in 2019 in Yemen and is being adapted for Lebanon and Syria. When Tearfund UK first started exploring the possibility of providing psychosocial support in Yemen, it had not intended to create a new modality. After all, there were a number of interventions that had demonstrated evidence in similar contexts. After consultations with communities, it became evident that the intervention had to encompass the following key elements: (1) community-based; (2) faith-sensitive; (3) can be implemented by lay persons; (4) strengths-based; and (5) addresses symptoms of distress, depression, and anxiety. This chapter will present the context in which the intervention was designed, the development process and rationale for the modality. It will also discuss the underpinning values of the approach, impact and the lessons learned along the way.

DOI: 10.4324/9781003192978-24

CONTEXT

Prior to the Arab Spring of 2011, Yemen was already experiencing a Houthi insurgency and water insecurity. Pro-democracy protests in 2011 resulted in President Ali Abdullah Saleh leaving office in 2012. However, unrest continued, and in late 2014 the Houthis' uprising escalated and Houthis took over the capital, Sana'a. This resulted in the transitional leader fleeing to Aden and the situation turning into a civil war in March of 2015. By 2021 about 80 per cent of Yemeni were in dire need of humanitarian assistance (OCHA, 2021). Yemen has the largest food-insecure population in the world, with tens of thousands living in famine-like conditions and another five million at risk of starvation. The underlying drivers of the crisis continue to persist, leading to insecurity, protracted displacement and a lack of basic services and this is further compounded by the effects of the COVID-19 pandemic. The country also continues to grapple with disease outbreaks such as cholera, diphtheria, and measles, and natural disasters like flooding.

Mental health

The WHO estimates that mental disorders (i.e. depression, anxiety) affect about 22 per cent of conflict-affected populations (Charlson et al., 2019). About one in five Yemeni are struggling with a mental disorder (UNFPA, 2020). The suicide rate is believed to have risen by 40 per cent between 2014 and 2015.

Prior to the conflict, about 90 per cent of men and 50 per cent of women chewed khat three to four hours per day and 5–20 per cent of children under 12 consumed it daily (Al-Mugahed, 2008). An assessment conducted by Tearfund UK in 2019 found that the dependence on khat, especially among adolescents and young people, has increased since the conflict began. Khat, a plant-based stimulant, causes euphoria followed by depression, characterised by irritability and poor appetite. It may also lead to psychosis and persistent hallucinations and negatively affect a person's sleep (Al-Mugahed, 2008). The chewing of khat is socially and culturally acceptable and few recognise its negative effects. Khat is often consumed at social gatherings and not participating in khat chewing can lead to social exclusion. Khat expenses also negatively affect household dynamics and social relationships.

The mental health system in Yemen

Mental health is highly stigmatised and poorly understood in Yemen, and there are limited mental health services. Prior to the crisis, Yemen only had four psychiatric hospitals and by 2017 only 40 psychiatrists remained in the country serving a population of about 28 million (WHO, 2017). Some public hospitals have established outpatient mental health clinics, but most have budget constraints or staff shortages. About 90 per cent of primary health clinics lack the capacity to provide mental health and psychosocial support (IMC, 2019) and fewer than 40 per cent of secondary health facilities provide mental health and psychosocial support services. The COVID-19 pandemic has caused a number of the existing mental health services to close. Additionally, there is a shortage of mental health workforce.

PATHWAY TO THE NEW INTERVENTION

Tearfund UK is a Christian aid and development agency that has been providing funding to local organisations in Yemen to address food insecurity and communicable disease outbreaks.

As the situation evolved into a protracted crisis, field assessments indicated an increasing need to move beyond basic material support to tackle the deteriorating psychosocial wellbeing of Yemeni. Through a series of consultations in 2019, it became clear that a multi-sectoral response was necessary and more holistic approaches would be more effective.

Needs assessment and secondary analysis

The assessment was conducted in Taiz governorate where the local partner was providing food assistance and had a strong presence. Taiz is one of the most volatile areas in Yemen; it has experienced intense fighting since the onset of the crisis, and the shifting frontlines and natural disasters have resulted in multiple waves of displacement.

Chronic daily stressors associated with lack of employment, inability to afford basic needs, along with the constant insecurity and protracted displacement were affecting psychosocial wellbeing. Parents were increasingly irritable, and children were displaying increased anxiety, regressive and disruptive behaviours, and an inability to concentrate in school. Incidences of sexual harassment, exploitation and abuse were on the rise, resulting in women and girls being fearful to leave their homes, with increasing feelings of isolation and disconnection. Men spoke of feeling powerless and hopeless as they were unable to fulfil their traditional role of protecting and providing for their families. Both men and women also reported having difficulties connecting with their feelings. Persons with mental health concerns are highly stigmatised and there is a general lack of understanding of the signs (IMC, 2019). Additionally, Yemenis have a collectivist culture that emphasises the needs and goals of the group over the needs and desires of each individual. All of these factors are likely to affect the willingness and ability of an individual experiencing mental distress to seek help.

It was evident from the assessments and discussions with local staff that Yemenis had existing coping skills that could help them manage the adversities they were experiencing. Coping strategies commonly identified by both men and women included prayers, connecting with families and friends, and engaging in enjoyable activities. However, displacement, disruptions and ongoing stressors had made it more difficult to employ these coping strategies.

Why groups?

The findings of the assessment suggested that a group modality led by lay persons from the targeted community appeared to be most appropriate for this context. A large proportion of the population were displaying some symptoms of psychological distress, and a groupwork approach would enable large numbers to receive support in a relatively short period of time, with efficient use of the limited resources available. A non-specialist intervention was also considered appropriate given that estimates suggest that 80 per cent of people in conflict-affected areas recover without specialist mental health services when they are able to access appropriate support (Charlson et al., 2019).

Group approaches recognise the value of every participant, and offer a judgement-free space for voices to be heard and experiences to be validated. Additionally, groupwork can assure individuals that they are not alone and that other individuals share similar problems and struggles. Also, sharing one's experiences offers the opportunity to both receive and to give support. This is particularly valuable as members have different personalities and backgrounds, so are likely to view a situation from different perspectives. Moreover, the act of helping others has been shown in recent research to greatly enhance an individual's wellbeing (Lishner and

Stocks, 2017). It is a central principle of mental health and psychosocial approaches in emergency settings that individuals and communities have inherent strengths, resources and positive attributes and should be at the centre of the helping process.

Since Yemen is a collectivist culture, relationships with other members of the community play a central role in one's identity. Social support has been found to be a key element of wellbeing, especially in adverse situations. Group approaches to therapy acknowledge the centrality of relationships in the Yemeni culture, creating positive shared experiences among the members and re-establishing social connection and relationships that may have been disrupted by displacement and distressing events. Groupwork is particularly pertinent in this context because both women and men expressed difficulties in relating to their own emotions, and through explaining one's feelings to others, and hearing how they explain their experiences in turn, self-awareness can be increased. It also led to improved communication skills. Hearing how others have successfully overcome similar challenges can potentially be encouraging and could motivate group members to model positive behaviour changes.

We were also aware that group modality has its disadvantages. Confidentiality is one of the biggest concerns raised by the community, particularly because all the group members, including the group facilitators, are from the same communities. Hence, it was critical for the project team to establish the importance of confidentiality prior to an individual joining a group. Members of the group also had to establish their own rules in the first session on how they would manage a situation in which confidentiality was broken. Secondly, in any group setting there will always be some voices that emerge as more dominant than others and take up more time and space. This can lead some members of the group to feel alienated or may encourage silence. Therefore, it is important that the facilitators are trained on how to manage such group dynamics to create a positive environment in which all voices are heard and valued.

VALUES

The overarching goal was "Men and women have improved overall wellbeing and coping mechanisms." This is based on the theory that when men and women exposed to acute and/ or chronic stress are (a) provided with a safe environment to discuss and support each other, (b) develop improved understanding of mental health, and (c) can find compassion for self and others, reactivate and learn new coping skills, rebuild social connection and re-establish routines and rituals, they will have improved functioning and overall wellbeing. To achieve this, Connecting Hearts and Minds was developed with the following underpinning values:

Human rights and equity

Humanitarian activities and interventions should promote human rights of all affected persons and protect them from human rights violations, especially those who are marginalised. Due to pre-existing inequalities, particular groups like older persons and persons with disabilities are more affected in situations of conflict. Crisis also has a gendered impact, for example women and adolescent girls often pay a high price for harmful and discriminatory gender norms, including gender-based violence, while men and boys face elevated risks linked to arbitrary detention and forced conscription, among others. Therefore, my team and I were very aware that because crises do not affect everyone equally, we must strive to promote equity and accessibility for all. This can only be achieved when we design interventions that take into consideration gender, age, disability and the intersectionality of different identities.

Faith-sensitive

The local partner frequently emphasised the importance of being sensitive to the culture, context and an individual's religious tradition, beliefs and affiliation. This is especially important in the Yemeni context because people rely heavily on their faith as a coping strategy in times of adversity. It is also a fundamental right of every individual to practice their faith freely. That means that the modality we employ must include elements that take into consideration the influence and importance of an individual's faith on their wellbeing. Faith is a term used to describe religious tradition or affiliation and associated beliefs and should be regarded as inclusive of diverse religious groupings (Ager et al., 2018).

As a faith-based organisation, Tearfund UK values and sees the potential of faith in contributing to individual and community wellbeing. From the beginning we made a distinct effort to have a faith-sensitive model rather than a faith-based model. The distinction is important: a faith-based model is rooted in a particular sacred text, whereas a faith-sensitive approach recognises the importance of faith to an individual's wellbeing and coping and is deliberately incorporated throughout the intervention. This is not just because Tearfund UK has its roots in a different religion but also because there can be different faith traditions and expressions within a religion. Therefore, it was critical that we understood the religious views and practices of the communities we worked in and facilitators were respectful and sensitive towards members' religious and spiritual experience, since people relate and express their faith differently depending on gender, area of origin and personal experiences. Our responsibility is to build on relevant and appropriate coping mechanisms. We did so by ensuring that the intervention included prompts to have members of the group reflect on how their faith had supported them, and working with them to find ways of re-establishing important routines and rituals connected to their faiths (i.e. Friday prayers, Salat). The model also integrated the concepts of empathy and compassion which are central to most religions so as to cultivate empathy and translate that into compassion for oneself and others. Research has shown that empathic and compassionate people have more satisfying relationships and are more connected to, and understood by, their families and communities (Seppala et al., 2013).

Community-led

Participation is a core principle, and it means putting people at the centre of decision-making. Hence, from the beginning, the project team actively engaged the community in the design process. The engagement process was also used to build consensus among the community. The focus group discussions with community members helped us determine both the number of sessions and the length of each session. Community members indicated that sessions should not interfere with daily work and household responsibilities and should be held in a location that was easily accessible. During the initial review of the curriculum and in subsequent adaptations, Yemeni colleagues were quick to point out the need to ensure the model was suitable for people with low levels of literacy, such as women in rural areas and older people. Hence, sessions were designed to be experiential and included pictorial references. Finally, because of the stigma associated with mental health, volatility of the context and difficulty in obtaining approvals, it was vital that our intervention targeted communities in which the local partner had established relationships, and the community had expressed a desire to improve their psychosocial wellbeing.

Strengths-based

People react differently to crisis events, largely dependent on how severely they were impacted and the existing assets and resources they have. By emphasising people's agency and existing capacities instead of their deficits, we are able to build on what is already going well. Externally driven programmes may lead to inappropriate support and have limited sustainability. Therefore, our intervention needed to build on the individual and community's existing capacity and resources. Our role as facilitators was to engage the participants to reflect on, identify and recognise their own strengths and resources and to utilise these to support themselves and potentially others.

Sustainability

Due to the limited professional mental health workforce, we needed a model that could be delivered by lay persons from the community. By doing so we would also be working through individuals that the communities had a trusting relationship with, and the skills and knowledge would remain in the community after the intervention ended. To avoid creating a situation where the lay facilitators became overburdened with the community's mental health issues after the project ended, we also ensured there were group supervision sessions so they could learn to support each other after we left.

Quality and evidence-based practices

Having experienced many ineffective and unstructured psychosocial support programmes in different humanitarian contexts, it was important that the intervention was evidence-based, rooted in good practice and built on the skills learned in each session. Therefore, the design of the intervention included elements of cognitive behavioural therapy (Eskici et al., 2021) and Acceptance and Commitment Therapy (Geda et al., 2021). The project was also designed around rigorous data collection to measure the effectiveness of the intervention and to capture wider learning to improve the modality. The optimum number of sessions to effectively treat symptoms of depression is eight while anxiety continues to improve with more sessions (Forde et al., 2005). Hence, the total number of group sessions was fixed at nine.

Do no harm

We assessed for protection risks and unintended harmful effects at the design stage and throughout implementation. Targeted communities should not have experienced displacement in the previous six months and should not be at high risk of displacement. This is to ensure that the participants were not in acute need and the sessions would not be disrupted. Service mapping was completed to ensure higher levels of care were available and within travel distance of the targeted communities. When people with impaired decision-making capacity or individuals who could pose a potential risk to themselves or others were identified, they were referred for further clinical assessment and specialised care. For instance, we were working in communities that had reasonable access to the psychiatric clinic in Taiz city and were able to establish an agreement for referrals. We had clear inclusion and exclusion criteria but remained flexible so that individuals with more complex needs could be included when they had been clinically assessed by a local provider and/ or with the approval of the clinical supervisor. The ethical decision to include some high-risk individuals was not taken lightly as I understood the potential risks and stress it could have on the community facilitators. However, the local partner and I also noted that the programme could be a pathway to seek further support. The project team was structured to ensure good clinical supervision and support to both local staff and community facilitators. The local partner and I wanted to be sure that our team, who themselves were facing many of the same challenges and may experience vicarious trauma, were adequately supported.

Contextual adaptation

This intervention underwent three cycles of adaptation, including a review by an Arab psychologist with contextual experience, and testing the entire intervention with local Yemeni staff, the community facilitators and two groups of ten individuals in the community. Feedback was solicited at each stage and the curriculum adapted accordingly. This included revising terminology and activities so they were more appropriate for the context. For example, part of the adaptation involved the rewording of an entire section on the consequences of stress events on brains, as Yemeni colleagues highlighted that focusing on brain science in this context can sometimes result in parents blaming themselves.

Learning through experience and doing

Prior to training to become facilitators of this intervention, local staff and community facilitators completed all nine sessions as a participant. The idea was for them to experience the intervention first-hand so they could better relate to what the participants would be going through. Also, it was an opportunity for us to model how the intervention should be delivered and the best practices of facilitation. A Yemeni colleague shared that because he had experienced the benefits of the session as a participant first, he felt more convinced and committed to deliver it. Then they received training on how to become a facilitator, which included learning through reflection, whereby they prepared and led some of the sessions with the guidance of the clinical supervisor. This allowed them to practice and role play, and learn to deal with potential challenges and different individuals in the group.

IMPACT

As of December 2020, more than 400 men and women had completed Connecting Hearts and Minds. Over this period, data were gathered on the effectiveness of the intervention using standardised assessments administered at intake and end of the group sessions and also at every session to track progress. In this section, we will present and reflect on the evidence obtained on the impact of the intervention on the wellbeing of participants.

The intervention has demonstrated effectiveness in reducing depression and anxiety symptoms and improving functioning and wellbeing. At the baseline assessment, 86 per cent and 83 per cent of the participants were presenting symptoms of depression and anxiety respectively. By the end line, among those with presenting symptoms, 97 per cent had decreased symptoms and improved functioning. The intervention also had a 94 per cent regular attendance (defined as participants who had not missed more than two sessions).

Power of connecting with others

> I have seen a change in his behaviour with his family and neighbours. He is taking part in
> family life and started playing and visiting relatives.
> (neighbour of 38-year-old male participant)

Prior to attending the sessions, participants shared feelings of isolation and having no or limited engagement in any form of social activities. Social connection is a big part of the Yemeni culture and one of the coping mechanisms that had been disrupted by displacement and insecurity. The sessions became a regular opportunity for participants to re-engage and connect with other members of the group. During the course of the intervention, some participants who had stopped seeing their families started meeting up with them again. Gradually, participants started reporting feeling less isolated. Facilitators also worked with them on identifying routines and rituals (i.e. Friday social gathering after prayers, visiting relatives or neighbours for tea after meals, and daily prayers as a family) that were important to them and their families and integrating these back into their lives.

Most important was the significance of journeying with others. The group offered a space for safe social engagement and renewed participants' sense of belonging in the world. It helped reduce their feelings of isolation which, in turn, encouraged them to reconnect with people they cared about. The strong relationships established in a few of the groups also resulted in meetings and get-togethers after the sessions ended.

Managing feelings and emotions

> Frankly, I used to be angry and intolerant with the children for a trivial reason, but now I am another person.
>
> (56-year-old male participant)

Family violence, including intimate partner violence and child abuse, became more prevalent during the crisis. In 2019, the United Nations estimated that violence against women and girls in Yemen had increased by 63 per cent since 2015. Women and men participants with children shared that they had trouble managing their anger and were physically or emotionally abusive towards their children and each other. This led to children avoiding home for long periods of the day, which in turn increased the risk of their exposure to other forms of child protection concerns (i.e. recruitment into armed groups, sexual exploitation, and child labour). Members of the group reported finding ways to manage their negative feelings and have more patience and empathy for themselves and their family members.

Faith and its benefits

> Thanks to the programme, which has the merit, after Allah, for transforming my life from misery and sadness to one that is beautiful and calm.
>
> (30-year-old female participant)

Faith is an important factor among members of the groups. However, humanitarian agencies tend not to engage and leverage faith and faith actors because religion is often politicised and at times perceived as a driver of conflict. However, faith is very much intertwined with culture; by ignoring a person's faith humanitarian agencies ignore a large part of the affected individual's identity.

Research has shown that religion is a protective factor for mental illness (Oman and Lukoff, 2018; Rutledge et al., 2021) and can be critical to many people's healing. Members of the group referred to their faith in sessions and some turned to their faith to make sense of what they are experiencing. Many members of the group also identified faith as a comfort, and faith practices (such as prayers, speaking to religious leaders) as a primary coping mechanism. In general, religious rituals provide structure, regularity and predictability and encourage compassion and gratitude. Regularity and predictability re-establish a sense of stability and normalcy after lives have been disrupted by violence and/or displacement, while compassion and gratitude may elicit positive emotions. Faith practices, such as Friday prayers, can re-establish social connections for some participants. Instead of avoiding religion, groupwork can be strengthened through supporting participants to decide to what degree and in what ways they want to connect with faith. It may enhance their sense of self and can be an empowering experience.

Practice and modelling

> Initially she attended the sessions as though she was forced. ... Then she began practicing physical activities and was happier.
>
> (45-year-old female participant)

A number of participants shared that the first three sessions were the hardest period of the intervention as they struggled to find motivation to attend the sessions. After these initial sessions they found it much easier to continue. The initial challenge and eventual change in attitude could be attributed to a number of factors. Some of the participants were exhibiting depression symptoms, so finding the motivation to break out of the cycle and start doing something different was often one of the most difficult steps. To address this issue, at intake participants were asked to identify potential challenges and barriers. The staff then worked with each participant to identify strategies to overcome these, including seeking help and including exercise in their routine. In the initial stages of the intervention (first three sessions), great emphasis was placed on the idea that change is possible and that seeking help from others is acceptable. Throughout the sessions there was a strong focus on behaviour activation and psychoeducation on the symptoms. Relaxation and mindfulness techniques were practiced at the start and end of each session and members were encouraged to use them regularly. Lastly, the PHQ-9 and GAD-7 assessments and mood check-ins were conducted at the start of every session, which may have helped participants become more aware of what was affecting their symptoms and mood. Upon reflection, it appears the sequencing of the session is critical and the repetition along with regular reflection allows participants to practice the skills they learn.

Empathy and compassion for self

> I learned to put my problems to the side and to deal with myself kindly.
>
> (19-year-old female participant)

The sessions worked to support participants in accepting their difficult thoughts, memories or feelings. Data collected from 2019 through 2021 indicated that participants found the session which focused on this particularly helpful. During this session, participants worked on identifying and acknowledging their problem/s, and the impact on their feelings, behaviours and thoughts. The goal was not to get rid of the problems, but for the problems to become something group members could live with without causing further hurt or harm. They can eventually learn how to manage these painful thoughts and feelings more effectively. This was followed by a session on compassion for self and others where participants learned the importance of extending the care and empathy they have for others towards themselves.

LEARNING AND CONCLUSION

The team working on Connecting Hearts and Minds learned the importance of allocating sufficient time during the planning process to conduct a needs assessment, analysis of the context and community consultation. The participation of the community enabled the team to identify the key priorities and the most appropriate groupwork approaches in the Yemeni context.

The competence of the lay community facilitators was a key factor in the success of this intervention. Facilitators needed to fully understand the modality, be able to remain faithful to the model and know how to manage high-risk situations. The selection and training of lay facilitators required a substantial time investment, which can be challenging when most humanitarian funding is only for one year. Humanitarian agencies have an ethical obligation to create an environment and supervision structure where local staff and facilitators are well supported, especially given that lay facilitators have often had similar experiences to programme group members.

Security in humanitarian settings is fluid and volatile, so it is necessary to reflect on how the intervention may be impacted and plan accordingly. The mapping of available services (e.g. psychiatric services, individual counselling, gender-based violence and child protection actors) allows the selection of appropriate target areas, as well as referral systems to be put in place for high-risk (i.e. suicide, psychosis) and protection situations. By the second cycle of the project, an emergency budget line for transportation or payment for acute specialised care was included.

Communication and preparation with the target communities was also an important element of successful programming in this context. This included managing expectations as to what the project team was able to provide; and ensuring participants understood what would be involved in the programme, including the principle of confidentiality and its limits.

Lastly, MHPSS programming must be sensitive to the faith aspect of participants' lives, in order to build on existing resources and capacities and identify potential risks and harms. People within and between communities express and experience faith differently, and a faith-sensitive approach allows participants to choose whether and how they engage with faith issues. An analysis of expressions of faith, along with other issues such as gender, coping strategies and the ways in which faith intersects with mental health, should be the starting point for any agency wanting to ensure that a therapeutic groupwork intervention meets the needs of a conflict-affected population.

REFERENCES

Ager, W., Horn, R., and Ager, A. (2018) *A Faith-Sensitive Approach in Humanitarian Response: Guidance on Mental Health and Psychosocial Programming.* Geneva and Birmingham: LWF and IRW. Available at: https://interagencystandingcommittee.org/system/files/faith-sensitive_humanitarian_response_2018.pdf (Accessed: 26 January 2022).

Al-Mugahed, L. (2008) 'Khat chewing in Yemen: turning over a new leaf'. *Bulletin of the World Health Organization,* 86(10), pp. 741–742. doi:10.2471/BLT.08.011008.

Charlson, F., Ommeren, M., Flaxman, A., Cornett, J., Whiteford, H., and Saxena, S. (2019) 'New WHO prevalence estimates of mental disorders in conflict settings: a systematic review and meta-analysis'. *Lancet,* 394(10194), pp. 240–248. doi:10.1016/S0140-6736(19)30934-1.

Eskici H.S., Hinton D.E., Jalal, B., Yurtbakan T., and Acarturk C. (2021) 'Culturally adapted cognitive behavioral therapy for Syrian refugee women in Turkey: A randomized controlled trial'. *Psychological Trauma, Advance Online Publication.* doi:10.1037/tra0001138.

Forde, F., Frame, M., Hanlon, P., Maclean, G., Nolan, D., Shajahan, P., and Troy, E. (2005) 'Optimum number of sessions for depression and anxiety'. *PubMed,* 101(43), pp. 36–44.

Geda, Y., Krell-Roesch, J., Fisseha, Y., Tefera, A., Beyero, T., Rosenbaum, D., Szabo, T., Araya, M., and Hayes, S. (2021) 'Acceptance and commitment therapy in a low-income country in sub-Saharan Africa: A call for further research'. *Frontiers in Public Health,* 9. doi:10.3389/fpubh.2021.732800.

International Medical Corps (2019) *Mental health and psychosocial support assessment: Needs, services and recommendations to improve the wellbeing of those living through Yemen's humanitarian emergency.* Available at: https://app.mhpss.net/wp-content/uploads/2019/08/imc-yemen-2019-mhpss-assessment-1.pdf (Accessed 23 January 2022).

Lishner D. and Stocks, E. (2017) 'Helping and well-being', in Maddux, J. (ed.) *Subjective Well-Being and Life Satisfaction.* New York: Routledge, pp. 184–209.

OCHA (2021). *Humanitarian Response Plan: Yemen.* Available at: https://reliefweb.int/sites/reliefweb.int/files/resources/Final_Yemen_HRP_2021.pdf (Accessed: 26 January 2022).

Oman, D. and Lukoff, D. (2018) 'Mental health, religion, and spirituality', in Oman, D. (ed.) *Why Religion and Spirituality Matter for Public Health: Evidence, Implications, and Resources*. New York: Springer International Publishing, pp. 225–243.

Rutledge K., Pertek, S., Abo-Hilal, M., and Fitzgibbon, A. (2021) 'Faith and MHPSS among displaced Muslim women'. *Forced Migration Review*, 66, pp. 24–26. Available at: https://www.fmreview. org/sites/fmr/files/FMRdownloads/en/issue66/rutledge-pertek-abohilal-fitzgibbon.pdf (Accessed: 26 January 2022).

Seppala, E., Rossomando, T., and Doty, J. (2013). 'Social connection and compassion: Important predictors of health and well-being'. *Social Research*, 80(2), pp. 411–430. doi:10.1353/sor.2013.0027.

UNFPA (2020) *Against the odds, delivering mental health support in Yemen*. Available at: https://www.unfpa. org/news/against-odds-delivering-mental-health-support-yemen (Accessed: 26 January 2022).

World Health Organisation (2017) *Mental Health Atlas*. Available at: https://www.who.int/publications/ i/item/9789241514019 (Assessed: 26 January 2022).

CHAPTER 21

SEW TO SPEAK

Common Threads Project psychotherapy circles

Rachel Cohen

Our deepest human experiences – whether of love, terror, loss, awe, or despair – seem to defy words. We often use the term 'unspeakable' to refer to atrocities that are generated by war and human rights violations. The term is fitting because life-threatening traumatic events are primarily experienced and retained in non-verbal channels, rather than in the verbal domain. Why would we expect survivors to be able to speak to us about their pain? Yet, with clipboards in hand, well-meaning practitioners greet those who have suffered brutality and hope that they will narrate their story for us in words. But what if this is not even possible? How must it feel to be approached this way? There is a compelling case to be made that in order to process the experience of violence, we need to access expressive channels that exist in the realm beyond words. This is the basis for the integrative approach of Common Threads Project (CTP) (Cohen 2013a).

It is estimated that about one in three women worldwide are exposed to sexual and gender-based violence (SGBV) in their lifetimes, often with devastating physical, social, economic and psychological consequences. The need for modalities to support recovery from SGBV is especially urgent in areas of armed conflict, where rape is a pervasive weapon of war and a tool of genocide. This brutality devastates individuals and families, terrorizes communities, and contributes to the displacement of entire populations. Millions of Rohingya, Yazidi, Bosnian, Syrian, Nigerian, Congolese, Rwandan and Colombian girls and women amongst others have been victimised in the past two decades. Their perpetrators are often treated with impunity, and victims are stigmatised, rejected, and silenced.

Our aim is to fill a gap in long-term psychological recovery from SGBV in the humanitarian context. It is essential not just to offer crisis intervention, but to help those wounded by sexual violence achieve the transformative, enduring healing they deserve. These methods need to address all dimensions of human experience affected by trauma: the body, the emotions, cognition, social relationships and the spirit. We set out to develop an integrative model informed both by neuroscientific understandings of trauma and traditional practices that have healing power.

In 2022, CTP works in collaboration with local community partners in Nepal, Bosnia, the Democratic Republic of Congo (DRC), and with refugee and immigrant communities in the United States to develop programmes that are culturally resonant and sustainable. Our role is to offer a treatment model that can be adapted, to provide training, supervision and mentorship for the facilitators who lead the psychotherapy circles, and to encourage them to adapt the approach to fit their own community's needs.

Before they begin the circles, CTP offers intensive experiential training to local mental health staff to familiarise them with the methodology and to provide a lived experience of all dimensions of the programme. They learn art therapy activities, practice sewing, make story cloths, and engage in somatic exercises. Once the intervention begins, CTP continues to mentor and supervise the facilitator-therapists as they master the skills needed to conduct the circles. We take inspiration from a ubiquitous ancient practice in which women across many diverse cultures have found relief and support: collective sewing circles where women stitch narrative textiles to depict their experiences of oppression. Whether enslaved women in the American

DOI: 10.4324/9781003192978-25

South, mothers, partners and sisters of 'the disappeared' during the dictatorship of Pinochet in Chile, Hmong people surviving genocide in Laos, Bosnian weavers following the genocide in Srebrenica, black women living under Apartheid in South Africa, mourners sewing squares for the AIDS quilt – all those have gathered together in groups to support each other and to stitch their stories (Cohen, 2013b video).

PSYCHOLOGICAL RATIONALE FOR STORY CLOTHS

Therapists working with those who have endured human rights abuses have a great deal to learn from these naturally occurring examples. Sewing groups have intrinsic therapeutic capacities:

1   When whole communities have been devastated, the collective experience provides a connection and solidarity that is so essential for healing.

2   The sewing circle provides emotional safety. When the hands are busy and eye contact is not expected, participants feel freer to disclose to each other and express. A participant in Ecuador says, "It's here we can share what we keep hidden".

3   Hand stitching promotes needed self-regulation for those who are experiencing the neurophysiological effects of severe stress. The repetitive rhythmic action of sewing is meditative and calming for a nervous system that has had to function on high alert in order to survive. The sewing helps to keep one grounded in a state of equilibrium when considering memories that are painful and overwhelming.

4   Expression in images allows for direct representation of experiences that may be hard to convey in words. This can be especially important for people who have suffered political silencing or where stigma and taboo prevent them from speaking their truths. Verbal constriction is common in those who have endured chronic violation.

5   The slow, gentle pace of hand sewing matches the gradual work of long-term recovery. The process takes a great deal of time and patience. Each intricate stitch brings one a little closer to wholeness.

6   Having an opportunity to put one's inner pain "out there" into an object where it can be seen and touched can bring much relief. A woman in the Ecuador programme said "I feel like I've rid myself of a heavy load, a load I carried. It's passed now. I am getting rid of things that I had carried in my heart".

7   Displaying a story cloth allows for the possibility of *bearing witness* that can be an important element of the healing process in human rights abuse. Those who see the story cloth can affirm "I hear you, I believe you, I stand with you".

8   Participants in sewing circles tell us that making something beautiful of a horrific experience helps them to transform the pain. A sense of mastery and pride can replace feelings of helplessness and shame.

One CTP participant said:

> The pain we were going through was inside our hearts for a very long time, but we were unable to pour it out in any form. This was a shared pain.... I have tried to reflect the situation because the situation is indescribable. But with this [story cloth] I felt quite relieved.

Neuroscientific knowledge about the nature of severe traumatic experience validates the therapeutic value of creating story cloths. When we face mortal threat, the verbal/analytical centres of the brain in the cerebral cortex automatically shut down allowing the autonomic nervous system to activate in the service of survival. Energy shifts to privilege sensorimotor and visual processing, as the individual scans the environment for opportunities to escape threat.

Traumatic events are held and processed in the body, in the autonomic nervous system, in visual images, and in sensations, not in words. Life and death events are encoded and stored differently than other memories (Van der Kolk, 2014). Because they are essentially non-verbal it makes sense to employ a non-verbal channel when accessing these experiences. In a story cloth circle, women begin with images and over time are able to put these experiences into words so that the stories can be processed and reinterpreted.

AN INTEGRATIVE MULTIDIMENSIONAL APPROACH

CTP has developed an intervention that borrows the tradition of story cloth-making and blends this with a number of other modalities that address the complex recovery needs of women and girls who have endured abuse. We seek to embed the therapeutic protocol within a holistic array of other services that go beyond the psychological – to also address medical, legal, educational, socio-economic, and social needs of participants. Group psychotherapy is seen as only one aspect of the healing process and cannot occur in a vacuum.

Because profound human rights abuses such as sexual violence inflict wounds on the body, the emotions, cognition, interpersonal relationships, and the spirit, we believe that all these dimensions of human experience need to be addressed in an effective psychological healing process. This understanding has led us to build a multidimensional protocol for therapeutic groups.

The CT intervention is not designed for people in acute crisis. Psychological first aid and other crisis intervention tools would be more appropriate (WHO, 2011). The deep work of recovery requires a level of stability that is not present in the immediate aftermath of an assault. We employ a screening process to determine whether a woman is in a position to tolerate this type of therapy.

THERAPEUTIC METHODOLOGY OF THE HEALING CIRCLE

Safety

From the outset, activities are designed to create a sense of safety and security. Members of the group engage in therapeutic games to develop a sense of connection and trust with one another. The games continue to build a sense of community cohesion throughout the programme. Play encourages participants to reclaim joy, laughter and exploration. Each session opens with warm up and energising physical games and ends with a closing circle ritual. This structure also provides security and predictability.

Rules of confidentiality and privacy are essential for establishing safety in the group. These are emphasised from the beginning.

Connection

We believe that collective trauma merits a collective healing process. Targeted violence and systematic cruelty may produce protective ruptures in basic trust that need to be gradually re-established by the experience of safe and supportive relationships. In the initial phase of CTP circles, the facilitators teach empathic listening skills to ensure that group members can feel heard, supported and understood by one another. They practice "mirroring" exercises in movement, in art activities, and in words.

As the group sessions proceed, women find a sense of commonality and begin to open up to each other: Gradually they build trusting relationships. A group member in Nepal recounts:

"We came closer to them next week and closer next week. Since then, I have understood their feelings and they understood me."

In her ground-breaking book, *Trauma and Recovery*, Judith Herman emphasizes that "The solidarity of a group provides the strongest protection against terror and despair, and the strongest antidote to traumatic experience" (1997, p. 214). It is our experience that women who have endured stigma and isolation related to SGBV find great relief in the group experience.

> I never thought that I would be able to talk with others about my private difficulties. … Honestly, I didn't! For me this is a big step! I feel better, I see now that my problems are not the biggest, I am not alone. … Life is still difficult but when you are not alone it is easier to deal with everything.
> (a CTP participant in Nepal)

Psycho-education

Within the first couple of sessions, the facilitators provide psycho-education about the biopsychosocial consequences of severely distressing events. It is important that the participants appreciate that their symptoms are normal responses to abnormal circumstances, and that these physiological responses arose to promote survival. Many feel relieved to discover that they are not "crazy" and that others in their situation are also having difficulties with sleep, mood, concentration, heightened startle reactions, or episodes of re-experiencing. A participant in a Nepal circle told an interviewer: "it was then where I realised that I wasn't the only one suffering but, my friends too were on the same road".

Experiences of joy/play

One might assume that psychotherapy is serious gloomy work. But evoking positive emotional states is an essential element of recovery. A participant in Bosnia commented "I can't explain to you what a wonderful time we had here. I remember the most that we were always smiling, laughing, learning new things. I feel powerful, I am full of energy now." In CT circles, participants engage in play and games where they can experience joy and laughter again. Every session begins with a circle game, dance, or song, often contributed by a member of the group. The experience of laughter and joy improves the neurochemistry in the body, fosters group cohesion, and affirms that the experience of pleasure is again possible. Play provides a safe way to reconnect with parts of the self that may have been left behind in the wake of fear and self-protection. One member of the group explains "Sometimes I am kidding that after each session here I feel like I have wings. This means a lot for me" (participant from Bosnia).

Somatic work

Before considering emotionally challenging memories, participants learn specific skills to manage triggers and re-experiencing. Drawing upon techniques from Somatic Experiencing (Levine, 2015), Sensorimotor Therapy (Ogden, Minton and Pain, 2006), and Polyvagal work (Dana and Porges, 2018), we follow a 'bottom-up' approach to healing, wherein participants tune in to their embodied experiences and learn how to regulate their nervous systems so that they can feel safe and connected to others. There are weekly somatic exercises to help restore equilibrium in the body, orient to the here and now, and modulate levels of autonomic nervous system (ANS) activation. Participants practice awareness of ANS responses, regulated breathing, muscle relaxation techniques, guided imagery, containment, and sensory grounding to manage intense emotional and body states that arise for them. This lays the groundwork for the safe processing of distressing memories later on in the recovery work.

Frequent repetition of somatic exercises in the group setting is key so that participants can internalise them and use them for coping in daily life. Participants tell us that after a great deal of practice, they do use these techniques outside of the sessions:

> In some moments I feel eternal tensions, I am like upset … that feeling when you think that something bad will happen to you … I practice breathing exercises and soon after I am calm, I am better, I don't feel fear…

> (participant from Bosnia)

Art activities and self-expression

In the early sessions of the healing circle, facilitators introduce therapeutic art activities to encourage the participants to explore the use of art materials, to become comfortable in non-verbal expression, and to experience freedom in the creative process. For example, participants may explore colours or shapes to embody various mood states. They may create spontaneous markings to engage in a visual dialogue with a partner. At another point, the women will paint mandalas as a meditative experience. In a later exercise, they may denote sensations mapped onto an outline of their body. All along, the emphasis is on the process and not the product they are making. They acquire the capacity to appreciate their expressive work (their own and everyone else's) with open curiosity and without judgement.

As they become more fluent with art activities, they begin to depict some personal stories or memories in images. They are given prompts such as "this is what I cannot put into words", "this is a moment I will never forget", or "this is what I need you to know". They may take turns sharing these drawings with a partner or small group in a carefully guided progression so as not to overwhelm either the listening partner or the creator of the sketch. One of these drawings becomes the sketch for their story cloth.

Making story cloths

Participants in the circle learn and practice a variety of simple embroidery stitches as another self-soothing activity. They have an opportunity to stitch the border of the story cloth first, using this as a metaphor for the containment that is needed for the gradual exploration of personal stories. Once the participants have established a sense of safety and are more skilled at self-regulation, they are ready to lay out the content of their story cloths, working from one of the drawings they have done in response to the prompts. Typically, they create a background scene (landscape or indoor environment) cutting and placing pieces of cloth on a backing as a cloth collage or applique. The women sew and talk in small groupings.

Art therapist and CTP trainer Lisa Garlock describes the soothing practice of stitching:

> These actions are also rhythmic, creating vibrations in participants' bodies as they pull thread through fabric. There is a rhythm, too, in moving around for setting up and cleaning up the space, often an important ritual that marks the beginning and closing of art therapy groups. In both art therapy and story cloth groups there is also a meta-rhythm, an ebb and flow to the conversations that transpire; there are times of total silence as participants become absorbed in their process, and then there are times when questions are asked, stories are told, and people interact on various levels.

> (2016, p. 60)

Facilitators help participants learn various ways of depicting human figures in their story cloths, either embroidered or using appliqué figures to represent people in the scene depicted. Because we have found that the women and girls enjoy sewing small dolls and playing with them, this has become a regular practice in subsequent groups. They have opportunities to use the dolls in imaginative enactment of scenes with one another as another element of expressive therapy.

As the participants work on sewing their story cloths, they may disclose different elements of their stories as they are ready to do so, with a partner, a small group, or a facilitator. We find that if there is no pressure, circle members will speak about their experiences when they wish, at their own pace, and because they want to be understood – not because they are asked to do so.

When making a story cloth, the trauma narrative may be expressed visually through images on fabric, which enables the pathways to open so the stories can then be spoken. The process of sewing and working in a group allows the stories to unfold slowly, from before the trauma, during, and then afterward. Often the stories experienced by one individual resonate with others in the group, reducing the feeling of being the only one to have experienced traumatic events (Garlock, 2016, p.61).

Facilitators help the participants to stay aware of their nervous system responses to the narratives and to find "islands of calm" within the story cloth itself (i.e. "the cool shade under that tree feels ok," Or "that red chair is a comfortable place"). The women are invited to give words to parts of the story and to disclose the narrative in small, manageable sections. If needed, they are encouraged to return to their "safety" practices in order to tolerate the emotionally intense experience. Others in the circle offer empathic, supportive responses as they bear witness to one another's experiences. A strong sense of solidarity develops.

A circle member in Bosnia expresses how sewing the story cloth has helped her to find relief from the pain of her experience:

> It is difficult to explain … even if I was sad and upset, I also felt relief when I finished sewing of some parts … I don't know, like I left it on the canvas … It is still inside of me, but it doesn't control me so much.

STITCHING THE UNSPEAKABLE: TWO CLINICAL EXAMPLES FROM THE FIELD

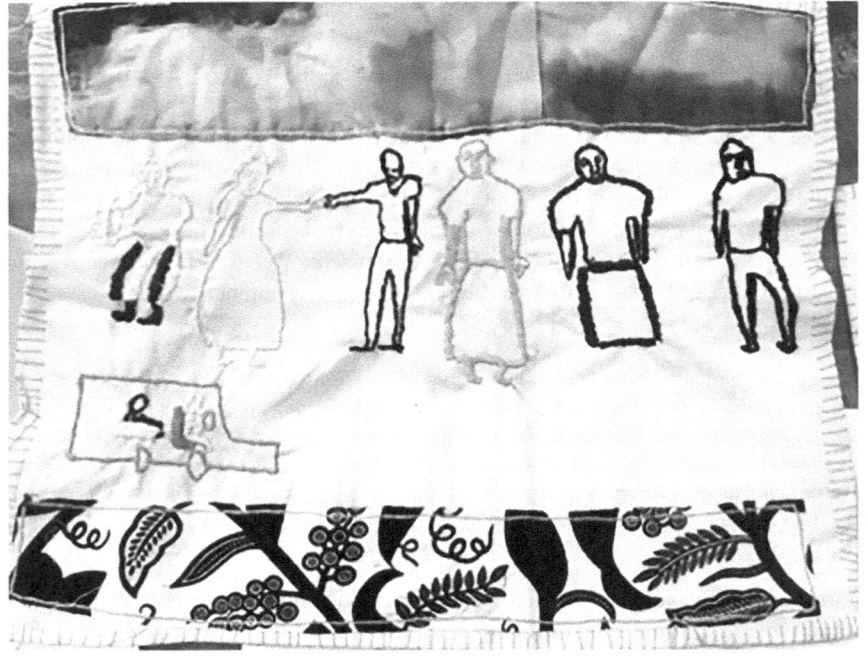

Figure 21.1 Sylvie's story cloth

This story cloth was made by a young woman in Eastern DRC, we will call Sylvie. After she was brutally raped and held captive for over a year, Sylvie's family and the perpetrator's family tried to force her to marry this man in order to "save face". With amazing courage, she defied them and escaped. You can see the perpetrator and his father chasing Sylvie in their vehicle. After she found refuge with our partner, Panzi Foundation, she joined a Kamba Moja (Common Threads in Swahili) circle, and made this story cloth, titled "Forced to Marry my Rapist". It told the story for which she had no words at the time (Figure 21.1).

As Sylvie works on the story cloth in her circle, it provides many opportunities for insight and growth, some of which are known to her, and some of which come without her awareness at first. There is mourning the loss of her baby who was seized by the perpetrator's parents. There is the fact that her own mother is portrayed without hands and feet – deprived of agency of any kind. As she works with this insight that the story cloth reveals to her, over time, Sylvie moves from anger at her mother for failing to protect her, towards a recognition of her mother's own helplessness. She expresses empathy and sadness about her mother's life circumstances and resolves to chart a different course for herself. When asked by her circle "sisters" about the figure she stitched of herself, Sylvie says, "I made myself invisible because no one really sees me." The facilitators took the opportunity to explore this feeling with the whole circle, inviting others to share their experiences and feelings about being invisible (Figure 21.2).

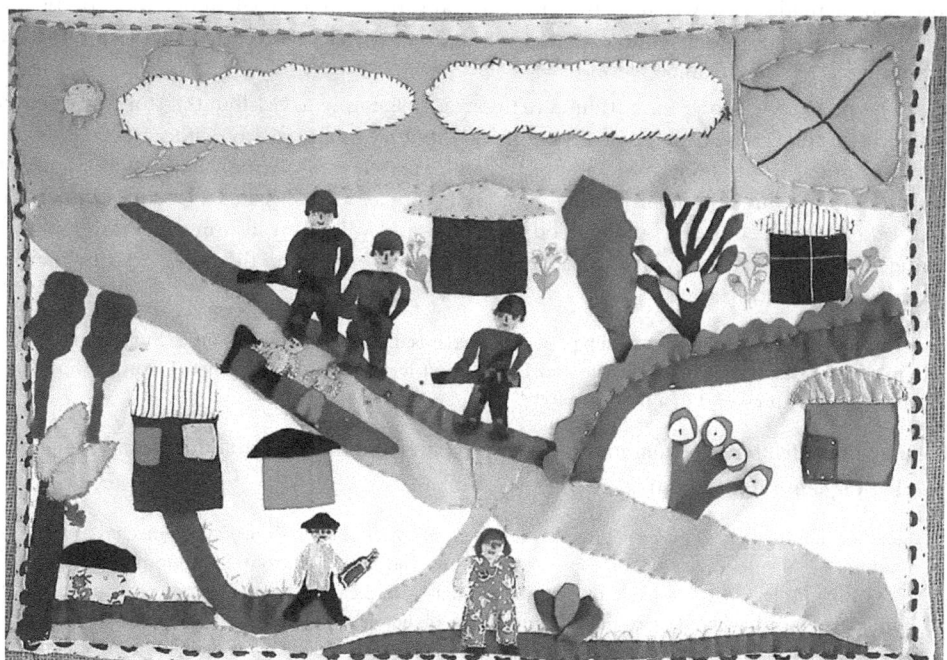

Figure 21.2 Maria's story cloth

This second story cloth was created by a Colombian refugee who had fled to Ecuador. She was responding to a drawing prompt "This is what I need you to know."

"Maria" (pseudonym) fled her home after an attack on her village by paramilitary forces in Colombia. She joined the CT group with other women in the refugee settlement just across the

San Miguel River. Maria created a story cloth that revealed what troubled her most about her circumstances. Though her family faced constant political violence, it was domestic violence that posed the greatest threat to her personally.

Most prominent in Maria's story cloth is the image of her children under attack on the river. If you look closer, you notice a man holding a bottle in the foreground. This is her husband, too drunk to help when she calls out to him. In the women's circle, she felt safe to disclose his violent rages, and acknowledge the fear she lived with every day. With the support of the circle and its facilitators, Maria found the strength to leave this relationship, and begin to rebuild her life. A year later she participated in an exhibition of the group's work and spoke out as part of the global 16 days of activism against gender-based violence. In 2014 the exhibition travelled to Geneva where it challenged representatives to the UN to take global action to end SGBV.

PHASE II OF THE RECOVERY PROCESS

After the first 12–14 weeks, most participants have completed their individual story cloth and the circle has begun to work therapeutically on the common themes that have emerged in the stories, such as loss, shame, survivor guilt, rejection, grief, self-doubt, etc. During the next phase, approximately weeks 13–26, the facilitators use their creativity and clinical expertise to design activities that will help the circle to gain insight and relief about their particular concerns. Participants engage in expressive art activities, reflections, discussions, and somatic reworking at a more advanced level.

The purpose of processing trauma memory is not simply to disclose the story, or to get it "out". It is rather to be capable of experiencing the story in a new way, without activating the threat response in the body, and without the felt experience of stigma, shame, self-blame, or guilt. Achieving this shift involves insight and self-compassion as well as a trusting connection with others so that one feels understood, accepted and valued. It also involves developing a changed (not a threat-survival response) nervous system response in the body. A participant in Nepal expressed it this way:

> I used to be disturbed while recalling my past incidents. I always thought about it. But this made us express our stories into a textile and now I don't feel very disturbed when I express those things. We expressed it in a piece of cloth.

Change in the felt sense of memories can be profound and may lead to other positive changes.
Pat Ogden summarises this process:

> Rather than becoming overwhelmed by the emotions of cognitive distortions connected to the trauma, clients discover that these can be contained and reworked from the bottom-up, that it is possible to feel grief and stay present or to laugh with pleasure as new empowering actions are experienced, where before there were feelings of helplessness and worthlessness. As clients slowly integrate these new experiences of old events, they are able to formulate a narrative that makes sense of the past.
>
> (Ogden, Minton and Pain, 2006)

During this second phase, the circle participants now create collective story cloths. Either in subgroups within the circle, or as one large group, they design and stitch a story cloth based on a common theme. These collective story cloths help to shift the group's focus from the past onto the present and the future. Some collective themes have been "This is what we will no longer tolerate", "These are our hopes for the future" or "This is what we feel proud about".

Commenting on a collective story cloth made in 2017 during Phase II by a circle in Bosnia-Herzegovina, a participant explained:

> After so much time we spent here together I think this was a great idea, now we have a wonderful memory, no matter that our story is about our war experience … and you know, whenever I take a look at our work, I feel some special energy, I see all of us together … that is very special!

Another group member adds "This has unique meaning for all of us. Not all of us are good at sewing but it is not important. It is important that all of us said something on this cloth."

During the later weeks of Phase II, the circle also prepares itself for independence from the facilitators. To practice for this, participants are given opportunities to lead activities alongside the facilitators.

Meaning-making

One of the significant challenges of moving forward from a horrific experience is being able to "make sense" of what has happened and to reclaim hope, purpose and a future. The world may seem so fundamentally shattered that it is difficult to restore a sense of meaning. Some participants report that they need to restore their spiritual core.

The CT approach tries to reach beyond the reduction of symptoms and aspires to a deeper level of change. The aim is not only survival but reclaiming a sense of purpose and meaning. The capacity to share their stories with one another is an essential step in that direction: "Sharing the traumatic experience with others is a precondition for the restitution of a meaningful world" (Herman, 1997, p. 70).

One of the ways the women in CTP find meaning is in being able to help one another. This is exemplified by a statement from a Bosnian participant:

> I think I am somehow better person now. … You know, I have learned how important is to listen others, to understand them and to help them in certain situations. … Before maybe I was much more focused just on myself and my life. … Now, I think it changed…

The strong feelings of solidarity within the circle often awaken a new awareness. Instead of placing blame for their predicament within themselves, as they have so often been socialised to do, the women may identify with the systemic sources of their suffering. This may lead to a sense that solutions to the problem of SGBV are located in collective action. For some, engaging in this struggle brings a sense of meaning and purpose.

> Social action offers the survivor a source of power that draws upon her own initiative, energy, and resourcefulness but magnifies these qualities far beyond her own capacities. It offers her an alliance with others based on cooperation and shared purpose.
>
> (Herman, 1997, p. 207)

A research team in Nepal summarised their findings in this way:

> Participants were relieved from memories of their painful past. Past incidents used to disturb the participants … following them like a shadow. In CTP they learned many exercises, which helped them get relaxed. Not only did they have the courage to express their feelings and share with each other, they were able to control their anger as well. Mainly it was found that they gained self-confidence to raise voices against injustice, mentally felt more at peace and overcame

depression, learned to make friends and developed positive thinking. They found a new way of building relationships with others, gained respectful life and learnt to respect others.

(TPO Nepal, 2015)

PHASE III: A COMMUNITY MOVING FORWARD

The addition of Phase III was initiated by the participants in the early circles. They had formed a new community and needed to stay together. They felt that this was their new family and chose to continue to support one another. From the participants we have learned to encourage this continuity.

Phase III circles are defined by their members' priorities: some circles have focused their energy on income-generating activities together, some have engaged in advocacy, participating in local women's rights campaigns, others have organised public exhibitions of their story cloths, some have provided support to subsequent circles as they begin their healing journeys. All have felt a strong sense of group cohesion. Herman notes that for a significant minority of survivors of SGBV, working for social change becomes a final step of the healing process:

> Most survivors seek the resolution of their traumatic experience within the confines of their personal lives. But a significant minority, as a result of the trauma, feel called upon to engage in a wider world. These survivors recognize a political or religious dimension in their misfortune and discover they can transform the meaning of their personal tragedy by making it the basis for social action. While there is no way to compensate for an atrocity, there is a way to transcend it, by making it a gift to others. The trauma is redeemed only when it becomes the source of a survivor mission.

(Herman, 1997, p. 207)

OUTCOMES OF COMMON THREADS PROGRAMMES

In the work of CTP, we have observed that even in the most challenging circumstances, deep and effective recovery is possible. By enlisting the remarkable healing power of the group itself, by engaging the participants' creativity and strengths, by allowing the recovery process to unfold at a gradual pace, by making use of both non-verbal and verbal channels for expression, by working to restore the body's system of equilibrium, we find that significantly improved mental health functioning and well-being is attainable. Our experience has been that true collaboration with local partners, intricate and thorough supervision of the clinical process, and adaptations for cultural resonance are key factors in success.

An especially powerful outcome is when local partners take full ownership of the intervention. In Nepal, for example, trained local facilitators have become supervisors, trainers and managers for the project. Former participants have become co-facilitators. The local staff have developed their own Center of Excellence for Sajha Dhago (Common Threads in Nepali). They are leading the way forward to expand their reach across other communities. Preliminary studies have shown that Common Threads methods are effective in mitigating the psychological consequences of sexual violence. Quantitative analysis of standard self-report measures indicate that depression and stress related symptoms decrease significantly over the course of the intervention (Common Threads Project, 2019).

Qualitative results

In interviews with participants, they report transformative changes across many domains of their lives. The group came to occupy an important place in their lives: "I feel relieved when I come here. I feel that this time is for me. I mean I feel like I exist."

A qualitative review of participant comments indicates that improving self-regulation, daily coping skills and self-care helps to build confidence and instil the sense that one can be in control of oneself and one's future. The shattered self-esteem and depleted sense of agency that can result from severe violations of human rights are rebuilt through the group process. Instead of feeling ashamed, powerless, and socially isolated, survivors develop self-respect, affirm their strengths, and restore their capacity for effectiveness in the world.

The following six themes emerged as important to many women in more than eighty interviews collected from participants in Ecuador, Bosnia, Nepal and The DRC. These are commonalities in the experience of the programme across diverse cultures:

Connection with others

> They listened to us, they understood us. I know they cannot do anything, but even if someone listens to you that is a great thing.

> I feel we are like a big family, like I have more sisters and that is really encouraging – that moment when you find out that whatever happens you have a group with whom you can share it!

> After listening to other's pains, our suffering seemed less. Our pain gradually decreased. I feel like a free bird with a positive outlook.

Improvements in relationships

> I used to get angry at the smallest things and would beat my daughters in frustration. Even though I used to feel guilty about it, I could not control myself. I realized that my anger's in check now, I don't fight with my husband and don't beat my daughters – these changes were better for my mental health.

Symptom reduction

> I was feeling terrible, heavy, desperate, disoriented. I didn't have strength for anything, in my home and at my work. What I used to do was to cry. Today I feel like a new person. I feel lighter, with more strength to work and to have my own business.

> I used to drink alcohol. I couldn't sleep and I used to drink but after coming here I have stopped drinking.

Creative self-expression

> We started feeling that we are someone. Our inner confidence came out and we felt that we have some force ... slowly with paper and common threads when doing the work we transferred it to paper and cloth – what we felt made tears roll out of our eyes. So all the healing came out and we felt very light.

> I've told my story, expressed myself on that cloth. I am proud of my work.

Overcoming shame

> I didn't used to speak like this, I used to feel fear. But now I don't feel fear and shame to speak

Sometimes I was ashamed of what happened to me before. Honestly, I was! I was not able to speak about it. … Now I see how good is when you share what happened to you with somebody who also survived something difficult.

I heard some stories and I also have had painful experiences … but I think there is no reason to be ashamed of that. Now I am clear … what happened to me is not my fault.

Self-efficacy

Previously, when we had problems, we used to run away. But after coming to CT program, we came to know that we should not run away from our problems. We realised that rather than running away from problems we should develop solutions to them.

When I came here, I realised that my existence too matters, and I should take care of myself and think about myself as well. I had many changes in myself. Like, I started taking care of myself as well.

I thought that I can't do anything but now I feel I can do something.

CONCLUSIONS

By using the extraordinary power of the group, the human capacity for creative expression, and the wisdom of what the body knows, an effective pathway to healing can be achieved. CPT is still working to refine and improve this integrative methodology, learning from the women in our circles, and their skilled and dedicated facilitators. Because it is a trauma-processing intervention, great care must be used in order not to cause harm. Those who conduct the healing circles must be highly skilled in clinical work with survivors, and closely supervised as they master the CTP approach. We hope that this model can be available for more girls and women in similar circumstances. We have seen that the use of story cloths as part of a comprehensive healing programme can reduce suffering, restore dignity and promote agency for survivors of sexual and gender-based violence. Atrocities cannot be erased from any personal or collective history. Those who have lived these experiences will always walk with them. As healing practitioners, we can accompany them and stand in solidarity. Then they can be the strongest advocates for systemic change, and together we can work to end the occurrence of SGBV.

REFERENCES

Cohen, R. (2013a) 'Common Threads: A recovery programme for survivors of gender based violence', *Intervention: Journal of Mental Health and Psychosocial Support in Conflict Affected Areas*, 11(2), pp. 157–168.

Cohen, R. (2013b) Common Threads video. Available at: https://vimeo.com/84129707 (Accessed: 14 June 2022).

Common Threads Project (2019) Unpublished Pilot study. Available at: bit.ly/2NjOnXc. (Accessed: 14 June 2022).

Dana, D. and Porges, S. (2018) *The Polyvagal Theory in Therapy: Engaging the Rhythm of Regulation*. New York: W.W. Norton.

Garlock, L. (2016) 'Stories in the cloth: Art therapy and narrative textiles', *Art Therapy*, 33 (2), pp. 58–66. doi:10.1080/07421656.2016.1164004.

Herman, J. L. (1997) *Trauma and Recovery: from Domestic Abuse to Political Terror*. New York: Basic Books.

Levine, P.A. (2015) *Trauma and Memory: Brain and Body in a Search for the Living Past.* Berkeley: North Atlantic Books.

Ogden, P. Minton, K., and Pain, C. (2006) *Trauma and the Body: A Sensorimotor Approach to Psychotherapy.* New York: W. W. Norton.

TPO Nepal (2015) *Focus Group Discussion for Common Threads Project* (unpublished).

Van der Kolk, B. (2014) *The Body Keeps the Score: Brain, Mind and Body in the Healing of Trauma.* New York: Viking.

World Health Organization, War Trauma Foundation and World Vision International (2011). *Psychological First Aid: Guide for Field Workers.* Geneva: WHO. Available at: https://www.who.int/publications/i/item/9789241548205 (Accessed: 14 June 2022).

CHAPTER 22

VOICING THE UNSPOKEN

Support Our Sisters: a model of groupwork for women affected by
female genital mutilation

Peggy Mulongo

This chapter presents a model of groupwork, Support Our Sisters (SOS), which was developed with and for women affected by the practice of female genital mutilation (FGM).

The context in which the groupwork has been implemented, the pathway to its development, the values underpinning the SOS groupwork approach, and a description of the model will be discussed in this chapter. I have also reflected on its effectiveness on women's emotional wellbeing, to inform existing knowledge around groupwork for women affected by FGM internationally.

Support Our Sisters was established by New Step for African Community (NESTAC) in 2011, as part of their programme of health and wellbeing initiatives. NESTAC is a UK-based non-governmental organisation (NGO) in Greater Manchester in the north of England. NESTAC works with diverse ethnic groups, including refugees and people seeking asylum and their families.

The Greater Manchester region has a high incidence of FGM, specifically within the migrant population of women seeking asylum (GMCA, 2019). This is 'home' to the SOS Project, which I initiated, having worked with women and girls affected or at risk of undergoing FGM since 2009. SOS offers a range of psychosocial interventions within community-based clinics, including peer-led support and community development around the practice of FGM.

SOS aims to break the taboo of FGM practice and highlight its mental health impact, encouraging women to speak out, and not to remain silent about their experiences. FGM is a criminal act that needs to be openly discussed, regardless of its cultural complexity and the shame it engenders. By voicing the unspoken and sharing their experiences with other women, women can take a significant step towards a healing process.

My own refugee experience and knowledge of FGM were strong motivators for developing the SOS project. As a cross-cultural mental health practitioner, I have particularly focused on working with women and girls who have/are experiencing mental distress as a result of gender-based violence.

UNDERSTANDING THE CONTEXT OF FGM PRACTICE

The World Health Organization (WHO) describes FGM as all procedures that involve the partial or total removal of external genitalia or other injury to the female genital organs for non-medical reasons (2016). FGM has no health benefits, often damaging the normal functions of the organs that have been removed or changed, and negatively affecting its victims physically, mentally and sexually (WHO, 2008).

FGM has been classified into four types, known as Type 1 – clitoridectomy (involves partial or total removal of the clitoris); Type 2 – excision (refers to partial or total removal of the clitoris and the labia minora, with or without excision of the labia majora); Type 3 – infibulation (refers to the reduction of the vaginal opening by sealing, sewing this); Type 4 – consists of all other

DOI: 10.4324/9781003192978-26

harmful procedures that may happen to the external female genitalia for non-medical reasons (WHO, 2018).

FGM is practiced on girls between the ages of five and 14 years, or before they get married, for a variety of sociocultural reasons. It is often justified as a rite of passage into womanhood, to preserve a girl's virginity, or for social acceptance (WHO, 2018). Although FGM has been further reported in some other countries, the African continent has the highest prevalence of FGM, with 30 countries reported to undertake the practice in 2021. FGM is a global issue, and in 2021, 200 million women and girls have survived at least one form of FGM (Wood et al., 2021).

Seeking protection to escape FGM

FGM is a serious breach of human rights. In the UK women and girls seeking asylum who escape this practice from their home country are entitled to claim asylum and be granted protection (WHO, 2018). However, there is limited statistical evidence in the UK for successful asylum applications on the basis of FGM, and the UK has been criticised for refusing FGM claims (Burrage, 2014).

In the UK it is an offence to aid, abet and practice FGM under the Female Genital Mutilation Act (2003). This was reinforced under the Serious Crime Act (2015), which includes further extended extra-territoriality for FGM, whereby the asylum context can be addressed. The Serious Crime Act could therefore be considered as a critical response in effectively safeguarding vulnerable women and girls from asylum-seeking families at risk of FGM.

The UK government actively tackles the practice of FGM by supporting local and national campaigns (WHO, 2018), collaborating with key stakeholders and using the media to demystify this harmful procedure. As this welcomed joint force programme has gradually developed, it has contributed to raising awareness of FGM and has provided a platform for women who have undergone FGM to participate in public debates and share their experiences about FGM and its harmful impact.

FGM AND MENTAL HEALTH, THE IMPACT ON WOMEN

Whilst the physical health consequences of FGM are well documented, knowledge regarding the impact it has on emotional wellbeing has been slow to develop, with a dearth of studies exploring therapeutic interventions that could benefit women and girls (WHO, 2018; Reisel and Creighton, 2015).

Between 2010 and 2021, several studies acknowledge that FGM is associated with mental health problems, citing mainly post-traumatic stress disorder (PTSD), anxiety and depression (Smith and Stein, 2017). In 2018, WHO published a comprehensive report on FGM and mental health, which highlighted the importance of addressing, assessing and managing the mental health of women and girls affected by the practice. However, the focus was mainly on the benefits of individual therapy, rather than promoting groupwork as an alternative or complementary intervention. In 2021, there is little research on groupwork for women affected by FGM (Coho et al., 2019)

SOS women affected by FGM described symptoms of complex post-traumatic stress disorder (CPTSD). CPTSD is usually associated with childhood interpersonal trauma or chronic childhood stress, with the most common precedents being sexual trauma/s (Maercker et al., 2018). This is equally true for FGM, which is mainly practiced during childhood, often resulting in complex long-term trauma.

SOS women talk about the mental health impact of FGM

Women who have attended the SOS clinics have frequently talked about feelings of shame, often blaming themselves for being too frightened to speak out. Many describe having a negative body image and recall experiences of painful and/or "*embarrassing*" sexual intercourse with partners. Women have shared their anxieties around their marital problems, and the cultural beliefs and traditions attached to FGM in their communities.

> I was uncomfortable during sexual relations but could not discuss this with my husband, or with my friend. I could not talk about it; it was not good complaining. I was unhappy and did not like having sex, I am sure he was as well, but no one was speaking about it, no one.

Women described feeling frightened of not being re-infibulated following childbirth, and how for some this was linked to a loss of their cultural identity. They also talked about the potential for punishment in the form of being cursed or having misfortune fall upon the family or their daughters for non-obedience to FGM practice.

> I rushed to hospital each time my 5-year-old daughter was ill, thinking she was dying, because I refused that she has FGM. I always remember my grandma saying to me; it is an abomination, you've been told lies, you will lose your daughter. It is so distressful, I can't take it out of my mind.

Women explored feeling guilty for rejecting the FGM tradition in favour of "*Western beliefs*". Many described the impact of persistent family and community pressures to practice FGM and talked of how frightened they were of becoming socially excluded if they abandoned it.

> When I was pregnant and found out I was having a baby girl, I felt worried throughout my pregnancy. I don't want my daughter to have the same FGM, I knew it will happen. I had no one to talk to, I was very depressed. … Then I talked to my midwife, she didn't really know what to do. I considered terminating my pregnancy…

The majority of women outlined how their emotional distress was further intensified by the UK's FGM legislation. They described how they found the legislation threatening and stressful, and that they felt marginalised as a result.

> They think they understand. They think they are right, and they make the right decisions. … What do they know about us really? Why they use their power to make us abandon FGM? This is disgusting. … I am very angry, I feel sad and rejected.

> I don't understand why they want to show us how to raise our children. They say I am a bad mother because my daughter had FGM. We had no choice. … This is insulting and disappointing. They say FGM is wrong. … Themselves they do it and give it other names. It's so confusing. I heard about this surgery to change the vagina, and many women do it. … This is really ironic.

PATHWAYS TO THE DEVELOPMENT OF THE SOS GROUPWORK MODEL

SOS started as a three-year pilot project. The pilot was a coordinated specialist FGM mental health service delivered across Greater Manchester. The project provided a tailored psychosocial service for women affected/at risk of FGM. Clinics were set up within community centres in three areas of Greater Manchester known to have a high prevalence of FGM. While self-referrals were accepted, schools, social and health services, the police, and other NGOs referred women to the clinics.

Services delivered by the SOS project include provision of cross-cultural psychosocial individual therapy, groupwork, peer support, community engagement and empowerment of women to be active against FGM in their communities. The SOS clinics are delivered by cross-cultural mental health specialists, who are assisted by trained FGM peer mentors.

FGM PEER MENTORS

FGM peer mentors are volunteers from FGM-practicing communities, who have all had therapy for FGM within SOS and would like to support and empower their peers. Peer mentors are trained to develop basic cross-cultural counselling skills in order to support other women during groupwork. They work alongside SOS therapists and their role and input are pivotal to the project. The peer mentor training programme is run twice a year and consists of seven-weekly sessions of a full day's training.

Within the training, peer mentors develop a solution-focused approach through a learning process that uses real case scenarios. They build an understanding of all aspects of FGM, with a focus on the medico-legal and psychosocial impacts. Following the training, they assist women and families referred to the SOS clinics by offering emotional support. This support includes initial risk assessments; befriending; explaining safeguarding procedures; accompanying women and girls to attend FGM examinations; providing (bilingual) basic counselling to individuals with a low level of emotional need; and assisting SOS therapists to facilitate the groupwork.

> I thought I knew everything about FGM. During the awareness session, I heard the experience of other ladies in the group, I am so gutted. … I didn't know about types in FGM. … I thought FGM was the same in all cultures, was done for the same reason, but I found out it's not true. The FGM session was an eye-opener for me.

Peer mentors attend monthly clinical supervision provided by SOS therapists to ventilate their emotions, to ensure they stay psychologically safe and to avoid the effects of re-traumatisation. The peer mentor role is progressive, from 'junior' to 'senior', depending on the experience developed over time. Women are also provided with the foundation to progress into mental health/counselling careers and further education if they would like to develop further.

The peer mentor is a para-professional role and their involvement in groupwork for women affected by FGM is crucial. They are often described by group members as role models and are real proof of successful healing. Group members who do not speak English describe feeling *"valued, proud, understood and cared for"* when they are supported within the group by bilingual peer mentors. Interpreters are not needed at SOS, as the role of bilingual peer mentor has been developed over time and is fully incorporated in the delivery of the groupwork.

SOS NEGOTIATED CROSS-CULTURAL GROUPWORK

Feedback was sought from the women who attended SOS's group activities during the first years of the project and these consultations helped co-produce the developing groupwork model. During these consultations, it became evident that culture, art and spirituality were often used by group members as coping mechanisms to improve their mental wellbeing. Women talked about how when praying or engaging in activities such as singing, dancing, or knitting for their children, they felt stress-free. Women requested what they would find helpful: increasing the number of existing group sessions; considering women's socio-cultural and spiritual backgrounds in the groupwork delivery; reinforcing communication between peers; training women in developing basic counselling skills to help therapists during group sessions; being more creative during group activities. Women particularly wanted the opportunity to use art as a means of expression within a groupwork setting.

Following these discussions, a negotiated groupwork approach was developed that addressed all the themes and requests women had shared. This new approach combined Dialectal Behaviour Therapy skills training (DBT) (Linehan, 1993) and visual arts, creatively adapted as a therapeutic groupwork intervention.

DBT is known to be effective in treating those with a diagnosis of CPTSD. It has also proved effective in treating other mental health problems (Linehan, 2014), with some evidence demonstrating that it has been successfully culturally adapted (Cheng and Merrick, 2017). Given the complexity and long-term impact of FGM, DBT-based skills training was considered suitable for adaptation to the SOS context because in addition to addressing the impact of trauma, it explores self-concept and social interaction. It also has a strong motivational element and helps clients plan for the future.

The visual arts component of the groupwork included painting, drawing, photography, sculpture, cartooning, collage, graphic novels, 3D art, knitting, mixed-media art, installations, quilting and doll making (Casey et al., 2016). Incorporating visual art as part of the negotiated groupwork model enabled women to freely express themselves and to explain and reframe their emotions and experiences. We found visual arts to be a powerful therapeutic tool, which was positively welcomed and actively used by group members.

DBT skills training and embedded visual art activities were adopted to help women cope with their ongoing trauma, enabling them to reflect on their feelings in a creative environment that considered their culture and spirituality.

THE NEGOTIATED SOS GROUPWORK MODEL

The following model is a summary of the different stages in the integrated SOS groupwork framework that has been developed by the SOS team:

Stage one – individual therapy

All women referred for therapeutic groupwork would have initially benefited from one-to-one emotional support at the clinic. Following assessment, the frequency and number of sessions offered varies dependant on the level of distress and difficulty. Usually, women attend an average of three to six sessions. Sessions usually explore women's personal experience of FGM; self-developed coping mechanisms to manage related challenges and emotions; capacity to build positive thoughts and empowerment to move forward. Following women's final evaluation of one-to-one support, exit routes are discussed: (i) referral to alternative therapeutic interventions; (ii) referral to SOS groupwork (majority of cases – stage two); or discharge from the FGM clinic with a follow-up (stage three).

Stage two – groupwork

This is a twofold approach which consists of 12 weekly sessions lasting 90 minutes each with a maximum of 10 women per group. It is divided into two sections: the FGM skills building groupwork and the FGM groupwork activities. The SOS clinic runs two consecutive groups per programme, four times a year.

Psychoeducation / FGM skills building groupwork

The skills building groupwork is a starting point for all women referred to SOS groupwork and comprises of five weekly sessions. During the first two sessions, the SOS team and peer mentors welcome group members by introducing themselves, explaining their roles and the aims of the groupwork. This is an important phase, where group members learn about the groupwork they will be embarking on, as well as learning about the confidentiality of the group and the value of peer support. Group members' roles and contributions during this therapeutic journey are explored, so that women own the space and feel safe and confident enough to engage. Women are given the opportunity to ask questions to help them gain an understanding of the SOS groupwork approach. The third and fourth sessions begin once women give consent to be part of the process. Women are given homework at the end of each session, which is briefly discussed at the beginning of each group.

It is important that women develop a broad understanding of the interlinks between FGM, mental health, cultures, traditions and spirituality, which are covered during sessions three and four. These sessions are participatory, during which group members actively engage in educational activities delivered creatively by the SOS team, using various approaches that take into account women's cultural and educational backgrounds. Women build basic skills that help them improve self-awareness, awareness of others, as well as build self-confidence and improve self-esteem. During this process women often reflect on and learn the value of peer support. The team also creates opportunities for general discussion and for questions to be addressed. When women are distressed, they are supported by the therapists and group.

The fifth session is a review of this section of the programme, during which women's feedback and suggestions are recorded and exit routes are discussed: (i) progressing to groupwork; (ii) discharge from the programme, with an opportunity to be followed up (refer to stage three).

The majority of women continue to the groupwork, and very few are discharged from the programme after this stage of the process.

FGM therapeutic groupwork activities

This is led by the SOS team of therapists, assisted by peer mentors, to help women develop coping skills. The four components of DBT skills training (Mindfulness, distress tolerance, emotional regulation and interpersonal effectiveness skills) are incorporated into this groupwork. Mindfulness and distress tolerance skills help women to work towards acceptance of their thoughts and behaviours related to FGM. Emotional regulation and interpersonal effectiveness skills are used to help them work towards changing their thoughts and behaviours. Each session in this stage starts with a group mindfulness activity.

Seven weekly group sessions are delivered

In the first week, the programme is outlined, and women are supported to explore how they might actively participate in the activities during the groupwork. During the second and third weeks, women are encouraged to express their feelings through visual art, initially guided to be collectively involved in undertaking three specific art-based activities: (1) geographical map/ photo elicitation; (2) timeline; (3) self-portrait.

1   Geographical map/photo elicitation – a geographical global map is used to help women reflect on meaningful geographical environments to them and how they connect with those places. Women are asked to bring significant images (both positive and

negative), representing their culture, spirituality, traditions, or any other theme they would like to discuss with peers in the groupwork.

2   Timeline – individual timelines are given to women to help them represent in chronological order, events that have affected their lives positively and negatively, explaining how these events are meaningful for them.

3   Self-portrait – a blank self-portrait character is given to each woman to reflect on, and using key words, they are asked to describe their personality at that point in time.

These selected activities are linked with FGM-related issues and aim to help women reflect on the way FGM is affecting their mental health. Each activity is supported with open questions to encourage group discussions, individual and group reflections, and engagement in visual art activities. Examples of questions include: (i) What are the places in your local/social environments you liked or disliked the most; can you link these with significant events you can remember? (ii) What has been the impact of FGM throughout your life? Based on the negative events in your timeline, how do you think your mental health can be improved over time? (iii) Reflecting on your personality and character, in which ways has FGM affected your personality?

The fourth week is a group reflection exercise, whereby group members are invited to reflect together on the three art activities they previously engaged with. At this stage of the group process, women encourage and support each other as they each talk through their artwork. Women are then supported to think about their future aspirations and look at tools to help them move away from the negative thoughts that have built up over time as a consequence of FGM.

The focus during week five and six is on self-work, in that each group member is asked to produce a piece of individual artwork, following week four's reflective exercise. Art materials and tools are made available to women so that they can choose a suitable art form to help them create their own artwork. The visual arts most commonly used are drawing, painting, photography, collage and creative writing. Each woman is given some instruction to help them use the art form they have chosen. These art forms are used by group members to express their feelings around FGM, to portray how they visualise any acceptance and change of their thoughts and behaviours and describe any positive outcomes that have occurred as a result of the groupwork.

We have observed that visual art activities enable women to express themselves in different ways and provide a creative space for them to consider their cultural, traditional and spiritual beliefs, whilst expressing themselves and interpreting their behaviours. They communicate their hope and aspirations creatively, using art to reflect on the way they intend to change their negative thoughts and behaviours to more positive ones.

> Green and yellow are my favourite colours. Maybe because my mum loves the same colours, she says they are good luck colours in our culture. … She tried to protect me not to have FGM, but she couldn't. In the negative image, red means blood. This brings so many bad thoughts in my mind. Blood for FGM. … Blood for sacrifices. Also, we all have same blood colour, but we are not the same. I find this sad. We always look outside, not inside people. Finally, the dark colour is me, I am Black outside, people judge me, but they don't really know me. … I am working hard to be more positive in future.

In the seventh week, women are encouraged to share their artwork with other group members and to provide constructive feedback to each other. This activity encourages women to support each other as well as helping them to learn to listen to others. The SOS team then asks women to take part in an evaluation of the sessions, to help enhance future delivery.

After completing the group, women can choose to leave SOS, with the opportunity to have a follow-up meeting or they can decide to develop peer support skills through the FGM peer mentoring training. An average of three to four women per group usually join the peer mentoring programme.

Stage three – the support line

A telephone support line managed by the SOS team and supported by peer mentors is used to assist women who have been discharged during the different stages of groupwork. An online group is also available to reach those who are unable to physically access group sessions. Online group members are encouraged to take part in the visual art activities too, following the same programme offered in the groupwork. The online platform has been of great help during the COVID-19 pandemic.

REFLECTIONS ON THE IMPACT OF GROUP THERAPY – SURVIVOR FEEDBACK

Impact on women taking part in SOS groupwork

The SOS negotiated groupwork programme delivered at the clinics has been highly valued by SOS members, who have been appreciative of what they have gained emotionally from these sessions. Women's feedback is sought throughout the year via informal group discussions, quarterly feedback using evaluation forms and therapists also take notes of feedback received during the groupwork activities. Peer mentors are also consulted.

Women said they felt valued and part of the group; they felt safe and in control, as well as proud to have been associated in the planning of activities delivered in group sessions.

The majority of women who have completed the SOS programme have said that they felt empowered to freely express themselves, and to explain and reflect on their emotions. Many said that this was a new experience for them. They described how they had gained more knowledge of FGM, developed confidence in expressing themselves creatively and in showing empathy towards others and themselves. Furthermore, women talked about feeling a greater sense of stability with increased resilience, which they felt would equip them to move on with their lives as survivors of FGM. They also felt more confident to speak out in public and condemn the practice of FGM.

Many women described the groupwork as a significant part of their healing journey, where together they could recover from the hidden turmoil of FGM, as well as support and empower each other to voice their opinions.

> Since I was a child no one's seen my private part … when I had FGM done until I got married, I was tense when having sex, did not like it and I was ashamed all the time. I cannot believe that I can talk about sex now, discuss with other women like me, I feel free, understood.

> So, it's psychologically, they brainwash me and then now I realise that I've been brainwashed, and I can't enjoy my sex life, I'm not a full woman. Only God can help. … But I'm glad I can talk about it, I have a platform where I can get support from other women.

REFLECTIONS

As a cross-cultural mental health practitioner, I continuously learn from my practice and keep discovering the multitude of existing traditions and spiritual beliefs women share and learn from each other. During the life of SOS, I have observed several factors that have added value to the groupwork programme and ensured its positive impact on women: the team of mental health practitioners and trained peer mentors are ethnically diverse and bilingual, speaking several languages and dialects; many of the team have lived experience of FGM; they are all committed to groupwork and have an in-depth knowledge of FGM and cross-cultural mental health.

The SOS groupwork approach can be safely adapted by any therapist working with women affected by FGM within a community setting, or indeed by therapists working with women affected by other forms of gender-based violence within a diverse ethnic population. It is, however, important to emphasise the need to develop basic skills and expertise on cross-cultural awareness and therapeutic interventions, to be able to adapt this model. Therapists and NGOs could also consider running a peer mentoring training similar to the one delivered by the SOS clinic, to build capacity within the community.

For successful delivery of groupwork, it is essential to allow participants to express their emotions at their pace, acknowledging their past and present experiences and to value and prioritise their cultures/traditions during therapy, as well as any health beliefs attached to these.

SOS therapeutic groupwork provides a creative and innovative psychosocial intervention to women who have been affected by FGM. This has been demonstrated throughout the life of SOS as it has evolved, from individual support to groupwork, strengthened by the FGM peer mentoring team. The negotiated model that led to the SOS groupwork programme was developed from continuously listening to women's voices throughout the course of our therapeutic work and activities.

The SOS model demonstrates the value of a co-production model in groupwork which seeks to use practice-based evidence to develop a specialist therapeutic service for women affected by FGM delivered by a third sector organisation within the community.

REFERENCES

Burrage, H. (2014) The UK Home Office (Says It) has no Data on FGM Asylum Claims. Available at: https://hilaryburrage.com/2014/05/19/uk-home-office-has-no-data-on-fgm-asylum-claims/ (Accessed: 21 June 2021).

Casey, B. et al. (2016). 'Narrative in nursing research: An overview of three approaches', *Journal of Advanced Nursing* 72. doi:10.1111/jan.12887.

Cheng, P.H. and Merrick, E. (2017). 'Cultural adaptation of dialectical behavior therapy for a Chinese international student with eating disorder and depression', *Clinical Case Studies*, 16(1), pp. 42–57. doi:10.1177/1534650116668269.

Coho, C., Parra S.R., Hussein, L., and Laffy, C. (2019). *Female Genital Trauma: Guidelines for Working Therapeutically with Survivors of Female Genital Mutilation*. London, UK. Available at: https://www.dahliaproject.org/wp-content/uploads/2019/11/1924_Female_Genital_Trauma_Report_Web.pdf (Accessed: 16 May 2021).

Female Genital Mutilation Act (2003). London. HMSO.

Greater Manchester Combined Authority. (2019) Female Genital Mutilation in Greater Manchester: Prevalence Report. Available at: https://hummedia.manchester.ac.uk/faculty/qstep/student-stories-2018/wakeford.pdf (Accessed: 07 June 2022).

Linehan, M. (1993) *Cognitive-Behavioral Treatment of Borderline Personality Disorder*. New York: Guilford Press.

Linehan, M. (2014) *DBT Skills Training Manual* (2nd ed.). New York: Guilford Press.

Maercker, A., Hecker, T., Augsburger, M., and Kliem, S. (2018). 'ICD-11 prevalence rates of posttraumatic stress disorder and complex posttraumatic stress disorder in a german nationwide sample', *The Journal of Nervous and Mental Disease*, 206 (4), pp. 270–276. doi:10.1097/NMD.0000000000000790.

Reisel, D. and Creighton, S.M. (2015). 'Long term health consequences of Female Genital Mutilation (FGM)', *Maturitas*, 80(1), 48–51. doi:10.1016/j.maturitas.2014.10.009.

Serious Crime Act (2015) London: HMSO.

Smith, H. and Stein, K. (2017) 'Psychological and counselling interventions for female genital mutilation', *International Journal of Gynecology & Obstetrics*, 136, pp. 60–64. doi:10.1002/ijgo.12051.

Wood, R., Richens, Y., and Lavender, T. (2021) 'The experiences and psychological outcomes for pregnant women who have had FGM: A systematic review', *Sexual & Reproductive Healthcare*, 29. doi: 10.1016/j.srhc.2021.100639.

World Health Organization (2008). *Eliminating Female Genital Mutilation: An Interagency Statement – UNAIDS, UNDP, UNECA, UNESCO, UNFPA, UNHCHR, UNHCR, UNICEF, UNIFEM.* Geneva: WHO. Available at: https://apps.who.int/iris/handle/10665/43839 (Accessed: 15 January 2021).

World Health Organization (2016). *WHO Guidelines on the Management of Health Complications from Female Genital Mutilation.* Geneva: WHO. Available at: https://www.who.int/publications/i/item/9789241549646 (Accessed: 15 January 2021).

World Health Organization (2018). Care of girls and women living with female genital mutilation: a clinical handbook. Geneva: WHO. Available at: https://apps.who.int/iris/handle/10665/272 (Accessed: 21 February 2021).

CHAPTER 23

AUTHOR DISCUSSION
Together through talk

Two of the authors who contributed to the 'Together Through Talk' section of the book took part in this discussion: Peggy Mulongo and Weihui Wang. They were joined by Bryan Cheng, who was invited to contribute his experiences of the groupwork programme, Interpersonal Therapy for Depression, which is used widely in humanitarian settings. The discussion was facilitated by Rebecca Horn.

REBECCA: Welcome. I'm looking forward to the opportunity to learn more about the issues you've discussed in your chapters. I'd like to begin by inviting you to share the core message that you would like readers to take from your chapter.

WEIHUI: The key takeaway for me is the faith-sensitive part of our groupwork model. A faith-sensitive approach is different to a faith-based approach, because it's not rooted in any sacred text. It is about being sensitive to people's own faith or the lack of faith, however the participants choose to identify. In any groupwork we need to focus on strengths, and participants often identify their faith as a coping mechanism. However, sometimes as humanitarians we can be uncomfortable with the discussion of faith because we may be afraid to be seen as not neutral. Another key issue in the chapter is that because of the lack of mental health services in the contexts where I work, in order to provide services to the numbers of people who require them, there really needs to be investment in local communities. It takes time to invest in lay community facilitators, so this needs to be built into the planning and funding of groupwork interventions.

PEGGY: In terms of including participants in the delivery of groupwork, I think co-production is very important to outcomes when it comes to healing. In our groupwork the survivors have been continually consulted and included in decisions about how to improve the programme. We have an advisory group which includes professionals and those who benefit from the service, and together we are trying to co-produce what will be the best therapy for this group. This has also involved working closely and educating some participants who wanted to take on a peer mentoring role. This has been very powerful because the peer mentors develop counselling and other therapeutic skills, and are able to support others as part of the group therapy.

REBECCA: Thank you. Bryan, is there anything you've heard from Wei or Peggy that resonates with you in relation to IPT [interpersonal therapy] for groups?

BRYAN: Definitely. I think what resonated really strongly with me is what Wei mentioned about working with lay facilitators from the community. All of our projects have demonstrated that a lot of lay health workers can provide IPT, sometimes even better than a trained clinician. And that really increases sustainability because when we leave the region, the groups can continue. In fact a lot of our testimonies have shown that ten years after we left, the groups are still continuing to meet and there's still ongoing change and improvements to the communities.

REBECCA: So for all three of you a common theme is working with people who have experienced the issues of concern and empowering them to provide support to their fellow survivors. Bryan, you mentioned one of the positive aspects of that is sustainability. But I'm wondering also whether you think that there's any benefit to this approach in terms of the quality of the support that's being offered?

DOI: 10.4324/9781003192978-27

PEGGY: We've been running the peer mentoring program since 2014 and I can say that we've been learning since that time how to improve and how to sustain the quality. Training is one thing, but sustaining the quality of the service provided is another thing. There is always a certain level of supervision needed. With the peer mentors, for example, we have junior peer mentors and senior peer mentors, who are overseen by professionals. So we've created a kind of framework in terms of making sure that the quality remains and we keep working and improving it.

WEIHUI: I think when our local providers themselves have shared experiences, then their ability to empathise with the participants is really strong. In terms of the community, the big thing for us was trying to understand context and to adapt the programme accordingly. It's just good practice across all contexts to make sure that the community wants the service that is being offered, and that they are part of the decisions made, including the selection of the community facilitators. In our groupwork programme, community members were able to bring out aspects that, as a foreigner helping to design this project, I didn't necessarily fully understand. For example, like the nuances around the chewing of khat in Yemen, and how it impacts family life and how that in itself is a coping mechanism. And working through how to incorporate different interpretations of faith into the programme. Because we also learned that it's impossible to generalise Islam, participants practice their faith slightly differently and through sharing with each other members can see different ways to continue to connect to their faith. Some of the participants would say things like, 'I'm no longer connected to my community', or 'I'm no longer praying five times a day' and other participants would share ideas on how they continue to include faith rituals and routines.

REBECCA: I see some overlaps with how Peggy described co-production in the way that you talk about how the community members contributed to developing the content of the programme, in a way that felt right to them in their context.

WEIHUI: Yes, and I think the other thing is around risk. Because they are able to identify specific risks. Even simple things like the best time for sessions to be held for women, to work around childrearing expectations and other commitments.

REBECCA: Thank you. I'd be interested in whether any of you could say something about, with your particular programme, what you see as the strengths of a talk-focused programme in a group, rather than having that same approach on an individual basis?

BRYAN: I think my answer to this question overlaps quite a bit with what Peggy and Wei mentioned earlier. Especially the point about co-production and about how the group comes together to figure things out logistically. What I've seen in Group IPT is because, unlike in individual therapy, where there's no connection with others, we actually capitalise on the connection between group members. And, unlike here in the West, at least here in the States, when people come to a group at the clinic or the hospital, we discourage them from creating friendships within the group because it's a clinical thing. You go out and you try this with your own friends, you try to build connections outside of the group. But in all the regions that we work in – in Lebanon, Uganda, Ethiopia, Tanzania, Kenya, Peru – we actually capitalise on the group connections and say 'you can be friends here, in fact, it's great if you have supports', and I think that's actually a power or strength that the group has that individual therapy doesn't have. Especially with these types of populations that we work with, survivors of torture or survivors of intimate partner violence or gender-based violence, we see that the women become much stronger because they can lean on each other. For example, with childrearing practices, like Wei mentioned, the women in one group started figuring out how they could take turns babysitting each other's kids. And a lot of these groups ended up developing their own cash transfer programmes, they sought out new things, they started cottage industries as a group. But it all started because of groupwork, all this would be impossible if it was individual work.

REBECCA: Those are very powerful examples. So you've described how it's not just about social and emotional support, but actually developing practical support strategies as a group. Does that resonate with you, Wei or Peggy? Or are there other issues that you think are important in terms of group therapy compared to individual?

PEGGY: We work in different demographic and geographical environments, but there are some similarities. So yes, the therapeutic group, it's a support network. For the women we work with from different African, South Asian countries, having a support network is important. And what we've noticed as well, it's a tool for empowering women. With the approach that we use, all the women have been through individual therapy before they joined the group. And you can see the difference once they've joined the group. You can see that their well-being is improving every single day, just thinking that 'I'm not on my own, I thought that this was only my problem'. Sharing with others is powerful. And like Bryan was saying, supporting each other – What is happening with you? How can we help?

WEIHUI: I think Bryan and Peggy have touched on some really important things. The other thing that maybe it's important to highlight is the idea of the participants or the clients becoming helpers themselves. Increasingly there is more evidence showing that if you become involved in the helping process, you also improve your own wellbeing. The other strength of the group is the whole idea of re-establishing some kind of routines and rituals. I find this really important, because we forget how rituals are such a big part of our lives and the group setting allows for the group to share ideas of how those can be re-established. In fact, in itself the group is a routine and a ritual. Finally when you talk about your feelings and you reflect upon them while listening to other people's feelings, it encourages a different level of self-awareness. A lot of the time it's easy to give empathy to others but to show yourself empathy is very different. I think that the group setting allows for the participants or clients to be compassionate towards themselves in a very difficult situation.

REBECCA: Thank you. I would like to try to touch on the other questions before we close. The second one for Peggy and Wei is, 'has writing the chapter changed your approach to groupwork in any way? Or your reflections on your own groupwork?'

WEIHUI: On a personal level, it's really nice to be able to go back and look at all the testimonies. When we planned the programme I was very concerned that we were not using an established modality, because I really wanted to use IPT, Bryan, and I was pushing for that but it just didn't turn out that way. It was nice to get a little bit of affirmation that, even though it's something new, it's making its impact in a small way.

BRYAN: Or really a big way to those people's lives. You know, like it may seem small to us in the grand scale of project management, but to them it's everything.

PEGGY: I think for me, my approach to groupwork has not changed, as I've always considered this as essential, healing through sharing with others. It's just reinforced for me how important it is. The journey of writing the chapter and receiving all the feedback from editors made me appreciate further the power of collaboration. Just the fact of being in a book with other authors made me curious, already excited about reading their chapters and find out more about their approaches to groupwork, looking forward to reading the book.

REBECCA: Thank you. There's one final question, which is, 'what statements or messages can we come up with to encourage more groupwork opportunities?' And I guess this comes particularly from the perspective of non-humanitarian settings where groupwork is perhaps not prioritised in the way that it is in humanitarian settings or emergencies. What messages or statements would you offer to funders, donors, or policy makers or organisations to encourage them to support groupwork for people who've been through very difficult experiences?

PEGGY: In my case, I would say give a voice, listen. To bring change, you need to give the opportunity to listen to those who are experiencing difficulties, the survivors, those who have been through torture. So my statement would really be 'give a voice to the survivors, empower them to speak out, encourage safe and creative groupwork interventions that produce positive outcomes'.

BRYAN: I think it's high time that people move away from the medical model. A lot of times individual therapy stems from the medical model that we see as 'provider and patient', and you're treating the patient one on one, when in fact we're all social animals, we're part of communities, we're part of groups, we're part of family units, and so it is quite artificial to do that. Groupwork actually emulates the power of a community. And so when you create a community that becomes a therapeutic milieu for each person within the group, there's so much more to gain in a group change as opposed to an individual change.

WEIHUI: Bryan hit the nail on the head, it's literally that – people are not isolated beings. Socially, culturally, we are a collective and in some ways this tough experience and healing process can also be a collective experience. And there's so much power in collective experiences.

INDEX

Page numbers in **bold** indicate tables, page numbers in *italic* indicate figures.

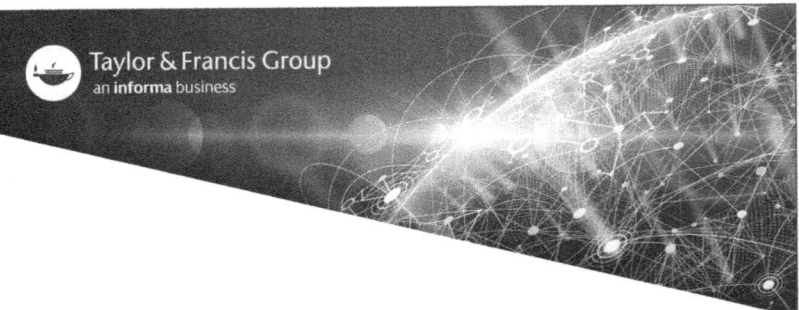
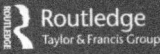
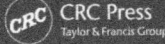